Managing long term conditions

Managing long term conditions

A social model for community practice

Edited by

Margaret Presho

*Senior Lecturer, School of Health,
Manchester Metropolitan University*

WILEY-BLACKWELL

A John Wiley & Sons, Ltd., Publication

This edition first published 2008
© 2008 John Wiley & Sons Ltd

Registered office
John Wiley & Sons Ltd, The Atrium, Southern Gate, Chichester, West Sussex, PO19 8SQ, United Kingdom

Wiley-Blackwell is an imprint of John Wiley and Sons, formed by the merger of Wiley's global Scientific, Technical and Medical business with Blackwell Publishing.

Editorial office
John Wiley & Sons Ltd, The Atrium, Southern Gate, Chichester, West Sussex, PO19 8SQ, United Kingdom

For details of our global editorial offices, for customer services and for information about how to apply for permission to reuse the copyright material in this book please see our website at www.wiley.com/wiley-blackwell.

The right of the author to be identified as the author of this work has been asserted in accordance with the Copyright, Designs and Patents Act 1988.

Library of Congress Cataloging-in-Publication Data

Managing long term conditions : a social model for community practice / edited by Margaret Presho.
      p.   ;   cm.
   Includes bibliographical references and index.
   ISBN 978-0-470-05932-6 (pbk. : alk. paper)   1. Long-term care of the sick – Great Britain.   2. Nursing – Great Britain.   I. Presho, Margaret.
   [DNLM: 1. Long-Term Care – organization & administration – Great Britain.   2. Community Health Nursing – Great Britain.   3. Cultural Competency – Great Britain.   4. Health Promotion – Great Britain.   WY 152 M2667 2008]
   RT120.L64M37 2008
   610.73′60941 – dc22

                                                            2008007174

A catalogue record for this book is available from the British Library.

Set in 10/12 pt Sabon by SNP Best-set Typesetter Ltd, Hong Kong
Printed in Singapore by Markono Print Media Pte Ltd

1   2008

Contents

List of contributors

Maureen Deacon PhD
Principal Lecturer for CPD and Framework Leader for the Framework for Continuing Professional, Personal and Practice Development (CP3d)
Continuing Professional Development and Post Graduate Studies Department
Manchester Metropolitan University
Elizabeth Gaskell Campus
Hathersage Road
Manchester M13 OJA

Garry Diack
Senior Lecturer
Continuing Professional Development and Post Graduate Studies Department
Manchester Metropolitan University
Elizabeth Gaskell Campus
Hathersage Road
Manchester M13 OJA

Eileen Fairhurst PhD MBE
Professor of Health and Ageing Policy Studies
Continuing Professional Development and Post Graduate Studies Department
Manchester Metropolitan University
Elizabeth Gaskell Campus
Hathersage Road
Manchester M13 OJA

Marilyn Fitzpatrick
Senior Lecturer
Continuing Professional Development and Post Graduate Studies Department
Manchester Metropolitan University
Elizabeth Gaskell Campus
Hathersage Road
Manchester M13 OJA

Diane Loggenberg PhD
Senior Lecturer in Psychology
Manchester Metropolitan University
Elizabeth Gaskell Campus
Hathersage Road
Manchester M13 OJA

Caroline Powell
Expert Patient Programme Manager/locality lead
Manchester Primary Care Trust
Manchester Community Health
Newton Heath Health Centre
2 Old Church Street
Newton Heath
Manchester M40 2JF

Margaret Presho
Senior Lecturer
Continuing Professional Development and Post Graduate Studies Department
Manchester Metropolitan University
Elizabeth Gaskell Campus
Hathersage Road
Manchester M13 OJA

Clare Street
Senior Lecturer
Continuing Professional Development and Post Graduate Studies Department
Manchester Metropolitan University
Elizabeth Gaskell Campus
Hathersage Road
Manchester M13 OJA

Ruth Thomas
Senior Lecturer
Continuing Professional Development and Post Graduate Studies Department
Manchester Metropolitan University
Elizabeth Gaskell Campus
Hathersage Road
Manchester M13 OJA

Introduction

Margaret Presho

With an ageing UK population, government commitment to reducing poverty and improving living standards, improvements in medical technology and increased life expectancy comes an increase in those living with long term conditions and some degree of disability. This book focuses on the management of long term conditions; not just by health care professionals but by patients themselves, as well as their families and carers. The authors who have contributed to this book strongly acknowledge that it is not only the older generation who live with long term conditions and this is illustrated in the inclusion of Chapter 7. Additionally, the vital role that both patients themselves and their families and carers play in managing long term conditions is valued and demonstrated in Chapters 3 and 4.

If you are hoping to learn how to manage specific long term conditions in the context of chronic disease management from a clinical, professional perspective, then this is not the book for you. Organizations such as the National Institute for Health and Clinical Excellence (NICE), the Scottish Intercollegiate Guidelines Network (SIGN), the British Thoracic Society, the British Hypertension Society, Clinical Knowledge Summaries (formerly NHS Prodigy), Asthma UK, Diabetes UK and other similar bodies can provide a range of clinical advice based on research, evidence-based practice and clinical expertise. Many of the chapters within this book will signpost you to similar organizations for further, or specific, information. However, this book will focus on the social model for health rather than the medical model, which is concerned with disease management. The aim of this book is to take a salutogenic approach to health; by this I mean an approach that explores how people living with one or more long term conditions may optimize their personal and social resources so as to improve the quality of their lives (or be assisted in doing so with their consent and collaboration).

The authors of this book come from a range of community nursing disciplines as well as from backgrounds in sociological and psychological research. Their academic and professional experiences, often combined with personal experience of long term conditions, and discussions with contemporary community practitioners have formed the foundations upon which this book is built. Experience of professional practice or community-based research has enabled the contributing authors to take into account some of the constraints that limit community practice as well as the political-, professional- and patient-driven incentives that motivate community practitioners.

The contributing authors want practitioners to consider what living with a long term condition means to those who experience it and how they as practitioners can contribute to improving the quality of patients' lives from both a physical and a psychological perspective. If you learn anything at all from this book, it is hoped that there will be a realization that health is much more than simply the absence of disease or provision of good quality (fit for purpose) health care services – although both of these aspects will have some role to play in improving the quality of patients' lives.

Each chapter has been written independently and could be used as a stand alone reference source; therefore some issues and themes will inevitably overlap, with their frequency of repetition possibly being directly correspondent to their acknowledged importance in the lives of those living with long term conditions. At the start of each chapter is a text box that outlines the key points contained within that chapter. Each chapter is ended with a list of references that have informed the chapter and that readers may find a useful resource for further reading. Please explore the book and, in doing so, consider some of the challenges that community practice presents as well as the rewards that practitioners can achieve in supporting patients living with long term conditions to improve the quality of their lives.

Chapter 1 explores the various models of care that have influenced the development of community practice within the context of managing long term conditions within the United Kingdom. The influx of North American philosophy on long term condition management and the way in which that fits (or not) into UK constructs of care provision are considered. The increase in use of technology to address care management is highlighted and there is some reflection on the potential effects of practice-based commissioning, although this is limited by the nature of the implementation process of practice-based commissioning across the country. Some role dilemmas and constraints of community practitioners are addressed (although this aspect is discussed in greater depth in Chapter 2), and the valuable role that patients, families and carers play in supporting the management of long term conditions is also reviewed. Finally, there is some mention of the single assessment process but as this is planned to be replaced by the Common Assessment Framework discussion is minimal.

Chapter 2 deals with the newly developed role of community case managers and community matrons, with a specific focus on how the existing infrastructure and implementation process have to some extent hindered role development and service delivery. There is some consideration of how policy has influenced practice, both in terms of driving and constraining service provision, although this aspect is covered in more depth in Chapter 11. Some of the tools used, and those currently under development, to case find and allocate resources are reviewed and a debate on the conflicting UK and North American care philosophies ensues. Education and training provision for those in and preparing to enter the newly established roles is highlighted and interprofessional as well as interdisciplinary contested issues are presented for contemplation. There is a focus on the social model of health as a foundation for practice and the thorny operational issues that this model elicits are aired. Perhaps more questions than answers are raised but the chapter is intended to stimulate practitioner reflection.

Chapter 3 discusses the vital role that patients and their support network have in promoting and maintaining healthy outcomes for people living with long term conditions. Concepts of health are discussed and the notion that heath is much more than the absence of disease, as advocated by the social model of health, is reinforced. The emergence of Expert Patient initiatives and the vital part that they play in supporting people in gaining autonomy, self-efficacy and empowerment is discussed; although the potential for patient–practitioner conflict is also acknowledged. There is also an explanation of the difficulties that measuring success of patient support initiatives can raise, given that they are often subjective and therefore not easily measurable. This is important given that the government is very much target driven and the fact that funding often goes hand in hand with the production of measurable results. An important aspect of this chapter is that it provides alternative perspectives on the notion of health, especially the notion of being healthy whilst concomitantly living with a long term condition.

Chapter 4 provides insight into the world of informal carers and the difficulties and rewards that they experience in providing care. The notions of care as a duty, as a burden, as a life experience and as a social phenomenon are explored and the expectations of society are challenged within this context. The social construct of disability is considered, as are the attitudes of the public to caring, illness and perceptions of value. It is acknowledged that carers have a valuable role to play in supporting the health economy and that their value is often ignored or made invisible by the government and its agents through policy and by the public through social expectations. The risks of caring are highlighted as economic, psychological and physical issues and the unequal distribution of caring roles between the two genders is presented for consideration. Finally, the practical resources and support networks that carers may wish to utilize are discussed as a road map for practitioners to help signpost carers with whom they may come into contact.

Chapter 5 is concerned with the National Service Framework for Long Term Conditions with a focus on learning disability issues. Living with a learning disability is shown as often being synonymous with living with a range of long term conditions whilst at the same time being afforded less access to care provision. The contribution of the seminal paper *Valuing People* is discussed and its limitations are indicated as a result of its status as a guidance paper rather than a legislative edict. Finally, the issue of health inequalities is given consideration and it is clear that those with learning disabilities are regarded as second class citizens from a range of perspectives; an issue that practitioners should take account of when planning and evaluating care provision.

Chapter 6 promotes mental health awareness as an issue for all practitioners and refers to the National Service Framework for Mental Health as a vehicle for enabling practice. The strong relationship between mental and physical illness is examined and the concomitant burdens that these two different experiences may have on people. The enduring nature of many mental health conditions is made explicit and the way in which those with mental health conditions are expected to conduct their lives to negotiate care provision and support is articulated. Issues of stigma, shame, identity and coping are all presented for reflection and practitioners are challenged to re-evaluate their perceptions of mental health problems. Living with a mental health problem is presented as a having a 'job' to fulfil with all its accompanying 'baggage'. This is a refreshing perspective on mental health issues that encourages practitioners to take into account the worldview of those living with such conditions.

Chapter 7 acknowledges the fact that not only older people but also young children live with long term conditions and, as medical technology advances, there will be a growing population of young people living with a long term 'disability'. The vulnerability of children with long term or complex conditions is reviewed, and their growing role as carers for others with long term conditions is presented for consideration. Policies that particularly affect young people are appraised and their influence on practice is reflected upon. The tripartite collaborative relationship between child, parent and professional is presented and the concomitant limitations and opportunities that this relationship avails are made explicit. Attachment theory, health inequalities, health inequity and social value are all taken into account within the context of the child with complex needs. The parent's perspective and the skill requirements of the practitioner are all considered in the light of legislative frameworks within which all adult parties concerned must operate.

Chapter 8 examines the psychosocial consequences of living with a long term condition. This chapter takes a different perspective in that it is viewed through the eyes of a psychologist. Quality of life or the well-being of those living with long term conditions is explored, not as a measure of disability, but rather as a means of maximizing a person's potential. Living with Parkinson's disease is used as an exemplar of living with a long term condition and, refreshingly, sexual well-being is offered as a point of discussion for those with long term conditions. This is an issue often glossed over when 'disability' and ill health are perused but when viewed from a salutogenic approach constitutes a vital component of a person's well-being. The psychological sequelae of living with long term conditions is scrutinized and, in particular, the potential iatrogenic impact of frequent contact with institutionalized care and health care professionals. The risks associated with health status disclosure and resultant stigma are reviewed and the 'dark side' of interpersonal relationships and altered identity for those with long term conditions is communicated in some depth.

Chapter 9 features the sociological concepts of home and the dearth of research on the redefinition of the home as a place of care by health care providers and policy-makers. There is discussion of risk assessments by practitioners redefining how and what a home should be; with a focus on home as a place of safety as determined by the practitioner rather than by the homeowner (patient/service user). This determinism confirms a paternalistic view of the home as a place to be deemed as safe only if supported by technology that assists the practitioner in their evaluation of and solution to perceived prevailing risk. In summary, care provision in the home by health professionals equates closely with medicalization of the home as a place of care and another, perhaps unrecognized, burden to be carried by those experiencing long term conditions. The home is viewed not as a private place for the homeowner but rather as a public space that one must qualify to inhabit when bound by the 'rules of health care professionalism'.

Chapter 10 considers the notion of cultural competence and asserts that this equates to professional competence given that a key component of the NHS Plan was that all practitioners be competent communicators. The underpinning tenet of this chapter is that the beliefs and values of cultures other than the practitioner's own should be valued and respected, especially where this is an important contributor to health outcomes. The notion of health literacy is also explored, as this has an important bearing on a person's ability for self-efficacy. Health inequalities are highlighted as having a key role to play in poor health outcomes and that it is those who are culturally disadvantaged that are most likely to be disadvantaged in terms of health. The practical aspects of language and cultural barriers are discussed across a range of domains, and tools to assist supporting practitioners and service users in bridging communication and ontological gaps are considered. Practitioners are invited to be reflexive and acknowledge their covert and overt prejudices so that they can look forward to ways of addressing cultural competence skills deficits.

Chapter 11 scrutinizes health and social care policy and the way in which policy-making decisions influence practice. This chapter challenges practitioners to become more politically active, at least at a local level, so that they are able to play a more proactive role as advocates for patients/service users rather than reacting to decisions imposed upon them that appear to adversely affect health outcomes. The issue of health inequalities and more particularly health inequity is addressed and it is emphasized how those most disadvantaged are most affected by policies that address the needs of the majority. The importance of community profiling is discussed, as is the link between profiling and the drive to reorient services to better address the needs of those living with long term conditions, if the outcome is to be greater independence for those with long term conditions. The single assessment process is identified as a tool to manage both service users' needs and to negotiate the health and social care interface. Whilst the name of the tool may change over time, the need for a framework for assessment and support of those living with long term conditions should look beyond the disease experienced and towards the best means (for the person) of achieving well-being and quality of life.

It is intended that the book be used as a resource to encourage critical thinking about long term condition management for those already engaged in community practice, or for those who intend to practise within the primary care sector in the near future. Nurses will perhaps find the content most applicable to their practice domain, although community case managers from a range of allied health professional disciplines may also find this a useful text. It is perceived that the contributions from authors with sociological and psychological research backgrounds, as well as from nurses across a range of disciplines, will appeal to the eclectic body of practitioners that constitute the community practice workforce.

Chapter 1

Frameworks for supporting patients with long term conditions

Marilyn Fitzpatrick

Key points

- A comparison of the similarities and differences between Wagner's USA model for improvement of chronic illness care and the UK NHS and social care long term conditions model
- Highlighting the constraints of the implementation of the UK model within the context of the social model of health
- Drawing attention to the potential professional misunderstanding surrounding the role of the community matron
- Exploring the contribution of technology to the management of long term conditions within community practice
- Examining the role that various patient support networks have in improving the quality of life for those with long term conditions

The move away from the traditional model of disease management, whereby patients were often passive recipients of care, is supported by government policy as prescribed in the White Papers *Our Health, Our Care, Our Say* (Department of Health (DOH), 2006a) and *Choosing Health: Making healthy choices easier* (DOH, 2004a), and the Green Paper *Independence, Wellbeing and Choice* (DOH, 2005a). This necessitates a proactive approach that focuses on the development of strategies to promote self-care, manage exacerbations of long term conditions, prevent complications and improve patient outcomes. This chapter explores the government's strategic vision for managing people with long term conditions, the concomitant impacts on NHS service delivery and the reconceptualization of the patient role. The influence of American models of long term conditions management is briefly explored as a precursor to a more detailed discussion of the NHS and social care long term conditions model (DOH, 2005b). Particular attention is afforded to ways in which the government's vision can be achieved and the impact that these have on patients, NHS staff, voluntary workers and the economy.

The development of a national policy on long term conditions management

The Department of Health (2005b) acknowledges the influence of the American generic chronic care model, developed by Wagner (1998), in its NHS and social care long term conditions model. Wagner's model contains six essential areas that need to be considered if effective care for people with long term conditions is to be achieved. These are comparable with the components of the NHS and social care long term conditions model (Table 1) which are individually addressed later in this chapter.

Information gathering, preceding and accompanying the development of the NHS and social care long term conditions model, comprised consideration of a number of reports including those published by the King's Fund (Weiner et al., 2001; Dixon et al., 2004; Hutt et al., 2004; Matrix Research and Consultancy & NHS Modernisation Agency, 2004; Corben & Rosen, 2005). The latter were commissioned to conduct a review of three US approaches to long term condition management piloted in the UK; these being Pfizer Healthcare Solutions, the United Health's Evercare model and Kaiser Permanente.

The Pfizer Healthcare Solution's InformaCare® approach uses technology to support patients and health professionals. The software incorporates national and local evidence-based guidelines and is tailored to local services. The philosophy underpinning the Pfizer approach is that of patient empowerment through support from case managers (Matrix Research and Consultancy & NHS Modernisation Agency, 2004).

Table 1 Comparison of the Wagner model and the Department of Health NHS and social care long term conditions model

Components of the model for improvement of chronic illness care (Wagner, 1998: p. 3)	Components of the NHS and social care long term conditions model (DOH, 2005b: p. 9)

Community and health system
Community resources and policies
Organization of health care
Decision support
Clinical information systems
Delivery system design
Self-management support
 	
Functional and clinical outcomes
Informed activated patient
Prepared, proactive practice team
	Infrastructure and delivery system
	Community resources
	Health and social care system environment
	Decision support tools and clinical
	   management information system (NPfIT)
	Case management
	Disease management
	Supported self-care
	Promoting better health
	
	Better outcomes
	Empowered and informed patients
	Prepared and proactive health and social care
	   teams

The second model to be evaluated was that of Kaiser Permanente, America's largest non-profit making integrated care organization (Kaiser Permanente, undated) that has demonstrated particular success in managing care for people with long term conditions (Dixon et al., 2004). Patients pay an annual fee and, in return, receive a comprehensive health care package. Unlike Pfizer Healthcare and Evercare, which utilize case management, Kaiser Permanente adopts a population-based approach to disease management. Feachem et al. (2002) undertook a comparison of Kaiser Permanente and NHS systems and found that the NHS performed less favourably in terms of outcomes for comparable inputs. Ham et al. (2003), who conducted a similar comparison but focused on hospital bed utilization, came to a similar conclusion. However, both studies were concerned with cost efficiency and performance and the patient experience was neglected, which is interesting given that the government purport themselves to be concerned with patient-centred services.

The third approach appraised in the Matrix study was UnitedHealth's Evercare model (which is in some aspects similar to the Castlefields model discussed in Chapter 2). The key components of the Evercare model are: (i) identification of high risk cases; (ii) preventative health care; (iii) intensive interventions to prevent deterioration; and (iv) care packages organized around the individual's needs. Case management is undertaken by advanced primary nurses (APNs) whose skills and clinical competence are comparable to those associated with the community matrons (Boaden et al., 2006). The Evercare approach is targeted at frail, older people and American studies indicate that it is successful in reducing emergency admissions by up to 50% (Hutt et al., 2004).

In 2003, UnitedHealth Europe introduced the Evercare approach to nine NHS Primary Care Trusts (PCTs) (Gravelle et al., 2007). The pilots were evaluated by Boaden et al. (2006) between 2003 and 2005 using a variety of methods including stakeholder interviews and analysis of hospital episode statistics on rates of emergency admissions and bed use. Whilst the Evercare approach was found to be popular with Evercare staff and patients in terms of perceived improved quality of patient lives, the rate of emergency admissions and bed occupancy failed to decrease. Gravelle et al. (2007) predict that the community matron initiative (see Chapter 2) will result in the same outcome, which is rather worrying given the huge resources that have been ploughed into it.

The NHS and social care long term conditions model

Evaluations such as those identified above were highly influential in the development of the Department of Health's strategic aim, which is to develop a systematic approach to supporting people with long term conditions. This includes: (i) creating new systems at a local level to maximize community resources and increase care provision in the home environment; (ii) ensuring that care packages are planned around the needs of the individual patient; and (iii) promoting self-care through patient empowerment (DOH, 2005b). Pivotal to the achievement of this aim is the need to establish an infrastructure that supports care delivery systems aimed at creating better outcomes. These three components form the basis of the NHS and social care long term conditions model (DOH, 2005b).

Establishing the infrastructure

Community resources, including statutory, voluntary and patient organizations comprise the first component of the infrastructure that underpins the NHS and social care long term conditions model. The Department of Health (2005b) has identified the development of appropriate services to support people with long term conditions as a priority. At the present time, the provision of services varies widely across the country. For example, the least affluent areas of England contain the lowest proportion of full-time general practioners (GPs) per 100 000 of the population (DOH, 2006b) and the provision of district nursing services varies according to geographical location (Audit Commission, 1999). New breeds of workers such as community matrons and case managers have been developed to address the needs of those with long term conditions, but these professionals cannot work in isolation; particularly as many do not provide 'out of hours' care. Collaborative working is therefore essential if the government's vision for long term condition management is to be achieved.

Voluntary and patient organizations complement statutory service provision and harnessing community resources is a prerequisite for supporting the model's success (DOH, 2005b). Social capital, whilst not explicitly mentioned in the NHS and social care long term conditions model, appears to be a relevant factor. The concept is multifaceted and difficult to define but there is a general consensus that it involves factors such as social participation, formal and informal social networks, and social cohesiveness (Harper, 2001; Morgan & Swann, 2004). Where social capital is established and flourishing, benefits to the community are apparent, although there is some concern that such a situation may be used to justify a decrease in the financing of welfare services (Harper, 2001). However, to provide equitable long term conditions services, sufficient community resources, regardless of whether they arise from social capital, voluntary services or statutory services, must be available to all regardless of an area's level of affluence or geographical location.

Action Learning Point

- Find out about social capital in your area.
- What informal social support networks are available for people with long term conditions?
- How could you raise awareness of these among your clients?
- How could you help them overcome any barriers to access?

Decision support and information systems form the second component of the infrastructure of the NHS and social care long term conditions model. Best practice in the management of long term conditions will be based on national and local guidelines and the use of information technology is promoted as the way forward in handling the information required for effective care management (DOH, 2005b). The implementation of summary care records, as part of the NHS Care Records Service is currently being undertaken by early adopter sites and will ultimately be rolled out across the NHS. Access to Summary Care Records will be limited to authorized health professionals although individual patients may view their records via HealthSpace (DOH, 2006c). The records of consenting patients will initially contain limited data such as current medication, adverse reactions and allergies, but it is envisaged that this will be expanded to include a wider range of information related to the patient's treatment including the results of diagnostic tests (NHS Connecting for Health, 2007).

Whilst the Summary Care Records initiative is in its infancy, it should ultimately prove useful to those working with people with long term conditions. Summary Care Records could be particularly useful to professionals undertaking first assessments as essential information could be gained prior to patient contact and utilized in the application of the Common Assessment Framework for Adults, proposed in the White Paper *Our Health, Our Care, Our Say* (DOH, 2006a). The single assessment process (see Chapter 11), introduced in the National Service Framework for Older People (2001), has been advocated as a model for the Common Assessment Framework for Adults but experience derived from the implementation of the care programme approach (DOH, 1999) and person-centred planning for people with learning disabilities (DOH, 2001) will also be utilized with the aim of developing an assessment framework that is applicable across the adult lifespan (O'Keeffe et al., 2007).

The final component of the NHS and social care long term conditions model infrastructure focuses on the health and social care system that is concerned with organizational issues such as the development of shared health and social care budgets, and practice-based commissioning (PBC) (DOH, 2005f). PBC involves the devolution of budgets from the PCT level to GP practices to be used to commission services. The Department of Health (2007) claims that its target of universal coverage of the PBC initiative was achieved by December 2006. However, Lewis et al. (2007: p. 1), as a result of their findings from a survey of GPs and practice managers, suggest that:

> 'in practice this means the creation of an environment in which PBC could flourish rather than one in which it is flourishing. As yet, active commissioning by general practice teams is not widespread.'

They explain that the purpose of PBC, in relation to the management of long term conditions, is to effect a change in emphasis from reactive care to preventative care that will subsequently reduce exacerbations of ill health and concomitant costs of treatment.

Any changes in service commissioning or delivery must be underpinned by a commitment to enhancing patient care and safety. The National Patient Safety Agency (NPSA) has developed a PBC risk assessment tool that is designed to help those involved in commissioning to ensure that a focus on patient safety remains central to the development process (NPSA, 2006). Consideration of risks to the patient must take priority but PBC also carries financial risks: for example, unpredicted fluctuations in service activities may result in budgets being exceeded. However, it is also true that budgets may be underspent, in which case the surplus can be used to develop other existing services (DOH, 2004b). Lewis et al. (2007) question whether the incentives to take on a commissioning role are sufficient to establish its widespread use in general practice; an issue discussed by others such as Mannion (2005) and Smith et al. (2005). The findings of Lewis et al. (2007)

indicate a high level of commitment to PBC and, although its impact on improving the quality of patient care was not immediately visible, respondents expressed optimism about the longer term benefits. PBC clearly is complementary to the ethos of the NHS and social care long term conditions model but it may be some time before its impact is truly determined.

> **Action Learning Point**
>
> - To what extent have general practices taken on the role of commissioning in your area?
> - Through discussion with colleagues and local PCT web-based information, make a list of examples that relate to which new services have become available.
> - Ask friends or family if they are aware of the changes and if they have experienced any improvements in service provision.

Developing the delivery system

The Department of Health (2005b) suggests that the delivery system is an appropriate starting point when developing strategies to support people with long term conditions but, arguably, community resources need to first be firmly established within the infrastructure of the NHS model. The delivery system is based on the Kaiser Permanente triangle which illustrates categories of care intervention determined by patient need. The three levels of intervention, in descending order of intensity of input are: (i) case management; (ii) disease-specific care management; and (iii) supported self-care. A core value underpinning each level of intervention is that of promoting better health by supporting people to make healthier lifestyle choices in line with the principles contained within the White Paper on public health (DOH, 2004a).

Identifying the 'high risk' population

The health of people with complex multiple long term conditions (level 3 of the Kaiser Permanente triangle) is subject to rapid deterioration, thus placing them at high risk of unplanned hospital admissions. The Department of Health (2005b) advocate that criteria for selecting patients for level 3 interventions should take account of the following factors:

- The frequency and duration of hospitalization.
- The number of existing medical conditions and associated problems.
- The number of medicines and level of concordance with prescriptions.
- The frequency of GP consultations related to their condition(s).
- High risk factors such the loss of an informal carer through bereavement or other circumstances.

The care of 'high risk' patients who meet these criteria will be managed by community matrons or case managers (see Chapter 2 for a detailed discussion of these roles). Their sphere of activity includes adopting a holistic approach to assessing health and social care needs, securing services on the patient's behalf and providing intensive interventions to improve quality of life. Where a high level of clinical intervention is required, patients should be assigned to a community matron (DOH, 2005e). However, it should be noted that the remit of the community matron also includes the political objectives of meeting public sector agreement (PSA) targets and reducing the use of emergency beds. Concerns have been expressed about the ability of community matrons to achieve PSA targets (Gravelle et al., 2007) but a recent report by NHS Employers (2006) suggests that they are instrumental in reducing hospital admissions. However, all exemplars in the report demonstrate a reliance on productive relationships with other professionals working in health and social care.

To orchestrate a reduction in acute bed occupancy, it is necessary to target those most at risk of unscheduled admissions. One way of doing this is to employ predictive case finding software such as the PARR (Patients At Risk of Re-hospitalisation) tools (DOH, 2006d). The PARR tool, originally introduced in 2005, has undergone a number of refinements. PARR1 and PARR2 rely on hospital inpatient data to predict the future admissions within the next 12 months and as such identify only those who have had contact with the acute sector within (normally) the past 3 years. To address this limitation the combined predictive model (the combined model), which utilizes a wider database, was released in December 2006. The combined model unites GP, outpatient and accident and emergency datasets with inpatient information and is thus able to identify people at risk of emergency admissions even if they have not yet experienced one (DOH et al., 2006d).

The value of combined model data as a means of case finding for community matrons is obvious but the tool could be of equal use to those who provide interventions at level 2 of the NHS and social care long term conditions model as it is able to stratify an entire population into levels of risk. The advantages of this in terms of long term conditions management are clear: preventative strategies can be aimed at those who are not yet presenting as complex cases but may do so without adequate support and intervention. However, in order for this to be feasible, the data need to be made available to those who work with 'level 2 patients'. General practice nurses will have access to such information but other community staff may have difficulty obtaining it. Therefore, strategies need to be established to facilitate sharing of relevant data.

The Department of Health (2005b) emphasizes the importance of collaboration and an integrated approach to care provision, although Singh (2005) reports that evidence on the effectiveness of multidisciplinary teams, in relation to clinical outcomes for people with long term conditions; is inconsistent. Hudson (2005: p. 381) takes up this theme and argues that:

> 'the scale of partnership ambition exhibited by the Government relates inversely to evidence of successful achievement. . . . In this respect, then, the LTC [long term conditions] policy tale is best located at the level of political rhetoric rather than daily reality.'

It is a question of debate whether this 'political rhetoric' will turn into 'daily reality' but it is clear that it will require a great deal of commitment by all involved in the management of people with long term conditions.

Multidisciplinary innovations in care delivery

One example of multidisciplinary commitment to the management of people with long term conditions is the 'virtual ward' initiative. This innovative way of preventing unplanned hospital admissions was first proposed by Dr Geraint Lewis, a specialist registrar, and developed by Croydon NHS (Croydon NHS, undated). Virtual wards mimic the reality of hospital wards in terms of management – the difference is that care is delivered in the home environment. Croydon's groundbreaking work is based on the development of two virtual wards, each of which 'admit' up to 100 high risk patients from a number of participating general practices.

Lewis (2006) explains that the 'wards' are led by a community matron who works in close partnership with patients' GPs. Staff allocated to these 'wards' include nurses, a pharmacist, social worker, occupational therapist, physiotherapist, mental health link, voluntary worker and ward clerk. Additional input is available from the palliative care team, alcohol service, dietician and specialist nurses. 'Beds' are allocated according to the required intensity of input and patients can be moved to a higher or lower category if their clinical circumstances change. Office-based 'ward rounds' are conducted on a daily basis and community matrons have direct telephone access to participating GPs. Patients in the lowest intensity 'beds' (those receiving monthly reviews) who have been stable for a number of months are discharged to the care of their GP. A full evaluation of the pilots is yet to be published but initial results appear very promising.

The role of technology in long term conditions management

Other ways of supporting people in the home environment include the use of assistive technology such as the Telecare system advocated by the Department of Health (2005c). Telecare provision is supported by a Government Preventative Technology Grant of £80 million (DOH, 2005c). A comprehensive range of services and equipment is available and the level of service can be tailored to individual needs. The government's ultimate aim is to ensure that by 2010, when the national framework agreement ends, all those who would benefit from assistive technology have Telecare systems installed in their homes. However, Wanless (2006) suggests that this ambition is unlikely to be achieved unless a very low level of service is established; given that much recent government health policy is based upon the advice of Wanless, such advocacy bucks the trend.

The Audit Commission (2004) identifies three components of the Telecare system: (i) providing information; (ii) monitoring the environment; and (iii) monitoring the person. At the most basic level, Telecare can provide alarm systems that alert a central response centre. In more advanced systems, sensors can be installed to monitor activity and trigger an alert if an expected activity fails to be undertaken within an agreed time. Action is then taken by the response centre on the client's behalf; for example by summoning a relative, professional carer or emergency service (see Chapter 9 for further consideration of the adverse effects that such invasive technology may potentially have on people's home environments).

At the top end of the spectrum is a comprehensive package of services and equipment that, in addition to providing basic alarms and environment monitoring devices, can provide medication alerts and convey data on a person's physiological status (NHS Purchasing and Supply Agency, 2007). 'Telehealth' is the term used to describe the more advanced systems used to monitor a person's health status (Cooke, 2007). Telehealth systems are deemed to be particularly useful in managing patients with a long term condition as they promote self-management whilst allowing the patient to remain in contact with health professionals (Audit Commission, 2004; DOH, 2005c). Patients are provided with equipment, for example, blood pressure monitors, peak flow meters and glucometers, for self-testing and the data are relayed to a health professional for interpretation. Hence signs of deterioration in a patient's condition are quickly recognized and appropriate preventative action can be taken.

Approximately 50% of patients fail to take their medicines as prescribed (DOH, 2005b). There may be a number of reasons for this, but where memory is an issue Telehealth can provide a medication reminder system. The Tunstall Lifeline 4000+ Medicine Reminder is currently under trial in Staffordshire PCTs (DOH, 2005d). An authorized carer records a medication reminder message on the patient's Lifeline unit, the machine activates visual and audible alerts at the time the medication should be taken, the patient presses a button to listen to the reminder and then presses another button (which connects them to the system's operator) to confirm that they have taken their medicine. If either of the last two steps is not completed within a specified time, an operator contacts the patient and takes appropriate action (Tunstall Group, 2007). Whilst this equipment has the potential to promote concordance with medication use, it will not be appropriate for all patients; for example, those who lack mental capacity or those with particular forms of hearing impairment.

In the situations described above, the use of technology is supported by personal interactions that can link patients, directly or via operators, to health professionals. This is particularly important as technology cannot replace human care provision (Brown, 2003). The patient's perspective appears to be somewhat neglected in the literature as most of this concentrates on cost efficiency and clinical outcome achievement (e.g. a reduction in emergency admissions). However, there is some evidence to suggest that users are generally satisfied with assistive technology (Chambers & Connor, 2002; Singh, 2005; Whitton & Mickus, 2007).

The effect on relationships between patients and professionals particularly merits further investigation as this is central to the care management situation. An ethnographic study by Hibbert et al. (2004) found that some nurses were concerned that it could adversely affect relationships with patients. The study highlights the barriers that exist when implementing changes in practice and the need to explore ways in which technology can enhance care delivery whilst supporting existing nurse–patient relationships.

It is apparent that Teleheath has huge potential in the management of people with long term conditions (DOH, 2007), particularly in relation to those most at risk of unscheduled hospital admissions – that is, those classified on the Kaiser Permanente triangle as requiring level 3 case management interventions. However, remote monitoring systems could prove very useful in disease-specific care management as well (level 2 of the Kaiser Permanente triangle).

Utilizing the skills of professional staff

Disease management requires a multidisciplinary approach and the application of disease-specific standards and guidelines such as those specified in the National Service Frameworks and National Institute for Clinical Excellence (NICE) guidance. Various health and social care workers have a role to play in supporting 'level 2' patients and the role of each merits detailed discussion. However, the Department of Health (2005e) suggest that general practice nurses, district nurses and specialist nurses can make a particular contribution.

General practice nurses play a significant role in the management of people with long term conditions (Mooney, 2000; Drennan & Goodman, 2004). Martin and Young (2006) report on a survey undertaken by the *Practice Nursing* journal (MA Healthcare Ltd) and the Royal College of Nursing that found that the general practice nurse contribution to managing long term conditions had increased as a result of the introduction of the Quality and Outcomes Framework (QOF) within the General Medical Services contract (NHS Employers & British Medical Association, 2006). The QOF provides general practices with financial incentives for achievement in four domains; one of which relates to the management of clinical conditions with an emphasis on common long term conditions. Participating practices (the majority) are required to establish disease registers and general practice nurses may contribute to the development of these in addition to carrying out other roles such as monitoring and supporting people with long term conditions (Morgan, 2005). They are likely to further develop their expertise in disease management and their position in the primary health care team places them in a prime position to share their knowledge with community-based colleagues (Saville et al., 2005), such as district nurses who are normally GP attached with responsibility for the more vulnerable members of the practice population, in particular those who cannot attend the practice, for example, housebound and elderly patients who are more likely to have a range of long term conditions.

The main client group of district nurses comprises people with long term conditions (Audit Commission, 1999; Wilson, 2005). The Department of Health (2005b) postulated that district nurses were the group most likely to make the transition to community matron. Hence, it follows that those who have remained in the district nursing role are likely to have existing expertise in managing the care of people with long term conditions. The Royal College of Nursing, Association of District Nurse Educators and Queen's Nursing Institute (2005) present a clear case for district nursing involvement in the long term conditions agenda by highlighting district nursing knowledge and skills of relevance to case management. Morgan (2005: p. 6) also examines the contribution of district nurses and asserts that:

> 'patients with long-term conditions have a special need for the skills and knowledge of district nurses, enabling them to make a unique contribution to the care of this vulnerable group.'

District nurses are the key providers of nursing care in the home (Audit Commission, 1999; Goodman et al., 2003). This affords them the privilege of gaining an intimate insight into the patient's health needs as well as the ability to glean information about environmental, personal and social circumstances. The nature of their work affords them opportunities of personal contact with relatives, neighbours and carers, and hence permits them to assess the availability of support networks. Although few district nurses have experience of care brokerage, they are skilled in mobilizing resources, have a wealth of case management skills (Drennan & Goodman, 2004) and a history of managing the care of patients with a wide range of long term conditions (Olver & Buckingham, 1997).

The political agenda for long term condition management has imposed widespread changes in the delivery of community health services and has major implications for district nursing (While, 2005). Morale amongst district nurses has been reported as low and feelings of uncertainty exist regarding their future role (Queen's Nursing Institute & the English National Board for Nursing, Midwifery and Health Visiting, 2002; Pratt, 2006). None the less, district nurses are embracing the challenges resulting from the impact of government policies and concomitant service reconfiguration (Queen's Nursing Institute, 2006) although it clear that they need to be more vocal in staking a claim in the long term conditions management agenda (Morgan, 2005; While, 2005).

The same may be true for specialist nurses who may find that the patients that they once had responsibility for are being case managed by community matrons. The vision of the Department of Health (2005b) is that all professionals who contribute to a person's care will work together in productive harmony but, as Hudson (2005) points out, this may not manifest in reality. Issues of territorialism and accountability will need to be resolved before effective partnership working can be established. Unlike North American organizations that employ all nursing and allied health care professional staff caring for patients with long term conditions subscribing to the organization, British nurses and their allied health professional colleagues are employed by different sectors of the NHS (social services and voluntary sector) and are therefore controlled by different budgets, different priorities and differing philosophies. The government stance is that community matron and nurse specialist roles are not interchangeable (Meadowcroft, 2006), but concerns have been raised by some multiple sclerosis specialist nurses that funding priority will be given to community matron posts (Multiple Sclerosis Trust, 2006). The Parkinson's Disease Society, Multiple Sclerosis Society and the Royal College of Nursing (2006: p. 16) acknowledge these feelings of unrest and advocate that:

> 'The Department of Health must make a statement that reinforces the valuable role of and need for disease specific specialist nurses as well as community matrons. Without this commissioners will not understand the importance of these distinctly different roles.'

It would also be prudent for the Department of Health to explicitly acknowledge the value of district nurses, whose role is afforded only a cursory mention in government literature on long term conditions. Although the work of district nurses is not disease specific, it is concerned with the provision of care across the spectrum of interventions outlined in the NHS and social care long term conditions model (Morgan, 2005). Together with community colleagues from other areas of practice, they possess the potential to make a particular impact in the promotion of self-care.

Action Learning Point

- Identify other professionals in your area who contribute to the long term conditions agenda.
- How does their work differ from your own? Are there any areas of overlap?
- How could collaborative working be developed to improve the patient experience?
- What barriers might exist and how might they be overcome?

Supporting self-care and self-management

Supporting self-care is advocated by the government as the way forward in managing long term conditions. The supported self-care (level 1) category of the Kaiser Permanente triangle comprises between 70% and 80% of the long term conditions population (DOH, 2005b). The demands of these patients on NHS and social services may not be as pronounced as those categorized as level 3 or level 2 patients but, if neglected, their conditions may deteriorate and their level of dependency may increase. Hence, interventions need to be aimed at slowing the progress of a disease, providing more effective ways of managing exacerbations, and helping people to fully participate in their treatment and cope with any limitations imposed by their condition. Where appropriate and with the patient's permission, families, friends and carers can be included in self-management plans.

The concept of patient empowerment is closely linked to self-management, which has been shown to improve health outcomes (Embrey, 2006). However, it is important to remember that some people may be reluctant to take more responsibility in the management of their condition and may prefer to maintain a level of dependency on others. The reasons for this are diverse but factors such as age, gender, level of education and social class have been noted as influential factors (Corben & Rosen, 2005). Cultural issues are also important: a recent study funded by the Joseph Rowntree Foundation found that some ethnic groups are more likely than others to embrace the concept of self-management (Salway et al., 2007).

Health and social services are urged to develop strategies to support self-care and self-management (DOH, 2005b, 2006e) and some of these elements are further discussed in Chapters 3, 4 and 10. The Department of Health (2006f) claims that some self-care strategies can reduce NHS expenditure on medicines, reduce GP consultations by up to 69%, and produce a decrease in emergency admissions and bed occupancy, although the latter is contested by Gravelle et al. (2007). The financial benefits reaped from reducing reliance on statutory services by assisting people to self-manage their conditions are obvious, yet in order for self-care strategies to be successful they must be sold in terms of benefits to patients and their families. One way of doing this is to stress the associated gains in relation to obtaining a greater degree of independence in managing their condition(s), but, as previously noted, not all patients seek to be independent.

Self-support networks

The Department of Health acknowledges that people will self-manage to varying degrees but advocates that promoting optimal self-management should be the goal of NHS service providers. In order to achieve this, it will be necessary to identify the information needs of patients and respond accordingly, establish the availability of patient education and training programmes, and invest in staff training to ensure that professionals understand the principles of self-care and are aware of self-support networks (DOH, 2006e). More information about these aspects of managing long term conditions can be found in Chapter 3.

Patients with a long term condition require sufficient and timely information. This is particularly true for the newly diagnosed, but Corben and Rosen (2005) found that the NHS was failing in this area. The Department of Health (2006e) fails to acknowledge this inadequacy and claims that people are more likely to trust information acquired from informal sources. Patients will should benefit from information produced by professionals that, in the main, is clinically focused. However, health professionals need to be aware of a range of information services so that they can direct patients to the most appropriate sources, including voluntary and public support networks.

A huge range of support networks exist, many of which may be particularly useful for people with long term conditions. The use of support networks is advocated by the Department of Health but findings from a systematic review of the evidence of the clinical effectiveness of self-care support networks (Woolacott et al., 2006) suggest that their overall value is questionable. This is not to say that all support networks are unsuccessful in their attempts to support their target population. The study by Woolacott et al. (2006) was concerned with clinical effectiveness and this may be at odds with the reasons why people join support networks (as outlined in Chapter 3).

The Expert Patient Programme

Helping people to acquire the skills and knowledge required for self-management is given particular prominence in the government's proposals for developing strategies to promote self-care. The Expert Patient Programme (EPP) (DOH, 2001), based on work undertaken at Stanford University Patient Education Research Centre, is one example of a NHS-based initiative devised to help patients gain skills in managing long term conditions. By November 2004, 98% of PCTs had participated in the pilots and a total of 1300 programmes had been delivered to approximately 17 000 people with long term conditions (Squire & Hill, 2006).

The duration of the programme normally spans six to seven weeks and the predetermined content is derived from the Stanford University manual (Expert Patient Programme, 2005). The distinguishing features of the EPP are that it is developed from the experiences of people with a long term condition and it is almost exclusively facilitated by tutors who are themselves living with a long term condition. The main aim of the EPP is to promote improvement in a patient's condition and prevent deterioration (DOH, 2001). Programme interventions are designed to develop patients' knowledge of their condition and treatments with the intention of increasing their capacity for effective self-management. The original programmes were disease specific but a generic model (Box 1) is generally favoured as many people with long term conditions share common problems (Expert Patient Programme, 2005).

Box 1: Typical content of a generic Expert Patient Programme (Wilson & Mayor, 2006: p. 17)

- Overview of self-management and chronic illness
- Making an action plan
- Relaxation/cognitive symptom management
- Anger, fear and frustration
- Fitness and exercise
- Better breathing
- Fatigue
- Nutrition
- Living wills
- Communication
- Medications
- Making treatment decisions
- Depression
- Working with the health care team

The final report on the national evaluation of the EPP, undertaken by Rogers et al. (2006) from the National Primary Care Research and Development Centre (NPCRDC), reveals some interesting data. The findings indicate mixed responses regarding the value of the programme but, overall, participants were positive about their experiences. Some reported increased motivation although the researchers suggest that this may not be sustained once the course has ended. Opportunities for social contact and a sense of support resulting from group membership were highly valued. The content of the course was appreciated by the majority; however, the course did not suit all and almost one-quarter expressed the view that the course was too basic.

Existing self-management behaviours appeared not to be influenced and the NPCRDC researchers postulated that this may be related to the generic nature of the programme. Aspects of the programme content were viewed negatively; in particular, the inclusion of living wills (also known as 'advanced statements' or 'advanced directives') (Dimond, 2004) was seen to be inappropriate and relevant to only a small minority of participants. The reasons for negative feelings towards the inclusion of living wills are only vaguely addressed in the evaluation report but it was noted that the topic was emotive. Under the Mental Capacity Act 2005, a number of requirements have to be met in order for a living will to be legally valid. One requirement is that it must be written by an adult with capacity; the document will come into effect only in the event that that person reaches a stage where they lack mental capacity (Fullbrook & Sanders, 2007). It may be that the EPP course participants preferred to focus on the 'here and now' of managing their conditions rather than confront the possibility of future mental incapacity that may render them unable to make decisions about their care and treatment.

In light of the findings regarding the perceived value of programme content, Rogers et al. (2006) recommended that the topic of living wills should be excluded from future EPP courses. Additionally, a recommendation was made that the living wills session be replaced by one that focused on social services and community support. It was thought that particular attention needed to be given to welfare and benefit systems as these are highly relevant to those who are either unable to work or intending to resume paid employment.

It was found that no reduction was achieved in the utilization of community health and primary care services but that some savings were apparent in relation to the use of overnight hospital and day case resources. Whilst financial gains for statutory health services are evident, Wilson and Mayor (2006) suggest that it will be some time before a significant impact is made because, as yet, only a small proportion of the long term conditions population are accessing the programmes. Cost savings for the NHS are obviously welcome but ethical issues are raised if these are gained at the patient's expense. Rogers et al. (2006) report that patients were financially disadvantaged by attending an EPP due to an increase in out of pocket expenses. As people with long term conditions are likely to be socially disadvantaged (Wheller, 2006), and hence living on reduced incomes, this finding is particularly worrying and may need to be addressed in order to promote recruitment to the programme. Kennedy et al. (2005) found that early EPPs were dominated by white, middle class participants so recruitment of a wider population is likely to be particularly challenging.

Despite the noted limitations, the EPP clearly offers real and potential benefits for participants and, furthermore, it appears to be cost effective. However, given the main findings of the national evaluation, a number of improvements will need to be made if the intended impacts of the programme are to be fully realized. It remains to be seen whether or not the EPP will continue as other strategies to promote self-care may be equally, or more, effective. The government recognizes that not all people will wish, or be able, to develop self-management skills to the extent promoted by the EPP. However, it asserts that most people will want to be involved in decisions about their care and treatment.

Strategies to promote self-care through shared decision-making

Concordance is the term used to describe the process of helping people to make informed choices about their care options. It is normally associated with the prescribing of medicines but, as Oakley (2007) points out, it is equally applicable to situations where other medical interventions may be deemed necessary or desirable. Concordance pivots on the concept of informed choice, which relies on the provision of information that is evidence-based, culturally sensitive and relevant to the needs of individual patients. The importance of providing timely and appropriate information is addressed in the first of the 11 quality requirements set out in the National Service Framework for Long Term Conditions (DOH, 2005g).

The Long Term Conditions Framework focuses on neurological conditions but contains guidance that is applicable to the provision of services for people with other long term conditions. In addition to promoting the EPP, it advocates 'newly diagnosed courses' (DOH, 2005g: p. 22) that should arise from a collaborative partnership between statutory sector health professionals and voluntary organizations. Minimal information is given on the nature of these courses and the role of the voluntary sector is not made explicit. However, in common with the EPP, they are likely to take advantage of the knowledge, skills and experiences of voluntary workers and consequently contribute to a reduction of NHS expenditure.

Conclusions

This chapter has considered how the NHS and social care long term conditions model (DOH, 2005b) attempts to make provision for those experiencing long term conditions but highlights the shortfall within the existing system that may constitute a barrier to its effective implementation. The barriers are mainly concerned with inappropriate planning within the context of community service reorientation, a theme that will be revisited in other chapters within this book. Additionally, some of the new role responsibilities for community case managers and community matrons have been investigated and appear to have been left open to interpretation at a local level. This aspect has resulted in misunderstanding and suspicion amongst other existing community practitioners and has been confounded by lack of structured preparation for those new roles. The disadvantages and benefits of various North American models of community care provision for those with long term conditions has been briefly explored with the notion of the Expert Patient Programme as an element that can be seen to have positive benefits for patients with long term conditions, especially those who are willing to take responsibility for self-care. However, it is acknowledged that this enthusiasm and capacity does not extend to all those experiencing long term conditions, in particular the more vulnerable members of society. The prospects for technology and decision support systems have been examined as a means of enhancing the options for those living with a long term condition. This has been discussed in particular as a means of avoiding emergency hospital admission, although moving hospital equipment into the home environment could be construed by some as an invasion of privacy and medicalization of the activities of daily living. Such technologies could be seen as a move towards the mechanization and dehumanization of health care.

Politically motivated decisions and their impact on health care provision have been alluded to within the context of the community matron's role as a backcloth for the implementation of frameworks focusing on the management of long term conditions. The financial benefits of patients self-managing their conditions, a move towards preventative health care interventions and reducing hospital occupancy, being the main drivers for the implementation of the model, are all considered within this chapter. Finally, the notion of peer support from others experiencing long term conditions as well as the generation and profile raising of various voluntary and public patient support networks as a means of promoting self-care within the community of those with long term conditions have been taken into account. Since the inception of the NHS, patients and practitioners have experienced many changes, including some ideas that have been recycled under a different banner. The shift towards community care began more than 15 years ago but the move back to the promotion of self-care and prevention of hospital bed occupancy may signify either the welcome rebirth of the NHS in its originally intended format as a 'sickness prevention' service or a return to the days when the disadvantaged found access to health care provision particularly difficult to obtain. Practitioners engaged in community practice must ensure that the latter does not become reality.

References

Audit Commission (1999) *First Assessment: A review of district nursing services in England and Wales.* London, Audit Commission.

Audit Commission (2004) *Implementing Telecare: Strategic analysis and guidelines for policy makers, commissioners and providers*. London, Audit Commission.

Boaden, R., Dusheiko, M., Gravelle, H. et al. (2006) *Evercare Evaluation: Final report*. Manchester, National Primary Care Research and Development Centre.

Brown, S. (2003) Guest editorial: next generation telecare and its role in primary and community care. *Health and Social Care in the Community* **11** (6): 459–462.

Chambers, M. & Connor, S. (2002) User-friendly technology to help family carers cope. *Journal of Advanced Nursing* **40** (5): 568–577.

Cooke, R. (2007) Introducing: Telehealth and Telecare. *British Journal of Community Nursing* **12** (7): 307.

Corben, S. & Rosen, R. (2005) *Self-management for Long-term Conditions: Patients' perspectives on the way ahead*. London, King's Fund.

Croydon NHS (undated) Introducing Virtual Wards. http://www.croydon.nhs.uk/sections/frame.html?sec=182 [accessed 12 July 2007].

Department of Health (1999) *Effective Care Co-ordination Mental Health Services. Modernising the care programme approach*. London, Department of Health.

Department of Health (2001) *The Expert Patient: A new approach to chronic disease management for the 21st century*. London, Department of Health.

Department of Health (2004a) *Choosing Health: Making healthy choices easier*. London, Department of Health.

Department of Health (2004b) *Practice Based Commissioning: Promoting clinical engagement*. London, Department of Health.

Department of Health (2005a) *Independence, Wellbeing and Choice*. London, Department of Health.

Department of Health (2005b) *Supporting People with Long Term Conditions. An NHS and social care model to support local innovation and integration*. London, Department of Health.

Department of Health (2005c) *Building Telecare in England*. London, Department of Health.

Department of Health (2005d) *Examples of Self Care Devices and Assistive Technologies to Support Self Care*. London, Department of Health.

Department of Health (2005e) *Supporting People with Long Term Conditions. Liberating the talents of nurses who care for people with long term conditions*. London, Department of Health.

Department of Health (2005f) *Making Practice Based Commissioning a Reality – Technical guidance*. London, Department of Health.

Department of Health (2005g) *The National Service Framework for Long-term Conditions*. London, Department of Health.

Department of Health (2006a) *Our Health, Our Care, Our Say: Investing in the future of community hospitals and services*. London, Department of Health.

Department of Health (2006b) *Tackling Health Inequalities: Status report on the Programme for Action – 2006 update of headline indicators*. London, Department of Health.

Department of Health (2006c) *Report of the Ministerial Taskforce on the NHS Summary Care Record*. London, Department of Health.

Department of Health (2006d) *PARR1 and PARR2. A brief guide*. London, Department of Health.

Department of Health (2006e) *Supporting People with Long Term Conditions to Self Care: A guide to developing local strategies and good practice*. London, Department of Health.

Department of Health (2006f) *Self Care for People with Long Term Conditions*. London, Department of Health.

Department of Health (2007) Practice Based Commissioning: Implementation monitoring. http://www.dh.gov.uk/en/Policyandguidance/Organisationpolicy/Commissioning/Practice-basedcommissioning/DH_4136758 [accessed 12 July 2007].

Dimond, B. (2004) The refusal of treatment: living wills and the current law in the UK. *British Journal of Nursing* **13** (18): 1104–1106.

Dixon, J., Lewis, R., Rosen, R., Finlayson, B. & Gray, D. (2004) *Managing Chronic Disease. What can we learn from the US experience?* London, King's Fund.

Drennan, V. & Goodman, C. (2004) Nurse-led case management for older people with long-term conditions. *British Journal of Community Nursing* **9** (12): 547–553.

Embrey, N. (2006) A concept analysis of self-management in long-term conditions. *British Journal of Neuroscience Nursing* **2** (10): 507–513.

Expert Patient Programme (2005) *Stepping Stones to Success: An implementation, training and support framework for lay led self-management programmes.* London, Department of Health.

Feachem, R., Sekhri, N. & White, K. (2002) Getting more for their dollar: a comparison of the NHS and California's Kaiser Permanente. *British Medical Journal* **324**: 135–143.

Fullbrook, F. & Sanders, K. (2007) Consent and capacity 2: the Mental Capacity Act 2005 and 'living wills'. *British Journal of Nursing* **16** (8): 574–575.

Goodman, C., Ross, F., Mackenzie, A. & Vernon, S. (2003) A portrait of district nursing: its contribution to primary health care. *Journal of Interprofessional Care* **17** (1): 97–108.

Gravelle, H., Dusheiko, M., Sheaff, R. et al. (2007) Impact of case management (Evercare) on frail elderly patients: controlled before and after analysis of quantitative outcome data. *British Medical Journal* **334**: 31–34.

Ham, C., York, N., Sutch, S. & Shaw, R. (2003) Hospital bed utilisation in the NHS, Kaiser Permanente, and the US Medicare programme: analysis of routine data. *British Medical Journal* **327**: 1257–1263.

Harper, R. (2001) *Social Capital. A review of the literature.* London, Office for National Statistics.

Hibbert, D., Mair, F., May, C., Boland, A., O'Connor, J., Capewell, S. & Angus, R. (2004) Health professionals' responses to the introduction of a home telehealth service. *Journal of Telemedicine and Telecare* **10** (4): 226–230.

Hudson, B. (2005) Sea change or quick fix? Policy on long-term conditions in England. *Health and Social Care in the Community* **13** (4): 378–385.

Hutt, R., Rosen, R. & McCauley, J. (2004) *Case-managing Long-term Conditions. What impact does it have in the treatment of older people?* London, King's Fund.

Kaiser Permanente (undated) *Facts and Statistics.* http://newsmedia.kaiserpermanente.org/kpweb/fastfactsmedia/entrypage2.do [accessed 12 July 2007].

Kennedy, A., Rogers, A. & Gately, C. (2005) Assessing the introduction of the expert patients programme into the NHS: a realistic evaluation of recruitment to a national lay-led self-care initiative. *Primary Health Care Research and Development* **6**: 137–148.

Lewis, G. (2006) Virtual wards. (RCN annual District Nursing conference presentation.) http://www2.rcn.org.uk/pcph/forums/district_nurses/events [accessed 12 July 2007].

Lewis, R., Curry, N. & Dixon, M. (2007) *Practice-based Commissioning: From good idea to effective practice.* London, King's Fund.

Mannion, R. (2005) Practice based commissioning: a summary of the evidence. *Health Policy Matters* **11**: 1–4.

Martin, J. & Young, L. (2006) Practice nurses' terms and conditions: a survey. *Practice Nursing* **17** (11): 570–572.

Matrix Research and Consultancy & NHS Modernisation Agency (2004) *Learning Distillation of Chronic Disease Management Programmes in the UK.* London, NHS Modernisation Agency. http://www.natpact.nhs.uk/cms/363.php [accessed 12 July 2007].

Meadowcroft, R. (2006) How effectively workforce planning, including clinical and managerial staff, has been undertaken, and how it should be done in the future. (Written evidence submitted by the Parkinson's Disease Society (WP 53) to the Select Committee on Health.) http://www.publications.parliament.uk/pa/cm200506/cmselect/cmhealth/1077/1077we47.htm [accessed 12 July 2007].

Mooney, D. (2000) Managing chronic obstructive pulmonary disease in primary care. *British Journal of Community Nursing* 5 (11): 554–599.

Morgan, A. & Swann, C. (eds) (2004) *Social Capital for Health: Issues of definition, measurement and links to health*. London, Health Development Agency.

Morgan, M. (2005) New opportunities for district nursing: chronic disease and matrons. *British Journal of Community Nursing* 10 (1): 6–7.

Multiple Sclerosis Trust (2006) *Support for MS Posts. Way Ahead*, Vol. 10, Part 3. http://www.parkinsons.org.uk/pdf.aspx?page=7965 [accessed 12 July 2007].

National Patient Safety Agency (2006) *Risk assessment programme. Practice-based commissioning for patient safety*. London. NPSA.

NHS Connecting for Health (2007) *The NHS Care Records Service: A guide for the nursing community*. http://information.connectingforhealth.nhs.uk/default.aspx?ProductInfo=29486 [accessed 12 July 2007].

NHS Employers (2006) *Improving Services for People with Long-term Conditions through Large-scale Workforce Change*. London, NHS Confederation (Employers) Company Ltd.

NHS Employers & British Medical Association (2006) *Revisions to the GMS Contract 2006/07. Delivering investment in general practice*. London, NHS Confederation (Employers) Company Ltd.

NHS Purchasing and Supply Agency (2007) *National Framework Agreement for Telecare (including equipment, installation, maintenance, monitoring and response services)*, Version 2.2. http://www.pasa.nhs.uk/pasa/Doc.aspx?Path=[MN][SP]/ProductsandServices/Telecare/0707TelecareV2.2informationpack2july07.pdf [accessed 12 July 2007].

Oakley, S. (2007) Agreeing on treatment through shared decision-making. *Prescriber* 18 (4): 45–50.

O'Keeffe, M., Hills, A., Doyle, M. et al. (2007) *UK Study of Abuse and Neglect of Older People: Prevalence survey report*. London, National Centre for Social Research.

Olver, L. & Buckingham, K. (1997) Analysis of district nurse workload in the community. *British Journal of Community Health Nursing* 2 (3): 127–134.

Parkinson's Disease Society, Multiple Sclerosis Society & the Royal College of Nursing (2006) *Developing Integrated Health and Social Care Services for Long-term Conditions: Report from a symposium examining the interface between community matrons and specialist nurses for Parkinson's disease and multiple sclerosis*. London, Royal College of Nursing.

Pratt, L. (2006) Long-term conditions 5: meeting the needs of highly complex patients. *British Journal of Community Nursing* 11 (6): 234–240.

Queen's Nursing Institute (2006) *Vision and Values: A call for action on community nursing*. London, Queen's Nursing Institute.

Queen's Nursing Institute & English National Board for Nursing, Midwifery and Health Visiting (2002) *District Nursing: 'The invisible workforce'; a discussion paper*. London, Queen's Nursing Institute/English National Board.

Rogers, A., Bower, P., Gardner, C. et al. (2006) *The National Evaluation of the Pilot Phase of the Expert Patient Programme: Final report*. Manchester, National Primary Care Research and Development Centre.

Royal College of Nursing, Association of District Nurse Educators & Queen's Nursing Institute (2005) District nurses and the modern workforce. *Primary Health Care* 15 (3): 21–22.

Salway, S., Platt, L., Chowbey, P., Harriss, K. & Bayliss, E. (2007) *Long-term Ill Health, Poverty and Ethnicity*. Bristol, Policy Press.

Saville, M., Humphrey, C. & Mama, J. (2005) Supporting patients with long-term conditions. *Practice Nursing* **16** (10): 488–491.

Singh, D. (2005) *Transforming Chronic Care. Evidence about improving care for people with long-term conditions.* Birmingham, University of Birmingham Health Services Management Centre.

Smith, J., Dixon, J., Mays, N. et al. (2005) Practice based commissioning: applying the research evidence. *British Medical Journal* **331**: 1397–1399.

Squire, S. & Hill, P. (2006) The Expert Patients Programme. *Clinical Governance: an International Journal* **11** (1): 17–21.

Tunstall Group (2007) *Case Study: Medication compliance.* http://www.tunstall.co.uk/assets/literature/6_2_49Medication_Compliance_Staffordshire_MRI.pdf [accessed 12 July 2007].

Wagner, E. (1998) Chronic disease management: what will it take to improve care for chronic illness? *Effective Clinical Practice* **1**: 2–4.

Wanless, D. (2006) *Securing Good Care for Older People.* London, King's Fund.

Weiner, J., Lewis, R. & Gillam, S. (2001) *US Managed Care and PCTs: Lessons to a small island from a lost continent.* London, King's Fund.

Wheller, L. (2006) Limiting long term illness. In: M. Bejekal, V. Osborne, M. Yar & H. Meltzer (eds) *Focus on Health.* Basingstoke, Palgrave Macmillan, pp. 24–32.

While, A. (2005) Staking a claim to manage chronic disease. *British Journal of Community Nursing* **10** (4): 196.

Whitten, P. & Mickus, M. (2007) Home telecare for COPD/CHF patients: outcomes and perceptions. *Journal of Telemedicine and Telecare* **13** (2): 69–73.

Wilson, P. (2005) Long-term conditions: making sense of the current policy agenda. *British Journal of Community Nursing* **10** (12): 544–552.

Wilson, P. & Mayor, V. (2006) Long-term conditions. 2: supporting and enabling self-care. *British Journal of Community Nursing* **11** (1): 6–10.

Woolacott, N., Orton, L., Benyon, S., Myers, L. & Forbes, C. (2006) *Systematic Review of the Clinical Effectiveness of Self Care Support Networks in Health and Social Care.* York, Centre for Reviews and Dissemination.

Chapter 2

Case managers and community matrons

Margaret Presho

Key points

- Outlining the patient profile of those with long term conditions
- Exploring community case manager and community matron roles
- Identifying how USA models of care provision and case management differ from UK expectations
- Considering how government policy both constrains and drives the health and social care agenda
- Examining the public health role within the context of community matron and case management practice

Government expectations for practice

The Case Management Competences Framework (NHS Modernisation Agency & Skills for Health, 2005) details the educational and skills requirements deemed appropriate for practitioners supporting people living with long term conditions. For the purpose of defining the level of service provision required, people with long term conditions have been categorized into three separate groups. Those who fall into category level 3 are designated as requiring a high level of care with multiple needs usually requiring very skilled nursing input. Such high intensity needs are considered to be best met by community matrons who, in addition to having the skills required of a case manager, will also be capable of advanced clinical nursing practice. Hence only nurses can be designated as community matrons – a less than flattering title for male practitioners – whilst practitioners from a range of health-related disciplines can become community case managers. The range of skills required by both community matrons and case managers have been mapped against the Knowledge and Skills Framework of the Agenda for Change initiative (Department of Health (DOH), 2004a). This provides guidance for employers in determining levels of remuneration and role specification whilst also, to some extent, informing the public of professional role and service delivery expectations. Some Primary Care Trusts (PCTs) have not clearly defined the different roles expected of community case managers and community matrons, thus both titles may be used by different trusts to signify their interpretation of the level of service delivery that they expect and the remuneration that they intend to pay to the post holder.

People living with long term conditions who fall into category level 2 are designated as having less intense needs than those in category level 3 but still requiring an intermittently high level of service provision. The services required by this group, like those in category level 3, will be delivered by a range of providers. However, in order to prevent fragmentation of service delivery and to ensure that services are both timely and apposite, a case management approach is considered to be appropriate. Case managers will have skills across a range of domains but will predominantly co-ordinate rather than deliver services, although local needs and service organization will determine the balance of care management and care delivery provided. For this reason, it is expected that practitioners such as social workers, allied health professionals or nurses will take up the role of case management (NHS Modernisation Agency & Skills for Health, 2005).

Of those people with long term conditions who fall into category level 1, approximately 70% are considered to be self-caring although occasional support may be necessary. Support may be provided by input from family, friends and carers, Expert Patient Programmes (DOH, 2001a) or, in times of crisis, more intensive input from case managers or even community matrons. Given that there are more than 17 million people living with long term conditions (Coalition of Health Bodies, 2005) and that there is a government commitment that patients with complex long term conditions will be supported by 3000 community matrons or case managers (DOH, 2004b, 2005a), it is clear that criteria for referral to community matron and case manager caseloads needs to be carefully considered. It is also apparent that whilst Expert Patient initiatives have a strong role to play, people living with long term conditions have a huge responsibility for managing their conditions effectively if their own health outcomes, quality of life and life expectancy are to be improved.

Inequalities in health and inequity of access to service provision

The burden of chronic disease is greater in less affluent populations (DOH, 2004c; World Health Organization, 2006) and therefore the impact of managing long term conditions will be much greater in some primary care organizations than in others. This economic aspect is an issue that case managers and community matrons will need to proactively consider when drawing up their criteria for caseload admission and for determining the type and frequency of contact, especially where intensive, advanced clinical skills are not required. It should also be noted that less affluent populations are less likely to have sophisticated coping strategies, extended support networks or the financial means to enable alternative measures for coping with their condition such as private care provision or receipt of voluntary family-led care. Family and friends are more likely to be in paid employment with little or no opportunity for carers' leave or extended unpaid leave or may not be in a position to support a person with complex needs as they may also be living with one or more long term conditions themselves. Traditionally, caring has been seen as an aspirant human quality much lauded in the context of family relationships and, as such, promoted by government policy (National Health Service and Community Care Act 1990) but more recent policy acknowledges the social and economic burden of caring (DOH, 2001b). Should family or friends opt to become carers, they may find their social circumstances greatly reduced:

'Taking on a caring role can mean facing a life of poverty, isolation, frustration, ill health and depression. Many carers give up an income, future employment prospects and pension rights to become a carer.' (Princess Royal Trust for Carers, 2006: p. 2)

Hence an important element of the community case manager role is to provide effective professional leadership and work towards facilitating responsive changes in service provision to meet local needs. Also, the ability to work with multiple stakeholders and to engage both patients and their families and carers in health protection strategies are intended as key functions of the case manager and community matron roles. Yet, despite apparent government commitment to facilitate improved care provision for those living with complex long term conditions, discussion with practitioners in post reveals that services are difficult to co-ordinate due to cuts in primary care budgets, competition between health and social care providers for resources, and inappropriate and complex criteria for referral. All these result in delayed or refused acceptance by some services, competing priority agendas and patient reluctance to accept some supportive measures. Additionally, as general practitioners (GPs) become more aware of the potential of community matrons and case managers, caseloads are in danger of becoming overwhelmed unless specific referral criteria are applied for admission to caseloads. This latter aspect is of special concern now that primary care organizations rather than GPs are responsible for out of hours services. Some community case managers and matrons do not provide weekend or 'out of hours' services thus patients inevitably fall back on emergency services when a weekend or evening crisis arises. This service deficit will in turn impact on emergency bed admissions – one of the targets that community case managers and matrons were intended to reduce.

Discussion with community case managers has revealed how GPs in some areas appear to believe that once a patient has been referred to a community case manager's caseload, the GP is then absolved from home visits. One case manager had responsibility for the practice populations from five GPs and already had 80 patients with complex health problems on her caseload. She confirmed that as GPs become more aware of her role, the workload would increase and more stringent criteria for referral and active case management would have to be established. In addition, she added that as patients become aware of the support that can be provided by community case managers, they have an inclination to become more, rather than less, dependent upon her support. Such tendencies rather defeat the intended object of increasing independent living for those with the most complex long term conditions.

Conflicting reports about the success of the community case manager and community matron initiative from the government and independent researchers are perhaps making trusts reluctant to recruit, especially as budgets for community services are slashed to make up for overspending and funding inadequacies.

Action Learning Point

- Who is responsible for out of hours services in your practice area?
- Are community case managers or community matrons available for support 24 hours per day, seven days per week?
- Find out what the criteria are for referral to the case management practitioner and how patients might contact their case manager/community matron, particularly when faced with an 'out of hours' crisis.

Models for practice and case finding

The government envisaged that 3000 community matrons would be in post by March 2007 with caseloads of 50–80 patients, but by September 2006 only 366 community matrons were actually in post. This makes their intended remit hard to meet given that the number of people with long term conditions exceeds 17.5 million and an expected 5% of those (875 000) may require intensive support during any given period of time. The Department of Health claim that the discrepancy is due to people not entering job descriptions correctly in the NHS workforce census. However, given that the category of 'community matron' was clearly identified, the Department of Health's explanation appears rather limited. Clearly resources are not infinite but if more service provision is to be community-based and the intention is to manage the ambulatory conditions that largely represent long term conditions within the primary care rather than the acute sector, then funding levels and the workforce to deliver intended outcomes must be realistic enough to enable safe and effective care provision.

It is pertinent to remember that long term conditions fluctuate in their impact upon individual patients and vary in the same patient over periods of time. Obviously, an important aspect of practice for those in post is to define their caseloads using specific criteria to establish predictive risk of hospital admission. One mechanism for this is the Castlefields model; a further method is the use of the 'PARR + tool' (see www.kingsfund.org.uk for further information on these models). The latter is a case finding tool available to general practice and primary care organizations developed by the King's Fund, New York University and Health Dialog Analytic Solutions (2006) and the former was developed by the Castlefields Health Centre Team (DOH, 2005b: p. 15). An earlier version of the PARR (Patients At Risk of Re-hospitalisation) tool focused on specific conditions experienced by patients admitted as emergencies to hospital, whereas the later version, refined by response to user feedback, identifies all emergency admissions and has since been criticized by practitioners and PCTs for the greater number of false positive referrals identified using the threshold criteria.

Development of appropriate care models and risk assessment tools will be an evolutionary process as systems developed in the United States and adapted for use in the UK do not sit comfortably with NHS care delivery and management. One major reason for their incompatibility is that US systems are predicated on patient ability to pay. Given that UK patients do not pay at the point of contact and that less affluent populations are more likely to experience multiple and complex problems associated with long term conditions, then UK models of care must take into consideration how the wider determinants of health impact on patients with such conditions and use practitioners' time effectively to create opportunities for patients that enable equality of access to services and provide education on self-care, and access to available resources to improve the quality of the lives of patients. Hudson (2005) has identified other valid reasons for incompatibility between North American and UK health systems in the management of long term conditions. He cites how US nurses are employed directly by the health care economies responsible for patient care management and delivery whereas UK nurses are employed by a range of NHS PCTs and as such have varied responsibility and accountability issues. US nurses are concerned with preventing acute sector admissions by supporting patients in nursing homes whilst UK nurses are charged with maintaining independent living for those with long term conditions even of the most complex nature. In addition to these important different criteria, there are considerably more nurses per patient within the USA than is possible within the UK.

In a small North American study by Kane et al. (2001), Evercare, one of three North American companies piloted in nine PCTs across the UK, reported that one-third of their practitioners' time was spent on direct patient care and just under a third on indirect care, including liaison with formal and informal carers. How the remaining third of working hours were spent was not well articulated except to state that administrative duties were completed.

This chapter will explore the roles of UK community case managers and community matrons with reference to the NHS Modernisation Agency and Skills for Health (2005) Case Management Competences Framework, incumbent practitioner comments and published UK-based studies.

The government is keen to further develop services to support people with long term conditions to live independently in the community. Part of the process involved in enabling independent living and the prevention of institutionalization is to reorientate services to better respond to the changed needs of service users. Shared provider agendas and Common Assessment Frameworks are two potential means of enabling the reorientation process. So as to clarify the decision-making process that would enable individual patients to be properly assessed to determine their eligibility for continuing care, the Department of Health is currently devising a 'decision support tool'. This would enable identification of those eligible for continuing support so as to help prevent frequent readmission to hospital care and long duration stays where admission is unavoidable. The draft tool (DOH/Social Care Directorate/Continuing Care, 2007: p. 4) shown in Fig. 1 explores patient needs in 11 domains with patient requirements ranging from 'no need' to 'priority need'. The final version of the draft tool will eventually become part of the National Framework for NHS Continuing Healthcare. The domains to be considered by case managers, GPs, community practitioners, social workers, hospital discharge planners and any other relevant health or social care professional will potentially be those of: behaviour, cognition, psychological and emotional needs, communication, mobility, nutrition, continence, skin (including tissue viability), breathing, drug therapies and medication and altered states of consciousness. It is expected that where any need falls into one of the four priority categories, continuing care will be deemed necessary. Additionally, where two or more needs are considered to be in the severe categories of any of the 11 domains, then again continuing care will be required.

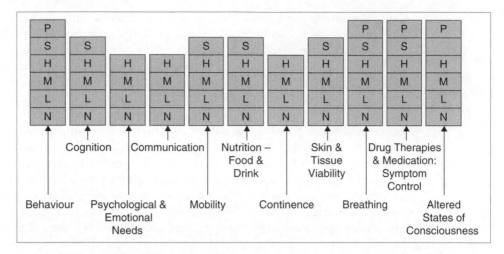

Figure 1 The draft tool (DOH/Social Care Directorate/Continuing Care, 2007: p. 4) for the assessment of patients to determine their eligibility for continuing care. N, no need; L, low need; M, medium need; H, high need; S, severe need; P, priority need.

In conjunction with this tool, it is intended that a fast track decision tool also be used for referral of those with short term life expectancy or in imminent need of palliative care. Existing and planned tools are or will be in place to determine those patients eligible or suitable for case management or more intensive support from community matrons with advanced clinical nursing skills. However, finding patients and assessing their needs is only part of the role in which community case managers and community matrons will be expected to engage. Other role expectations have been cited by the Department of Health and Social Services for Northern Ireland (2006) as care co-ordination, management of specific diseases according to protocol for high intensity service users, using advanced clinical skills for the care of those with heart failure, asthma, chronic obstructive pulmonary disease and diabetes, and the integration of health and social care provision. The King's Fund published a review of case management by Hutt et al. (2004) and cited the role as comprising case finding, screening, care planning, implementation, monitoring and review through improved cost effectiveness and efficiency of service delivery to improve the quality of life for those living with long term conditions.

Clearly within both of the above role specifications, case management and the role of the community matron are blurred and interchangeable. However, it should be noted that case managers can expect less remuneration than community matrons according to the *NHS Knowledge and Skills Framework Job Evaluation Handbook* (DOH, 2004d) and NHS Employers (2006), with case managers being awarded band 7 and community matrons band 8a. Of course trusts are not obliged to follow the guidelines provided by the Agenda for Change framework and can adopt pay scales, specify job roles and allocate job titles as deemed appropriate according to local need. Standardization of the role, remuneration, management expectations and practitioner skills are not universally applied across the country despite guidelines from the NHS Modernisation Agency and Skills for Health (2005) and NHS Employers (2006).

Many strings to their bow

The NHS Modernisation Agency and Skills for Health (2005) specify how both community case managers and community matrons should have leadership skills, be capable of identifying high risk patients, enable patient independence by supporting patient self-care and self-management, manage complex care co-ordination and complex long term conditions (including cognitive impairment and mental well-being) and also be able to manage end of life care whilst concomitantly working across organizational boundaries. Community matrons should also have advanced clinical nursing skills, although it is acknowledged that on the job training and education may be utilized to acquire both the latter and former skills, knowledge and attributes as both of the roles are new to UK health care professionals. It is also acknowledged by the same organizations that district nurses may already have many of the requisite skills and may be able to make the transition more smoothly than other health and social care disciplines.

Conversely, it has been stated that acute sector nurses may make the transition to community matron status more easily although the Queen's Nursing Institute (2005) have specified how additional skills would need to be acquired by those practitioners to enable novice to expert status within the context of community nursing. This is an issue that acute sector nurses have repeatedly raised concerns about when trying to make the transition from acute sector status to other community practitioner roles, such as health visiting or general practice nursing, when commencing community specialist practitioner (CSP) education preparation. Their concerns were acknowledged by strategic health authorities through the commission of a preparatory unit of study to address community issues prior to commencement of CSP degree level study, although this pre-course preparation has been replaced by longer CSP programmes of study. This acknowledged difficulty in acute to community sector transfer of skills highlights how it is important not only to have specific skills but to additionally have the skill of transfer, as well as a means of quickly learning the community practice landscape. The latter includes referral systems, isolated and remote team working in the absence of acute sector personnel and resource infrastructure, and also perhaps the micropolitics of community practice.

The Queen's Nursing Institute (2005) also articulated concerns that the role of community matron may cause conflict amongst nurses, although they did not specify what the nature of this conflict may be. Community practitioners, particularly district nurses, have complained how their educational preparation and leadership skills are being devalued by trusts appointing community staff nurses (with no additional qualification) to community case manager posts. Given that some PCTs do not differentiate between community matron and community case manager roles, district nurses do have a valid point. Perhaps the failure of the Nursing and Midwifery Council to publish guidance on post-registration education following their consultation in 2006 has contributed to the reluctance of trusts to invest money in adequately preparing people for the new community roles. The Queen's Nursing Institute (2005) additionally foresaw that community matrons may be alienated from community nursing services although, again, why this may occur is not made clear. The reasons explained above may well contribute to the potential alienation of those taking up new roles. However, surely patient care should be the focus of the newly developing role, not in-fighting amongst nursing disciplines.

Two key factors that have been recognized are the important (non-medical) prescribing role that community matrons may play, although, of course, this role is not unique to community matrons, and also the requirement for integration by community matrons of health and social care aspects of service provision. This latter perspective is perhaps a relatively new approach for community nurses even though district nurse team leaders have traditionally tried to marry the two disparate philosophies within the context of their care co-ordination role. The attempt to do this has been fraught with difficulty as differing agendas, competition for resources and diverse organizational goals have hindered their efforts. Reorientation of services including a shared budget and a common goal that focuses on independent living for those with long term conditions may assist in achieving integrated service provision. However, a bottom-up approach will not be successful in achieving this alone as there must be support from both senior management and the government to enable a social perspective on health that regards quality of life and functional independent living as aspirant qualities rather than increased life expectancy at all costs. In some areas of the UK, reorganization of community service provision with the implementation of care managers leading a multidisciplinary team that focuses on patient groups rather than specific clinical problems may provide a means of bringing together social care and health service provision. For example, within the field of learning disability practice, many nurses already work in multidisciplinary teams alongside their social care colleagues with service management being provided by a social worker.

The Queen's Nursing Institute's (2005) focus on role aspects very much reflects the vision of the Department of Health (2005a) on community matrons in their emphasis on clinical interventions, although it could be argued that the distinction between community matrons and case managers remains blurred given that both are intended to manage complex long term conditions as well as to co-ordinate care. It is possible that the confusion arose from the first announcement by the Department of Health (2004b: p. 38) of a new type of nurse known as a community matron who would manage complex patients using case management techniques with a promise of 3000 in post by 2008. Within the same chapter of the document *NHS Improvement Plan: Putting people at the heart of public services*, the DOH (2004b) advocates the input of emergency care practitioners in the prevention of readmission to hospital of those with long term conditions, and cites the use of ambulance service emergency care practitioners in applying appropriate first contact care skills to achieve this. This latter approach demonstrates how advanced clinical skills are not the prerogative of community matrons but rather the utilization of the right people with the appropriate clinical skills at the right time to prevent unnecessary hospital admission. Emergency care practitioners are not necessarily nurses and are also unlikely to be case managers; they are, however, responsible for the provision of packages and programmes of emergency and medical care as well as being responsible for the provision of advice to patients and carers. Interestingly they are paid at band 6 under the Agenda for Change agreement despite their ability to administer a range of drug therapies using patient group directives (NHS Employers, 2007). The role of the community matron and how it differs from existing community practice roles is, it appears, a difficult knot to untangle.

The patient perspective: well-being not ill health

Shield et al. (2005) explored the perspectives of older people, service providers and carers on community care skill requirements necessary for the provision of end of life care, as well as care and management of long term conditions. It emerged from their study that all stakeholders want a person with interdisciplinary skills that can function across organizational boundaries as a 'jack of all trades'. Although the study was carried out within the context of rehabilitation and inter-mediate care teams, the envisaged emerging role with its inherent skills, attributes and knowledge closely mapped against many of the qualities previously outlined as requisite for community case managers. The authors of this study concluded that educational preparation and training using a modular format would equate with entry-level foundation degree care workers at assistant or associate practi-tioner level, with possible development using the NHS skills escalator approach to achieve full honours degree status as interprofessional practitioners in the care of older people (it is acknowledged that not only older people experience long term conditions). This proposition embraces an approach that would negate the requirement for existing registered professionals to migrate into the roles outlined above by 'growing from scratch' a new kind of health and social care professional schooled into the philosophy of independent living for older people (or others with long term conditions) with a focus on quality of life. The medical model of health and its focus on disease management is thus pushed aside and replaced by the social model of health. This is a philosophy that concentrates on the wider deter-minants of health and consequently is more patient focused as the patients them-selves determine what would improve the quality of their lives and they do not appear to prioritize medical and nursing needs (Anderson et al., 2007).

The notion of educating support workers to a level that would enable appro-priate care provision for older people with complex conditions is at odds with government intent for providing clinical leadership, ensuring administrative and support services, and providing an authoritative presence for patient, families and carers as outlined by *The NHS Plan: A plan for investment, a plan for reform* (DOH, 2000) in their vision for the modern matron. These qualities are also per-ceived by nursing directors as constituting the role of the modern matron as reported by Ashman et al. (2006). The modern matron was, of course, originally intended for acute services although many of the skills and qualities outlined can be transposed to the role of the community matron. Critics could say that the acute sector modern matron's role did not focus on care of the older person, but it could be argued that older people and those with long term conditions represent the most vulnerable members of society, as do those acutely ill within secondary sector services and are therefore most in need of champions to represent their cause. In tracking the progress of the contribution of acute sector modern matrons in improving care provision for patients, the Department of Health (2002a) identi-fied that the modern matron's role was concerned with leading by clinical example, driving up the standards of patient care, setting and monitoring standards of environmental hygiene, meeting patient's nutritional needs, preventing nosocomial infection, using devolved budgets to improve patient environments, empowering nurses to take on extended roles, ensuring patient dignity, resolving problems for patients, families and carers, and ensuring adequate staffing levels for safe patient care. Almost all of these aspects could be relevant to community matrons and many to the role of the community case manager, whereas a practitioner operating at the level of assistant or associate practitioner would not ordinarily have the requisite skills, knowledge or attributes to realize many of these aspects without considerable experience, training and education.

There is certainly no cheap option for providing levels of care expected by professional regulatory and statutory bodies or for achieving the requisite skills and knowledge to meet the demands of patients with complex long term conditions. Furthermore, trying to directly transplant US health policy and practice into the UK health economy does not work for the reasons outlined earlier. Trusts that have attempted to cut costs by using support workers to fulfil the role expectations of health care professionals have been castigated by Sandall et al. (2007) in their recent report on maternity services. Their findings are also endorsed by Beasley (2007), the Chief Nursing Officer for the Department of Health who condemns the practice as unacceptable. It is in reality both unreasonable and unacceptable to expect untrained and unqualified staff to adequately support people with long term conditions. This aspect is clearly highlighted by Corben and Rosen (2005) in their exploration of patients' perspectives on managing long term conditions. They highlight how even doctors may not have the skills required to actively listen to patients' concerns, empathize with the patients' perspective and allow time to plan together for future management of long term conditions. They state that where those skills are not part of the doctor's repertoire then appropriate competence-related training should be provided (Corben & Rosen, 2005: p. 7). This caveat could be equally applied to other health and social care professionals. Once again, the medical model of health favoured by medicine and health professionals is rejected for a more social model that focuses on the patients' experiences and the reality of their lives when living with a long term condition. A clear element of the roles of both case managers and community matrons therefore lies in providing the patients, their families and carers with adequate information to enable them to take as active a part as possible in managing the person's condition in a way that optimizes quality of life.

Action Learning Point

- How are patients with long term conditions supported in your area?
- Other than case management, what roles do the voluntary, private and social services sectors play in supporting patients?
- Which patient support groups are active and do general practices in your area offer additional support to patients in addition to referral to carer centres?

The information highway: boon or barrier?

One way of ensuring that patients, families and carers have adequate information on how to best manage long term conditions is currently being piloted across one trust in the northwest of the UK, one of 20 pilot sites that are exploring the impact of 'information prescriptions'. This initiative is a response to the 2006 Citizens' Summit, a consultation exercise repeated by the Department of Health in March 2007 (DOH, 2007a). Within this context patients are intended to more easily find information about living with long term conditions from dedicated websites, as well as being signposted to appropriate books or journals, voluntary agencies and patient support groups, in addition to gaining advice on where to obtain benefits, how to engage in internet discussion groups and how to obtain home care services. This is a laudable innovation but there is a clear expectation that the individual or someone within their support network has internet access, health literacy, negotiation skills and some degree of mobility. The latter component is something that Expert Patient initiatives also expect as both practitioners and patients have commented in practice (see Chapter 3). It is also of interest to note that the government have now launched Expert Patient Programmes as not for profit community interest companies that can be commissioned by PCTs to deliver their services as required. Perhaps this means that more accessible services will be available to the housebound, but this remains to be seen as other aspects of NHS service provision that have engaged in commercial venture have fared less well economically, in particular those trusts that have embraced private financial initiatives (Private Eye, 2007). However, on an individual basis, patients having contact with a community matron or case manager will have direct access to equivalent information available from pilot sites and will also have an advocate to negotiate and initiate services on their behalf.

One element of patient contact that should be afforded additional attention by community case managers and matrons is that of health literacy. Health literacy is concerned with having the knowledge, understanding, motivation and application to use information in a health enhancing manner (Sihota & Lennard, 2004). Clearly this is an important aspect of care management if the patient (or their family) is to be expected to self-care (or support the patient in achieving self-care). Failing eyesight, poor educational experiences, reduced cognitive impairment inherent in conditions such as dementia or some people with learning disability, and limited ability to self-motivate or concentrate on tasks will inevitably impact on a person's capacity for health literacy. For example, some patients with enduring mental health problems may find reading or taking on board health education messages difficult due to their condition or the effects of prescribed medication; although, of course, these problems are not exclusively associated with specified health problems. Part of living with a long term condition is the need to prioritize what can be reasonably managed and what is important to function. Additionally, there is a recognized increase in levels of depression associated with living with a long term condition (De Souza & Dalgado, 2005; Arthritis Care, 2006; Diabetes UK, 2006; Whooley et al., 2007). Both of these aspects require recognition, and the latter needs positive management by care managers and co-ordinators regardless of their role titles. Helping patients to understand and make sense of what is happening to them within the context of their health problems is as important if not more important than ensuring appropriate aids and services are in place to maintain independence.

Pharmacy and flexible technology

An important aspect of information giving that is closely linked to the role of the community case manager and community matron is that of medication reviewer. Experiencing the effects of polypharmacy is perhaps an inevitable result of living with a long term condition but if properly monitored and managed this should not be so. Patients should not have to suffer the detrimental effects of multiple medications, be they iatrogenic or self-inflicted. Lay people cannot be expected to know that certain over the counter and herbal medications might have concomitant, confounding and detrimental side effects when they are taken together or in conjunction with prescribed medication. Additionally, they may be unaware that medication taken with alcohol or ill-timed pre- or post-prandial ingestion may adversely affect the medication, inactivate or reduce the intended effects of the medication, or exacerbate the intended or unintended effects.

The National Service Framework for Older People's Services (DOH, 2002b) advocated annual medication reviews for all aged over 75 years and six-monthly review for those taking four or more medications. Obviously the numbers of patients involved means that this load cannot fall upon community case managers or matrons alone, but it is clear that those experiencing long term conditions are much more likely to be taking four or more prescribed medications and that they would be the most likely group to benefit from a level 3 review – one that takes place on a face-to-face patient contact basis along with the patient's case notes as a reference point. Given that the General Medical Services contract does not specify the requirement for level 3 reviews (British Medical Association & NHS Employers, 2006), in trusts where level 3 reviews have been taking place, there has been a tendency for these reviews to happen in the context of complex or hard to reach patients (Celino et al., 2005). Whilst this may have been a missed opportunity for the General Medical Services, it is an ideal opportunity for community case manager or matron assessment of patients' experiences, as well as an intervention that could potentially be instrumental in improving patient health outcomes and preventing unnecessary hospital admissions. This is a further reason why assistant practitioners can not be expected to fulfil the role of community case managers and an aspect that highlights the importance of acquiring non-medical prescribing skills for those engaging in community matron and community case manager roles. Budget deficits within PCTs that negatively impact on education and training agendas, combined with the end of the government's commitment to fund non-medical prescribing courses, may well jeopardize the ability of professionally qualified community practitioners to meet medication review targets and subsequently detract from their ability to improve health outcomes for those with long term conditions.

A third strand of activity expected from health and social care professionals engaging with those experiencing long term conditions is that of making service delivery more flexible to meet the needs of patients. One such example of flexible service delivery may be achieved by PCTs embracing the disease management information toolkit (DMIT) (DOH, 2007b). This toolkit is designed to evaluate different intervention strategies and to encourage trusts to apportion the appropriate personnel with the means to instigate these interventions as a way of preventing hospital admissions or reducing hospital stays where admission is unavoidable. For example, where heart failure and coronary heart disease constitute a heavy workload within a PCT, it may be beneficial for the patients and more economically viable for the trust to allow community case managers and community matrons to arrange installation of telemonitoring equipment in patients' homes so that their condition can be monitored and early interventions activated before complications arise that would compromise patient health outcomes. However, it should be noted that this may compromise the patient's and family's notion of home as a private space. Alternatively, case managers may call upon the services of a specialist heart failure nurse to support them in managing the patient's condition. In addition, for those patients having already experienced a cardiac event, case managers may wish to refer their patients for cardiac rehabilitation as outlined by Beswick et al. (2004) and to support and motivate them in engaging with such interventions.

A further example of the use of DMIT can be seen when applied to patients having experienced a cerebral vascular accident (stroke). The toolkit demonstrates improved health outcomes for patients and fiscal savings for acute and community trusts where inpatients are managed in specialist stroke units (this aspect is, of course, beyond the remit of community-based practitioners), patients are scanned at an early stage to identify their eligibility for thrombolysis, those with transient ischaemic attacks (TIAs) and at risk of stroke are rapidly referred for surgery via a TIA clinic, and community care is managed by early supported discharge schemes. Some of these activities are associated with the roles outlined in the *NHS Plan: A plan for investment, a plan for reform* (DOH, 2000).

However, the overall complexity of these interventions demonstrates the requirement for strong clinical leadership with its inherent qualities, a sound knowledge base of the management of conditions that may be encountered within the community, and assessment skills that would be capable of rapidly distinguishing exacerbation from normal physiological processes expected when impacted upon by the natural progression of the condition(s) being experienced by individual patients. The health care professional must also be cognisant with the impact that any of these interventions will have on the patient and their family in determining, through negotiation, what is appropriate for that individual at that point of contact. It is important to realize, though, that these expressed needs will change over time, both because patients may experience different events during the natural course of their conditions and because the nature of long term conditions is such that symptoms will fluctuate in levels of intensity and remission over periods of time. Bearing these elements in mind, some community nurses, for example, may refer a patient to a team leader for assessment prior to involving other agencies and individuals with the care and management of that patient.

It is important that the referring health care professional supports the patient by acting as an advocate for the individual patient's expressed needs prior to agreeing to any interventions deemed necessary by the third party. Community matrons and case managers have a strong role to play in this context, as careful assessment of the patient and consideration of the opinions of the patient and their family or lay carers will ascertain preferences where choice is apposite or available. This role aspect will help to determine the best course of action for the patient, even if it is not the choice that the health or social care professional would have selected, nor one that is deemed most appropriate in the light of available evidence-based practice.

Public health practitioners: leaving the medical model behind

Case finding, patient assessment, clinical management of long term conditions, care co-ordination and cross-boundary working, non-medical prescribing and medication review, contribution to and lobbying for service reorientation, clinical leadership, political awareness raising, health and social care mediation and patient advocacy are all roles expected, to a greater or lesser extent, of the community matron and the community case manager although not necessarily in the order presented. One aspect of the role that is perhaps less obvious than those outlined above is the important public health role that these two new breeds of community practitioner will play in future care management and delivery. Improving the quality of patients' lives and encouraging independence in those with long term conditions are key functions of the practitioner role, whilst reducing emergency hospital admissions and improving preventative care within the community are major expectations of the government in reducing public expenditure of health care provision as outlined by Wanless (2002). Both reducing inequalities in health and improving health outcomes by the combined systematic efforts of individuals, society, professionals and the government contribute strongly to the public health agenda. Long term conditions pose a huge, personal, social burden on the affected individuals and their families with a particular impact on patients' self-esteem and self-efficacy. They also incur a personal financial burden due to the costs of medication, absence from work, loss of functional or employment capability and status, and the costs of caring. In addition, there is a cost to society that is both financial and social, through NHS and social care costs as well as loss of valuable and productive engagement with society by those temporarily or permanently severely affected by long term conditions. Enabling those with long term conditions to improve the quality of their lives, regain maximum possible independence and re-engage with society is a valuable contribution to the public health agenda.

Under the proposed Public Health Skills and Career Development Framework (Skills for Health & Public Health Resource Unit, 2007), community matrons may possibly be eligible to enter the voluntary public health register as level 6 practitioners and community case managers as level 5 assistant/associate practitioners in a skills escalator beginning at level 1 and rising to level 9. Both practitioners would be expected to use the core public health skills of population surveillance and assessment, assessment of interventions, programmes and services (and their appropriate application in practice), the development and implementation of policies and strategies, and leadership and collaborative working for health improvement. However, other specific public health skills may be used to a greater or lesser extent, depending on the level of employer expectation and the skills, knowledge and attributes that an individual practitioner may posses. As previously identified, some trusts have reviewed their need for community matrons and employed community case managers in their place. It is interesting that the role of the community matron is clearly defined by NHS Employers (2006) in their job evaluation profiles but there is no clear identification of the role of community case manager. Perhaps a lack of role definition is a reflection of PCTs trying to meet local needs that naturally fluctuate so to be prescriptive would stifle practice; alternatively it may be an entirely fiscal decision made by trusts in their attempts to keep within budgets.

Professor Rod Griffiths, President of the Faculty of Public Health, states that every government health reorganization agenda sees a diminishing public health workforce (McKenzie, 2006). Perhaps the birth of community case managers and community matrons and the publication of *Choosing Health: Making healthy choices easier* (DOH, 2004e) will prove a generative force for improving the public health function of community practice. Alternatively, practice-based commissioning may shift the focus once again from the social model of health with public health and its community-based approaches to improving health outcomes back to a more medical model approach of clinical disease management that obscures the wider determinants that impact on people's health.

It is clear that community case managers and more particularly community matrons have a role in disease-specific management but they also have a health education role in promoting self-care for patients with long term conditions. It is within the context of this latter role that public health concerns may be addressed. There may, for instance, be a focus on weight management with prevention of or reduction in obesity to assist in the management of diabetes, heart disease or musculoskeletal conditions. Alternatively, there may be a role in smoking cessation advice and support to address aspects of cancer management, coronary heart disease or micro- and macrovascular condition management. On a broader and less clinical scale the new community roles may prove instrumental in lobbying for improved housing, transport or improved health care access for their patients. In addition the roles may incorporate establishing community support groups or providing access to community-based initiatives that support patients' self-care capacity (such as the Expert Patient initiatives discussed in Chapter 3), as well as cardiac and pulmonary rehabilitation programmes, walking and exercise initiatives, healthy eating clubs or education opportunities that contribute to increasing health literacy and self-efficacy and redeployment opportunities. Practitioners may actively engage in any or all of the above activities; alternatively they may act in a signposting capacity, directing their patient group to others who may provide these services as an adjunct to the management of long term conditions within community practice.

Collaborative work and liaison with social care professionals already constitutes a substantial part of the community practitioner role and will do so even more in the future as the population ages and those living with long term conditions are encouraged to remain independent for longer. Community matrons and case managers may be sought for their professional opinion and to advise and support 'Partnerships for Older People' projects (DOH, 2005c). The roles of community case manager and community matron will inevitably evolve as the needs of patients and their carers fluctuate and change in the landscape provided by the prevailing political, demographic and economic backcloth. What will remain constant, even though clinical nomenclature may change, is that practitioners supporting those with long term conditions must remain responsive to the needs of their patient group and improve health outcomes with a focus on the quality of life for patients.

Action Learning Point

- Explore a quality of life model or a well-being model and consider a patient or group of patients living with long term conditions to assess the impact on their lives.
- Determine how you as a practitioner can improve a patient's quality of life beyond implementing nursing interventions or prescribing medication.

References

Anderson, K., Sylvester, C., Archer, S. & Alamdari, A. (2007) (eds) *Adult Social Services Statistics*. London, The Information Centre, part of the Government Statistical Service.

Arthritis Care (2006) *A New Deal for Welfare: Empowering people to work. Consultation response from Arthritis Care*. London, Arthritis Care.

Ashman, M., Read, S., Savage, J. & Scott, C. (2006) Outcomes of modern matron implementation: Trust nursing directors' perceptions and case study findings. *Clinical Effectiveness in Nursing* 9 (S1): e44–e52.

Beasley, C. (2007) Letter to all maternity services, 40. *Maternity Matters: Choice, access and continuity of care in a safe service*.

Beswick, A.D., Rees, K., Griebsch, I. et al. (2004) Provision, uptake and cost of cardiac rehabilitation programmes: improving services to under-represented groups. *Health Technology Assessment* 8 (41): 176.

British Medical Association & NHS Employers (2006) *Revisions to the GMS Contract 2006/07: Delivering investment in general practice*. London, BMA and NHS Employers.

Celino, G., Levenson, R. & Dhalla, M. (2005) *Evaluation of Room for Review – A guide to medication review: Part 1, the PCT and professional view*. Keele, Keele University, the Medicines Partnership.

Coalition of Health Bodies (2005) *17 Million Reasons: Improving the lives of people with long-term conditions*. London, NHS Confederation.

Corben, S. & Rosen, R. (2005) *Self-management for Long-term Conditions. Patients' perspectives on the way ahead*. London, King's Fund.

De Souza, E.A.P. & Dalgado, P.A.C. (2005) A psychosocial view of anxiety and depression in epilepsy. *Epilepsy and Behavior* 8: 232–238.

Department of Health (2000) *The NHS Plan: A plan for investment, a plan for reform*. London, Department of Health.

Department of Health (2001a) *The Expert Patient: A new approach to chronic disease management for the 21st century*. London, Department of Health.

Department of Health (2001b) *Carers and Disabled Children Act 2000: Carers and people with parental responsibility for disabled children, policy guidance*. London, Department of Health.

Department of Health (2002a) *Modern Matrons in the NHS: A progress report*. London, Department of Health.

Department of Health (2002b) *National Service Framework for Older People's Services*. London, Department of Health.

Department of Health (2004a) *The NHS Knowledge and Skills Framework (NHS KSF) and the Development Review Process*. London, Department of Health.

Department of Health (2004b) *The NHS Improvement Plan: Putting people at the heart of public services*. London, Department of Health.

Department of Health (2004c) *Chronic Disease Management: A compendium of information*. London, Department of Health.

Department of Health (2004d) *The NHS Knowledge and Skills Framework (NHS KSF) Job Evaluation Handbook*. London, Department of Health.

Department of Health (2004e) *Choosing Health: Making healthy choices easier*. London, Department of Health.

Department of Health (2005a) *Supporting People with Long Term Conditions: Liberating the talents of nurses who care for people with long term conditions*. London, Department of Health.

Department of Health (2005b) *Supporting People with Long Term Conditions. An NHS and social care model to support local innovation and integration*. London, Department of Health.

Department of Health (2005c) *Partnerships for Older People Projects*. London, Department of Health.

Department of Health (2007a) Tailor-made Information Will Help Patients Take Control of their Treatment. www.dh.gov.uk/cnobulletin. May 2007 [accessed 3 June 2007].

Department of Health (2007b) *Disease Management Information Toolkit*. London, Department of Health.

Department of Health and Social Services for Northern Ireland (2006) Case Management: A position paper. http://www.dhsspsni.gov.uk/case_management.pdf [accessed 20 May 2007].

Department of Health/Social Care Directorate/Continuing Care (2007) *NHS Continuing Healthcare: Draft tools*. London, Department of Health.

Diabetes UK (2006) Diabetes and Depression. http://www.diabetes.org.uk/Guide-to-diabetes/Living_with_diabetes/Coping_with_diabetes/Depression_and_diabetes/ [accessed 22 April 2007].

Hudson, B. (2005) Sea change or quick fix? Policy on long-term conditions in England. *Health and Social Care in the Community* **13** (4): 378–385.

Hutt, R., Rosen, R. & McCauley, J. (2004) *Case-managing Long-term Conditions: What Impact does it have in the Treatment of Older People?* London, King's Fund.

Kane, R.L., Flood, S., Keckhafer, G. & Rockwood, T. (2001) How EverCare nurse practitioners spend their time. *Journal of the American Geriatrics Society* **49** (11): 1530–1534.

King's Fund, New York University & Health Dialogue Analytic Solutions (2006) *Case Finding Algorithms for Patients at Risk of Re-hospitalisation PARR1 and PARR2*. London, King's Fund.

McKenzie, S. (2006) Crisis: Public health's haemorrhaging workforce. http://www.publichealthnews.com/news/showcontent.asp?id={70ABBFF0-FB69-4556-BD5B-B4AA77B7DB86} [accessed 19 July 2007].

NHS Employers (2006) Pay and Negotiations: Nursing and midwifery. http://www.nhsemployers.org/pay-conditions/pay-conditions-1991.cfm [accessed 20 May 2007].

NHS Employers (2007) Emergency Services: National profiles for ambulance services. http://www.nhsemployers.org/pay-conditions/pay-conditions-1989.cfm [accessed 28 May 2007].

NHS Modernisation Agency & Skills for Health (2005) *Case Management Competences Framework for the Care of People with Long Term Conditions*. London, Department of Health.

Princess Royal Trust for Carers (2006) Who is a Carer? http://www.carers.org/who-is-a-carer,118,GP.html [accessed 8 March 2006].

Private Eye (2007) 'HP Sauce' news. *Private Eye* 18 May. http://www.private-eye.co.uk/sections.php?section_link=hp_sauce&issue=1184 [accessed 1 June 2007].

Queen's Nursing Institute (2005) *Briefing: Community matrons*. London, Queen's Nursing Institute.

Sandall, J., Manthorpe, J., Mansfield, A. & Spencer, L. (2007) *Support Workers in Maternity Services: A national scoping study of NHS Trusts providing maternity care in England 2006: final report*. London, King's College London.

Shield, F., Enderby, P. & Nancarrow, S. (2005) Stakeholder views of the training needs of an inter-professional practitioner who works with older people. *Nurse Education Today* **26**: 367–376.

Sihota, S. & Lennard, L. (2004) *Health Literacy; Being able to make the most of health*. London, National Consumer Council.

Skills for Health & Public Health Resource Unit (2007) *Public Health Skills and Career Development Framework*, June 2007 consultation version. Bristol/Oxford, Skills for Health/Public Health Resource Unit.

Wanless, D. (2002) *Securing our Future Health: Taking a long term view*. London, HM Treasury.

Whooley, M.A., Caska, C.M., Hendrickson, B.E., Rourke, M.A., Ho, J. & Ali, S. (2007) Depression and Inflammation in Patients with Coronary Heart Disease: Findings From the Heart and Soul Study. doi:10.1016/j.biopsych.2006.10.016, http://www.sciencedirect.com/science?_ob=MImg&_imagekey=B6T4S-4NH6CWR-1-3&_cdi=4982&_user=4801305&_orig=search&_coverDate=04%2F16%2F2007&_sk=999999999&view=c&wchp=dGLbVlz-zSkzk&md5=1e561ecf4d3c813037238368afc34ab7&ie=/sdarticle.pdf [accessed 22 April 2007].

World Health Organization (2006) Commission on the Social Determinants of Health. http://www.who.int/social_determinants/en/ [accessed 1 March 2006].

Chapter 3

Empowering patients: the role of the Expert Patient Programme in promoting health amongst those with long term conditions

Clare Street and Caroline Powell

Key points

- Exploring patient empowerment, autonomy and self-efficacy
- Considering the concepts of health
- A discussion of the health gain, values, ethics and the contribution and limitations of the Expert Patient Programme
- A comparison of the key philosophical, ethical and theoretical principles that both confirm and challenge our knowledge and assumptions about the Expert Patient Programme and what constitutes work to promote health

'When you leave the clinic, you still have a long term condition. When the visiting nurse leaves your home, you still have a long term condition. In the middle of the night, when you fight the pain alone. At the weekend, you manage without your home help. Living with a long term condition is a great deal more than medical or professional assistance.' (Harry Clayton, Director for Patients and the Public, Department of Health (DOH), 2005a)

In this chapter we will argue that the Expert Patient Programme (EPP) represents the essence of health promotion work. Although it is not classically associated with prevention as people are already ill, suffering from a longstanding and limiting health condition, the nucleus of values and principles (patient participation, empowerment, informed choice, self-efficacy) that characterize the EPP are central to the promotion of health. A full appreciation of this emerges through an exploration of key underpinning concepts, in particular what is meant by 'health', or 'being healthy', and we will explore a particular concept of health, which we believe more comprehensively represents the nature of work to promote health, especially in the context of the EPP. We will start with an outline of the history of the EPP and related policy drivers and move onto an exploration of what 'health promotion' means for those who are already ill, in order to draw out the diverse and distinctive impact this programme has on people's health. In particular we will explore the social and psychological, as well as physical, benefits of becoming an 'expert patient' and the implications this has on our understanding of the nature of 'health gain' or 'health benefit'. Some examples are taken from local practice (personal details have been made anonymous). The limitations, both ethical and practical, of the EPP will also be acknowledged so that a clear and realistic picture of the contribution of EPP to the broad health promotion agenda can emerge.

History of the Expert Patient Programme

People with chronic health problems frequently lead lives restricted by their conditions, and while most day-to-day management involves self-care (DOH, 2005b), the contribution of patient support to improving the quality of life for individuals has been scrutinized for several years. Key work started in America with Kate Lorig and her team at Stanford Patient Education Research Center (PERC), Stanford University, California (formally known as the Stanford Arthritis Centre Education Office). They developed and evaluated patient education programmes during the late 1970s and early 1980s, investigating the links between patient education and health status. Out of this research emerged an understanding of the importance of a positive emotional state and the impact of patient control on an individual's overall state of health. These findings culminated in the development of the ideas that shaped the nature of patient participation through self-management programmes (Lenker et al., 1984).

The first successful programmes, although disease specific, were developed and delivered in 1982 by Stanford PERC and the Arthritis Self-Management Course (ASMC) and benchmarked the prototype for future self-management programs, including the generic Expert Patients Programme (Lenker et al., 1984). Voluntary sector organizations such as Arthritis Care, the Manic Depression Fellowship and Changing Faces worked closely with PERC to introduce self-management programmes within the UK during the 1990s. By the mid-1990s, the Long-term Medical Condition Alliance (LMCA) set up the Long Term Illness Project based on chronic disease self-management (CDSM). Both CDSM and the EPP are built upon the recognition that while people may have different conditions and diseases they share many experiences and needs associated with low self-esteem and difficulties in coping with everyday life (Patient Liaison Group, 2005).

Health care in the 20th century

In the second part of the 20th century, several major changes have taken place. People are now living longer (DOH, 2001, 2004a) with a concurrent increase in the numbers living with chronic health conditions – an estimated 17.5 million people (DOH, 2001, 2004b; Plews, 2005). This places considerable demand on health and social care resources as well as constraining the abilities of the individuals concerned (DOH, 2001, 2004a). Along with this has been a gradual shift in the nature of the relationship between health care professionals and patients (Baggott, 2004). With health care reforms focused on welfare pluralism, market forces and 'consumerism' there has been a growing emphasis on a patient-led NHS (Crossley, 2000; Baggott, 2004; Wanless, 2004; DOH, 2005c). Patients are no longer considered to be passive recipients of care, rather patients are regarded as 'experienced subject[s] who can contribute knowledge and take an active part in decisions' (Hardey, 1998, in Crossley, 2000: p. 84). These factors have focused government attention on the need for a better response to the management of chronic conditions. It is within this context that interest in the EPP has grown.

In July 1999 the government first announced its plans to establish an expert patients programme, in the health strategy White Paper *Saving Lives, Our Healthier Nation* (DOH, 1999a). This announcement was closely followed by the establishment of the Expert Patient Programme Task Force in October under the chairmanship of the Chief Medical Officer, Professor Liam Donaldson, which evaluated national and international research on CDSM programmes. The report *The Expert Patient: A new approach to chronic disease management for the 21st century* (DOH, 2001) concluded that the programme would add value to the provision of chronic disease management within the NHS. *The Health Act* (DOH, 1999b), *The NHS Plan: A plan for investment, a plan for reform* (DOH, 2000), *Future Partnerships, Primary Care in 2020* (DOH, 2003), *The NHS Improvement Plan* (DOH, 2004c), the *National Service Framework for Long-term Conditions* (DOH 2005b), the report *Supporting People with Long Term Conditions* (DOH, 2005a) and *Our Health, Our Care, Our Say* (DOH, 2006) all add to this focus and outline a commitment to empower people living with a long term medical condition to become key decision-makers in their own care. This support from government clearly signalled that health is not just the business of clinically qualified health professionals but should include community and primary care-based self-management packages of care and treatment (Patient Liaison Group, 2005).

Action Learning Point

- Identify any local EPP provision in your area.
- Contact your local EPP co-ordinator/manager to find out what is on offer in your locality (try your local Primary Care Trust or www.expertpatients.nhs.uk). Ask for any information on local evaluation of the EPP and referral pathways.
- Discuss the EPP within your team; are there any barriers to referrals into the programme or implementation within your local Primary Care Trust?

The EPP in England and Wales

The Department of Health introduced the generic EPP programme under licence from Stanford University in 2002 and the expectation is that the EPP will be implemented through all Primary Care Trusts (PCTs) by 2008 as part of level one – supported self-care (DOH, 2004b, 2005a). Level one refers to action aimed at enabling individuals to become active partners in their own care (70–80% of people in need of care for a chronic health problem fall into this category), underpinned by broader population-based health promotion activity to help individuals 'make healthier choices about diet, physical activity and lifestyle, for example stopping smoking and reducing alcohol intake' (DOH, 2005a: p. 10).

The EPP self-management programme has certain key features (Lorig et al., 1997). Based on our developing understanding that cognitive and emotional states, jointly and simultaneously, shape our overall state of health (Damasio, 1994), the EPP involves the development of cognitive skills but also coping strategies such as relaxation and the management of fatigue. Knowledge around generic health promoting activities such as healthy eating and exercise are included along with generic treatment matters relating to medications as only about 50% of medications are taken as prescribed (DOH, 2005a). Making treatment decisions and communicating with health care professionals are also key components of the EPP.

The EPP is a highly structured programme. It is delivered in six consecutive weekly sessions, with each session lasting two and a half hours. Two volunteer tutors lead 8–16 participants through a structured programme, delivered from a scripted manual covering topics relating to the key components mentioned above, such as relaxation, breaking the symptom/pain cycle, managing pain and medication, communication and cognitive symptom management. All tutors must themselves be living with and managing a long term condition, thus acting as role models to the programme participants (Taylor & Bury, 2007). The type of conditions that people will be experiencing include back pain, arthritis, asthma, diabetes, epilepsy, pulmonary disease, multiple sclerosis and heart disease.

Differences between the EPP and condition-specific programmes

The EPP is complementary to condition-specific programmes. The EPP is not concerned with educating patients about their condition or giving them relevant disease-specific information (Kennedy et al., 2004). Rather, the EPP makes a more holistic contribution to the promotion of health. Lorig et al. (1999) note that it may be difficult for people with a rare condition to access disease-specific programmes and the EPP provides equality of access to disease management education. People need knowledge of their disease and the disease process but there are more commonalities than differences in the experiences of those living with long term conditions (Patient Liaison Group, 2005).

People living with specific long term health conditions deal with similar issues to others with long term conditions on a daily basis (National Primary Care Research and Development Centre (NPCRDC), 2005). Regardless of type of disease, people experience fear, frustration and anger. Whatever the condition, individuals must adjust to changing capacities and capabilities, stress, low self-esteem and pain (Patient Liaison Group, 2005). The identification and sharing of these difficult emotions enable people to exit the insular concepts of the disease and can reduce stigmatization (Patient Liaison Group, 2005). A realization they are not alone and that such feelings are normal for people with long term health conditions can be liberating and effective in supporting the development of confidence and self-efficacy. From personal experience of running the EPP, this has been evident even from week one of the programme. Each member of the group introduces themselves, their condition and the problems they face in everyday living with their condition. Similar problems and concerns emerge during every course, regardless of locality of delivery and the specific nature of the problems that individuals live with (Plews, 2005). The generic, social and psychological foundations of the EPP provide an opportunity to explore these common difficulties and issues. The self-management principle is not intended to replace good health care provision (which remains essential), rather one of its aims is to provide patients with the necessary skills to make effective use of health provisions and treatment options available to enhance their lives, despite living with long term health conditions. Encouragement to utilize all available resources is fundamental to the programme.

Evaluation of the EPP: does it work?

The 'does it work' question is vital and there have been a series of evaluations of the programmes, starting with the work of Lorig and her colleagues. The success of CDSM and the EPP has been judged according to a range of benefits; disease/symptom-specific improvements, changes in the use of services and changes in a person's quality of life. Initial evaluations of the work in America, after follow-up between one and four years, indicated that participants could exercise for longer per week, manage their symptoms more effectively, experienced reductions in pain and disability and had improved communications with their physicians along with overall reduction in the use of health care (Barlow et al., 1998a, 1999; Lorig & Holman, 2003). A 40% decrease in demand for health care services and GP consultations in the UK has been noted in patients who participate in the EPP (DOH, 2005d).

Other data from the UK have been collected from participants (250 people) to gain an impression of perceived self-improvement (Patient Liaison Group, 2005). Participants were invited to complete a questionnaire three to four months after finishing a course. Their responses were compared with the data gathered from the same questionnaire, pre-course. The results indicated that participants reported improvements in various aspects of their overall health experiences:

- 10% reported greater compliance with medication regimes.
- 30% reported a significant reduction in depression and 'lacking energy'.
- 20–30% experienced a reduction in breathlessness and pain.
- 30–50% reported increased confidence.

Visits to GPs and outpatient departments were reduced by 9%, to A&E by 6% and there was a 17% reduction in days off work. Pharmacists were used more (15% increase in visits), along with accessing health information from other sources (6% increase).

Evaluating the outcomes of the EPP is clearly an ongoing matter and the Department of Health introduced the EPP as a pilot programme involving 298 PCTs between 2002 and 2004. The Department of Health commissioned a consortium of researchers from the University of Manchester, University of York, University of Bristol and the Rusholme Academic Unit to work with the National Primary Care Research and Development Centre (NPCRDC) to evaluate the pilot programme, including undertaking a randomized control trial (RCT).

RCTs are generally considered to be the most robust mechanisms for gathering evidence to answer the 'does it work' question, particularly in relation to health care intervention and are often referred to as the 'gold standard' in terms of evaluation studies (Raphael, 2000; DOH, 2004d; Tones & Green, 2004; Hillsdon et al., 2005; Pomerleau & McKee, 2005). RCTs, for instance, provide the only mechanism through which selection bias can be effectively managed. Once inclusion and exclusion criteria have been determined, the random selection of subjects to the intervention or control group ensures that any characteristics (age, sex, abilities, etc.) that may act as confounding variables (something independently affecting both the 'exposure' and the outcomes under scrutiny) are shared across the study sample (Unwin et al., 1997). Objective measures of health improvement/ health gain can be applied and the concomitant effect of natural remission or improvement of an illness can be monitored by assessing the health status of people within the control group (Unwin et al., 1997). Objective measures of health status are often attributed higher status than subjective measure of health by researchers and policy-makers when making judgements of success (Raphael, 2000).

Clearly, full RCTs are not always possible. It may be difficult, for instance, to find a suitable control group or area, and ethical concerns are raised when, by necessity, some individuals are denied access to an intervention that from existing evidence appears to be beneficial. RCTs rely on defining clear and objective outcome measures, usually linked to some shift in morbidity or mortality status (Raphael, 2000; Seedhouse, 2004). In other words the programme is judged a success only if demand on health care services or days off sick are reduced, or compliance with treatment is improved. Particularly in relation to health promotion work, the value of exclusively focusing on mortality and morbidity reduction, or other indicators that can be easily quantified, is increasingly being questioned (Perbedy, 2002; Raphael, 2000; Tones & Green, 2004; Green & South, 2006). Indeed, the recent report on the pilot EPPs included measures of reported changes in 'quality' of health/life, as well as changes to morbidity or morbidity-related behaviour.

The RCT of the UK pilot of the EPP involved allocating people with long term conditions to a six-week EPP course or to a waiting list for an EPP. Results on patient outcomes were collated after six months based on a hypothesized link between improved self-efficacy, changes in health states and consequent shifts in service utilization. These results have recently been reported and indicate a range of changes (NPCRDC, 2005, 2007; Rogers et al., 2006). For example, some improvement in self-efficacy and decrease in costs of hospital use were noted but with no contemporaneous change in the use of routine services (GPs, practice nurses and outpatients). However, overall costs of care provision did not increase (Rogers et al., 2006; NPCRDC, 2007). Quality of life measures (using QALYs and EuroQol – EQ-5D[1]) indicated that one additional week of perfect health over 12 months was achieved by participants of the EPP (Rogers et al., 2006; NPCRDC, 2007). Additionally, evaluation of the qualitative outcomes indicated that the EPP reinforced the value of people's existing coping strategies. Responses to the edu-

---

[1] QALYs or quality-adjusted life years is a formula designed to assess both the quantity and quality of life that can be achieved through a particular intervention. The EQ-5D is a brief, standardized, generic measure of HR-QoL (self-reported measures of health-related quality of life and functional status) that provides a profile of patient function and a global health state rating.

cational content varied. Some participants reported that it enabled them to review their current behavioural and treatment options but other educational content (e.g. living wills) had the potential to be disruptive and cause distress (NPCRDC, 2007).

Judging success and measuring health gain

The results from the pilot study evaluation suggest that participants attained a range of benefits and these included both objective and subjective measures of improvements in health status. Contemporary parlance would reference to this as a 'health gain'. 'Health gain' is defined as a measured improvement in the health of an individual person or a population group. It is plainly important to only offer interventions that 'do some good' or achieve their stated aim; otherwise money, time and effort are wasted. What is less obvious is what is legitimately considered to be a 'good' outcome or health gain. As mentioned earlier, there is a tendency for health gain to be linked to specific indicators of health status such as specific disease mortality or the prevalence of behaviours linked to mortality or morbidity, e.g. smoking or eating fresh fruit (National Assembly for Wales, 2001). It relates to an outcome that can be quantified.

Making judgements about health gain based solely, or primarily, on quantifiable measures can be problematic and is open to dispute. Amos (2002) asserts that this 'traditional' view of success (in terms of mortality and morbidity) stems from the narrow medical sciences/biomedical construction of health as the 'absence of disease' and, as Seedhouse (1997: p. 112) suggests, 'offers a disquietingly impoverished picture of human life, one in which not being diseased matters more than anything else'. Moreover it represents a conceptualization of health (something we will explore further below) that does not fully represent the nature of health 'gained'; for example, by participants of the EPP. Health gain in the context of the EPP was judged in functional, quantifiable terms but also in social and psychological achievements (e.g. increased self-confidence).

> 'The outcome most valued was the social support generated through sharing experiences, practical exchange of ideas and reduction in social isolation.' (NPCRDC, 2005: p. 3)

Social and psychological benefits are less easy to quantify and objectively measure but may represent vast improvements in an individual's health status. For example, the benefits or gains to be derived from an operation to unblock diseased coronary arteries obviously include an improved physical capacity and the potential avoidance, for the time being, of death; however, such benefits also include regaining lost capacities and choices such as the opportunity to return to work, or to re-establish a fulfilling sex life (Seedhouse, 2004). Making judgements about success based solely, or primarily, on changes to health that can be quantified in terms of shifts in mortality and morbidity fails to take enough account of the subjective nature of health and health gain and the general importance of people's perceptions of what constitutes a good outcome, or as Jones (2003: p. 4) states, 'Disease process is being mistaken for personal progress'.

This is very effectively illustrated by Case study 1.

> **Case study 1: Health gain – in the eye of the beholder?**
>
> An exchange during a PCT-led, protected learning event for GPs and practice staff in July 1995 illustrates the divergence in views regarding what constitutes a 'health gain'. The EPP manager and three volunteers were delivering a presentation on the benefits of the EPP and cited evidence of a 15% reduction in symptoms following involvement with the EPP (this data was extracted from Patient Liaison Group (2005)). A member of the audience retorted:
>
> 'A mere reduction of 15% was not of any real value in day-to-day medical terms.'
>
> This prompted an immediate response from one of the volunteers,
>
> 'You do not live with my condition or pain levels, don't you tell me that there is no value in me feeling 15% better, is that not my decision to see if that is of any value in my life?'
>
> Comments by JP from north Manchester.

Thus, perceptions of benefit are shaped by people's preferences and preferences are shaped by what people value in life. According to Seedhouse (1988), epistemological problems within health care stem from confusion over the meaning of health and its link to human value. It is often conceived of as if health were a 'thing' separate from other things we value in life. In Connor and Norman's (1996) book *Predicting Health Behaviour*, for instance, frequent mention is made of the link between behaviour and the value people place on health,

> 'individuals who . . . placed a high value on their health engaged in a greater number of health-promoting activities' (p. 69)

as opposed to people who place a low value on their health. Assessment scales have been developed (Lau et al., 1986) that explicitly ask people to compare the importance they place on health with other factors, thus ranking statements such as 'if you don't have health, you don't have anything' with 'there are many things I care about more than my health' and 'good health is only of minor importance in a happy life' (Norman & Bennett, 1996: p. 77). This sort of rating implies that we either value health or we value other things in life, that we do certain things for our health and other things for enjoyment, or achievement in life.

However, health and life are *not* separate things of value in our lives. Health can be an 'end' in itself but also a 'means to an end', enabling other things in life to be achieved. This depends, at least in part, on our perspective and our ambition. A doctor, for instance, may consider that health has been restored once a disease has been cured (health as the absence of disease), whereas the patient may consider this as the beginning of a lengthy process of restoration to a 'normal' life and the fulfilment of ambitions and goals (Seedhouse, 2001).

Moreover, what people value in life is not solely the avoidance of disease, illness or death (Mooney, 1998; Salkeld, 1998). This is an impossible ambition in any case, as wryly observed:

> 'The total number of deaths cannot change – one per person!' (Marmot & Mustard, 1994, in Pitts 1996: p. 1)

At a fundamental level what we value in life is our own existence and we value this because it holds the option for future choices (Harris, 1985), for example, the achievement of goals and fulfilment of potential. We also value intangible things such as friendship or creativity, principles, ideologies or aesthetics (Seedhouse, 1998), valuing something for its intrinsic qualities. We may value something for its utility (i.e. that it serves a useful purpose) but utility can also refer to the amount of satisfaction or pleasure gained from consuming a product or service, something that satisfies human wants (Salkeld, 1998). Benefits derived from work to promote health can therefore embrace a range of improvements such as anxiety reduction, reassurance and autonomy or simply the ability to make an informed choice. Indeed according to Salkeld (1998: p. 110), 'the goal of prevention is really informed choice' and health gain should not be confined to objective, quantifiable, disease-based change. Increased empowerment or sense of self-efficacy observed within EPPs symbolize such changes, and the nature of 'health gained' from the EPP is clearly less systematic and objective than classically claimed. JP's example in Box 1 certainly suggests that even if disease or pain continue, a level of change in the intensity of this experience is important and is perceived to be a valuable health 'gain'.

Concepts of health

> **Action Learning Point**
>
> * Consider the question 'Being healthy means . . .'. Discuss this concept with your colleagues.
> * Make a list of the key points. What are the similarities and differences? Do you think these are shared by all your colleagues and, particularly, your patients or clients? Who is correct?
> * Will the differing views on what constitutes 'being healthy' impact on your service delivery? Whose perspective will influence your practice?
>
> To help you here you might want to read some health ethics texts, e.g. Seedhouse (2000) and Cribb and Duncan (2002). Read the introductory chapters in books like Naidoo and Wills (2000).

The success and role of the EPP therefore necessitates an extension of our understanding as to what constitutes health and the promotion of health. Sociological theory, social constructivism (Berger & Luckmann, 1966), has contributed to an understanding that certain aspects of human reality, such as taken-for-granted assumptions about what constitutes 'health' or 'being healthy', are actually creations of and within a particular culture/society. They emerge from and represent certain dominant values within a given culture/society and so result from human choice, rather than existing as objective, indisputable facts about the nature of the world and life. The biomedical concept of health, which describes health as the absence of disease (Seedhouse, 1986, 2001; Naidoo & Wills, 1994, 2000; Ewles & Simnett, 1999; Raphael, 2000; Tones & Green, 2004), dominates Western cultural thinking about health (Seedhouse, 1986, 2001; Altschuler, 1997) but it clearly fails to capture the complexity of health experienced by, or lacking, amongst those with a chronic health problem. Other concepts of health are therefore just

as legitimate (Seedhouse, 2001). In addition, the EPP operates at a tertiary prevention[2] level (working with people who are already ill), rendering this perception of
health as an obsolete, unobtainable goal (Crossley, 2000).

For different reasons, the classic World Health Organization (WHO) definition
of health – health as a state of complete social, psychological and physical well-
being and not merely the absence of disease or infirmity (WHO, 1948)[3] – is also
an inappropriate way of perceiving 'health' in the context of the EPP. Individuals
who are already ill do not have 'complete' physical well-being, and may experience
both psychological and social limitations as a result of a chronic health problem.
Health and illness are coexisting states (Altschuler, 1997).

Tudor (1996) explores this idea of coexisting states in the context of mental
health and mental illness, suggesting that while health and illness are commonly
thought of as opposite states of being (Fig. 1), it is more appropriate to think of
illness/disease and health as two separate states (Fig. 2). Health and illness are
typified as two ends of one continuum. As an individual becomes ill, they auto-
matically and unequivocally become less healthy.

Figure 2 represents an understanding that health and illness/disease are coexisting states. An individual can be both healthy and ill. An individual, for example,
can experience an upsurge of symptoms relating to schizophrenia or deterioration
in their blood sugar control if they are diabetic, but with effective medication and
treatment this can be managed. They may simultaneously be training for a mara-
thon, getting married, holding down a fulfilling and worthwhile job, and thus may
be feeling 'alive' and 'healthy' in other respects.

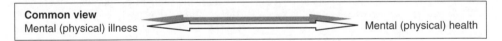

Figure 1 The common view of health and illness as opposite states of being.

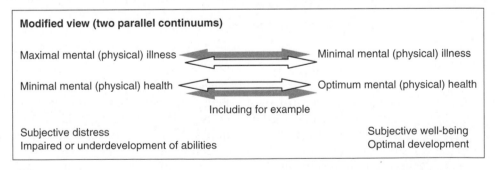

Figure 2 A modified view (two parallel continuums) of health and illness as two separate states.

---

[2] Tertiary prevention refers to action that seeks to limit the negative consequences of an existing/established condition, or to maximize remaining potential and thereby promote and create autonomy.

[3] Preamble to the Constitution of the World Health Organization as adopted by the International Health Conference,
New York, 19–22 June 1946, signed on 22 July 1946 by the representatives of 61 states (Official Records of the WHO,
No. 2, p. 100) and entered into force on 7 April 1948.

'I have breast cancer but the treatment is working and I have made some really important decisions about what I want to do with my life.' (I have a disease but I am happier and more content than I have been for years.)

This vision of health and illness/disease liberates our thinking concerning the nature of work to promote health for those who are living with a disease or illness. It alerts us to the fact that people can have 'dual citizenship' (Altschuler, 1997: p. 3) and that regardless of existing pathology all individuals have a capacity for being healthy. The work of Williams in the early 1980s and Sacks in the 1970s illustrates that health is perceived to exist even when people are considerably physically incapacitated. Williams (1983) found that people felt health could exist even when people had a serious illness. People were considered healthy if they 'had the power to "come through" or "come up"' (Williams, 1983, in Seedhouse, 2001: p. 51), and he reports accounts describing people with severe physical diseases (in one instance, gangrene of the leg) as 'being healthy' because of the strength they exhibited to survive this trauma.

Alongside this is the increasing recognition of the relationship between psychological and physical states and overall perceptions and experiences of 'health'. The dualistic vision of (wo)man described by Descartes (1596–1650), which separated 'body' from 'mind', is now largely discredited and makes no sense for individuals living with long term conditions (Altschuler, 1997). Damasio (1994), for example, cogently argues that somatic (of the body) experiences are part of our mental responses and vice versa. Physical problems, especially chronic ill health, can make us feel depressed and unhappy and this itself (psychological distress) can create physical symptoms throughout the body (Altschuler, 1997; Seedhouse, 2001). These ideas are highly relevant to work within the EPP, with people reporting a range of physical and psychological health problems as part of the entirety of their disease condition (Patient Liaison Group, 2005). Clearly what is needed, therefore, is a concept of health that captures both physical and psychological components and that can provide an effective and flexible vision of what constitutes health for those who are ill or diseased. It is helpful to take a broader view of health, which captures both an understanding of capacity and diversity, rather than defines a 'state of being' (e.g. not being ill or diseased). Both Seedhouse (1986, 1997, 2001, 2004) and Illich (1977) suggest that health be perceived of as achievement of autonomy, and one that recognizes differences in capacity and the attainment of biological potential, is more apposite (Seedhouse 1986, 1997, 2001, 2004).

'Health designates a process of adaptation. It is not the result of instinct but of an autonomous yet culturally shaped reaction to socially created reality. It designates the ability to adapt to changing environments, to growing up and ageing, to healing when damaged, to suffering and to the peaceful expectation of death . . . and inner resources.' (Illich, 1977: pp. 273–274)

'A person's (optimum) state of health is equivalent to the state of the set of conditions which fulfil or enable a person to work to fulfil his or her realistic chosen and biological potentials.' (Seedhouse, 2001: p. 95)

Seedhouse's ideas are informed by the importance of recognizing difference and diversity in matters of health. A concept of health must account for the complex and different (real and envisaged) dimensions of health. A particular form or 'state' cannot typify being healthy. He amply illustrates this in the following quote taken from the first edition of his book *Health. The foundations for achievement* (1986: p. 56):

> 'The idea that health is a specific, definable, fully describable state to which everyone can aspire equally is nonsense. It is as meaningless as the idea that there can be a perfect person. What would such a being look like? Individuals are occasionally described as perfect by people whose faculties of reason are temporarily clouded by romantic mists. A "Mr" or "Mrs Right" sometimes rides into a person's life. They are not, of course, everyone's choice of candidate for a perfect human being. The issue of health is similar. People are different – they have different ages, abilities, intelligences, disabilities, environments, ambitions, stresses, jobs and so on.'

In other words, as with 'romance', being healthy inevitably means different things to different people at different stages and times of their lives. What matters is that people are enabled to be as healthy as possible (and this will take many different shapes and forms). Health or 'being healthy' captures and represents hugely differing capacities and potentials and requires a different way of thinking about work to promote health than simply striving for the absence of disease, or even complete physical, mental and social well-being. Rather than considering health as a specific definable state, according to Seedhouse (1988, 1997, 2001, 2004), work to promote health is essentially about ensuring that the key foundations are as robust as they can be based on an assessment of the state of these foundations (do they have a home, do they have adequate information about a matter pertinent to their circumstances) and the person's internal physical and mental condition (e.g. what diseases/physical or mental problems they may have). The 'foundations' should be such that they support and enable the fulfilment of capacity or at least enable someone to work towards this goal. These foundations are explained below.

Foundations for achievement

Seedhouse's basic premise is that:

> 'A person's (optimum) state of health is *equivalent* to the state of the set of conditions which fulfil or enable a person to work to fulfil his or her realistic chosen and biological potentials.' Seedhouse and Buchanan (1997, p. 151)

The extent to which a person can function successfully (i.e. the extent to which a person is autonomous) is roughly the extent of his or her health. A person is enabled by the foundations to achieve chosen and biological potentials. The foundation boxes in Fig. 3 equate to the following central conditions:

Box 1   For good health, all have basic needs of food, drink, shelter, warmth and purpose in life.

Box 2   People also need access to the widest possible information about all factors that have an influence on a person's life (the nature and type of information will differ according to circumstances etc.).

Box 3   The skills and confidence to assimilate this information. Literacy and numeracy may be necessary. People need to understand information and

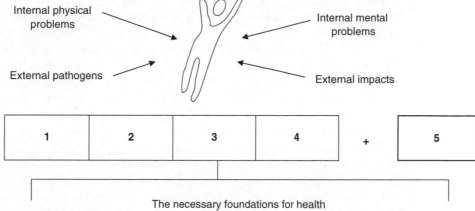

*'A person's (optimum) state of health is **equivalent** to the state of the set of conditions which fulfil or enable a person to work to fulfil his or her realistic chosen and biological potentials.'*

Figure 3 The necessary foundations for health.

how it applies to them and be able to make *reasoned and informed decisions* regarding actions they may take.

Box 4   Represents the importance of community. Individuals are never totally isolated from other people and the external world – being part of a community – is essential to good health (although the community may come in many different forms). In addition, people should not strive to fulfil personal potentials that undermine basic foundations of others. People must be aware of the implications of any actions and the basic duties that follow from living in community/society, i.e. how actions, behaviours and choices impact on others.

Box 5   Represents, for example, medical services and support, social services and improved facilities for disabled people. This relates to whatever is needed when a particular life problem becomes bad enough to impede significantly a person's movement on the platform formed by the other four boxes. The need for these 'special' services may be permanent or temporary.

In essence, Seedhouse's (1986, 1997, 2001, 2004) contention is that work for health is essentially about enabling individuals and groups to be as fully functioning as they choose and are able to be and that this can only be achieved if various obstacles that impede this 'full functioning' are removed. These obstacles exist when the above foundations are not solid. For example, a person who is homeless has a serious obstacle to achieving their full potential – for instance, they cannot get a job, they are more likely to become ill or a victim of crime and often live aimless and unfulfilling lives.

Foundations for achievement, need and the EPP

What Seedhouse (1986, 1997, 2001, 2004) aims to achieve with the foundations concept of health is a robust theory of health that can act as a framework for the analysis of (health) need, through the assessment of the state of each foundation. According to Liss (1990) the concept of 'goals' (desired/necessary achievement) is fundamental to the concept of need because need exists when there is a gap between two necessary conditions. These two necessary conditions are the actual state (AS), which can relate to an individual's physical, social and psychological state, and a goal (G), a desired, or required, state of being that enables fulfilment of potential. Needs emerge when something is missing or something is needed to fill the gap between AS and G. What is necessary to 'fill the gap' is unknown until the two conditions are understood (AS and G) and, as noted earlier, the foundations concept of health can provide this structure for assessment; identifying where, and how, foundations are weak.

Depending on circumstances, the foundations of a given individual may be sufficiently robust to enable autonomous functioning with little or no gap between AS and G, but for others, some or all may be weak and in need of attention. In other words not all foundations are equally relevant to an individual's needs at a given time and some may always remain more important than others. For example, someone who is living in a good home, is well educated, in a job they enjoy (with sufficient remuneration to pay the bills), with supportive and fulfilling relationships with others and in a good physical and mental health will likely have foundations, which for the time being, at least, are as solid as they can or need to be. Should such an individual break a leg or lose their job, though, this would change. At least one foundation would require attention. In the case of a broken leg, box 5 would need to be 'filled' and, with reference to unemployment, box 1 would be weakened. For individuals with chronic health conditions, several foundations may be weak. The state of conditions represented by boxes 2, 3, 4 and 5 may be particularly pertinent and in need of attention.

Filling need: strengthening the foundations

Clearly there are a variety of ways in which these foundations may be supported and improved. However, the specific nature of the interventions to achieve improvement requires consideration too and will vary according to circumstances (individual, social and cultural circumstances). Take the situation, again, in which someone has broken a leg. They are undoubtedly in need of some medical attention. The leg needs mending. Without this sort of therapy an individual's physical potential is truncated, as mobility may be severely restricted, disabling a return to work and so forth. Within a richer society, this medical attention would take the form of orthopaedic-based surgery, therapy and rehabilitation within both a tertiary and primary care setting. This is possible because the knowledge, skills and infrastructure enable the prescription of this treatment package. However, historically (for example before the development of effective surgical techniques) or culturally (in countries without the requisite resources), this specific package of care may not be possible.

Weakened foundations can be improved in a variety of ways and this depends on what is available and able to improve circumstances. Identifying such options requires both evidence of what will effectively do the job ('does it work?') and the priorities and resources made available through health and social care policy within a given country. The EPP is evidently one of those options and several foundations are at least in part fulfilled via the EPP. One example of the potential

**The Contribution of the Expert Patient Programme
to the Foundations for Health**

1	2	3	4		5
Basic needs may be met	**Information** Information about managing a chronic health condition, exploring choices, etc.	**Education** and the skills and confidence to make use of information. For example, developing self-efficacy skills	**Community** Being part of a group with similar problems. Learning and supporting each other, no longer being isolated		**Support services** Being able to maximize use of health care

Figure 4 The contribution of the EPP to the foundation for health.

contribution of the EPP to the promotion of health, using the foundations concept of health, is presented in Fig. 4.

Promoting health: promoting autonomy and empowering individuals

At this stage it is worth exploring in greater depth some of the other theoretical concepts that underpin the EPP and which establish its credentials as an effective means of promoting health. In particular, what will emerge is an understanding of the unique potential of the EPP to promote autonomy and enable individuals to fulfil their potential. According to Cribb and Duncan (2002) and Seedhouse (1986, 2001), health work is about creating autonomy and 'health promotion' has been defined as the 'process of enabling people to take control over, and improve their health' (WHO, 1986, in Koelen and van den Ban, 2004). The results from various evaluations of the EPP mentioned earlier indicate that this is indeed what participants are able to do and is cogently illustrated by CD's story below (Box 2).

Case study 2

When I attended the Expert Patients Programme I spent ten minutes outside the door, after 22 years of attending sessions with a clinical psychologist to deal with many issues as well as having unstable diabetes, cellulitis and liver problems, I didn't see what six weeks on a course could do, when my diabetes education session didn't help. But there I was, my psychologist said he didn't know what else to try, what did I have to lose?

I couldn't believe the way we all had different stuff wrong with us, yet we all had similar feelings and felt the same about how it stopped us living our lives. Over the six weeks my confidence grew, we made action plans every week and I achieved every one of them. I have never completed anything in my life. I am now a volunteer for the EPP and have been discharged by my psychologist. He was really pleased. My diabetes is quite stable, the information I gained from the EPP course helped me understand and put into practice what I learned on the diabetes course. I have even lost four stone. I never thought I was capable of talking in front of people but now I not only deliver EPP but attend events and help promote it to health professionals and the public; it saved my life, I have a *life* now which I live and not just exist.

CD, north Manchester

A core element of the EPP revolves around enhancing an individual's ability and self-belief (Wilson, 2002; Plews, 2005) with empowerment and autonomy being central themes. The notion of health as autonomy is extremely pertinent in the context of the EPP. Autonomy is from the Greek for self-rule and refers to an individual's capacity to choose freely for him/herself and be able to direct his/her own life. Autonomy is restricted by law, social tradition, autonomy of others and the circumstances of a person's life (age, class, financial position, physical capacities, ambitions and personality, etc.), but within these boundaries everybody has the potential to be autonomous – i.e. make choices and shape their lives to some extent. This ability is influenced by several factors including knowledge, understanding of options and ability to select appropriate goals and the existence of suitable environmental circumstances that enable individuals to act upon choices made, reflected in the components of the foundations concept of health.

The limited nature of choice is particularly apparent for someone with a chronic health condition. If an individual is physically incapacitated (e.g. through illness and disease), they do not have the same potential as someone with no malady. Living with a chronic, long term condition is likely to truncate and shape choices. As Altschuler (1997: p. 11) notes 'adaption to the discovery of illness demands radical reorganisation of individual and family life'.

Nevertheless, every individual has a capacity and potential. Mary Warnock discusses this notion in the context of her experience developing policy around 'special needs' education in the 1970s (Education Act 1972). This Act extended the entitlement to education to those who were severely disabled, as evidence increasingly indicated that education could make a considerable difference to the quality of life even of severely disabled children. Along with the evidence was a passionate moral persuasion that no child should be deprived of an opportunity for self-improvement and that people must never be treated as though 'what they have been and what they are, is what they will always be' (Warnock, 1998). To treat someone in this manner is to objectify and dehumanize, both them and us, as this doctrine accords the same qualities to people as to a machine (a predictable 'object'). Rather, Warnock (1998: p. 102) asserts that:

> 'humans . . . are able not only to learn from their past experiences . . . but consciously to envisage a future for themselves which may differ from the past. They are able not only to pursue the things they have learned to value highly and avoid those they have learned to hate . . . but they can form pictures for themselves of the universe as a whole and the part they wish to play in it. They can give themselves goals to pursue, which may be totally new and idiosyncratic, or which they have learned from people they have . . . met or read about, admired or loved . . . this ability to set new goals'.

In other words all individuals have the potential to make choices and set goals, to act as an autonomous individual, whatever the circumstances. The philosophy and content of the EPP is explicitly focused on enhancing and enabling choice.

Moreover, there is a connection between notions of autonomy and the importance of empowerment for individuals, with empowerment increasingly being regarded as a legitimate aim of health work (DOH, 2004a, 2005a, 2006; Kagan, 2006). Empowerment relates to an individual's ability to gain control over and deal with life's problems and reaffirm a sense of personal strength and value.

'Empowerment is self-determination' (Wallcraft 1996: p. 195) and personal empowerment exists when people feel in control of their lives or have control over their own affairs and are able 'to define their own needs and act upon that understanding' (Raeburn & Rootman, 1998: p. 65).

All individuals are able to be agents of their own destiny and have the capacity to grow and develop to live as full a life as possible. This is achieved, at least in part, through the giving and sharing of information, something which is central to the EPP.

'[This is] empowerment because the information provided to patients helps them to make informed choices. Based on the knowledge acquired and their own previous knowledge, patients can make decisions about their health, taking into account scientific, social and personal factors. This gives them the opportunity to exercise autonomy and self-government.' (Gastaldo, 1997: p. 129)

Empowerment, self-efficacy and the EPP

Improvements in 'self-efficacy' are a recognized outcome of participation in the EPP (Wilson, 2002; Rogers et al., 2006; NPCRDC, 2007). Self-efficacy refers to an individual's confidence and belief that one has the power to achieve a desired behaviour (Ogden, 2002) and is hence fundamental to 'empowerment'. Self-efficacy is recognized as the best predictor of behavioural intention and behaviour change (Schwarzer, 1992) and a 'vast body of evidence reveals that belief in one's efficacy to exercise control over health-related behaviour plays an influential role in health status and functioning' (Bandura, 2002: p. 304).

Essentially, self-efficacy emerges through opportunities for engagement and change (Bandura, 2000). This is not only in a practical sense, in terms of developing competencies and skills (improving what we are able to do) but also in terms of the confidence in our abilities to be autonomous (Wilson, 2002; Plews, 2005). Self-efficacy is developed 'in context', i.e. when the knowledge and skills can be utilized (Jones, 2003). Developing self-efficacy requires more than the provision of information, which Jones (2003) states can in itself be counterproductive. Preventative actions may be actively avoided if the individual feels overwhelmed and unable to utilize knowledge gained.

People's sense of self-efficacy can be developed in four main ways (Bandura, 2000):

1 Mastery experiences (overcoming obstacles).
2 Vicarious experiences (reference to appropriate role models).
3 Social persuasion (being told they have the capacity) and providing experiences of success.
4 Reducing people's stress reactions and correcting misunderstandings.

There are several characteristics of the EPP that contribute to the development of self-efficacy (Boxes 1–3).

What is evident so far is that the EPP can make a profound contribution to people's health, and provides a fascinating opportunity to explore and recognize the diverse and eclectic nature of 'health' and what constitutes health promotion work. Nevertheless, it is not an unproblematic solution to the health, health

---

Box 1: Mastery experiences: action planning and problem-solving

A central feature of the EPP revolves around developing skills of self-management. Essentially this means clarifying desired goals and identifying a variety of options for achieving these. Setting short-term goals and monitoring achievement of these is key to accomplishing important individual ambitions (Lorig et al., 2000).

Box 2: Vicarious experiences: lay tutors and group support

All EPPs are run by volunteer tutors who themselves have a long term condition and have been a participant in an EPP group. The group nature of the programme implicitly provides support for members and enables people to exchange ideas and to explore perceptions, understanding and behaviour. Groups provide individuals with the opportunity to explore achievements, difficulties and concerns enabling knowledge and confidence to develop (Katz et al., 2000).

Box 3: Reducing stress reactions and correcting misunderstandings: developing communication skills

Within the EPP emphasis is placed upon developing an understanding of the importance of communication. This includes listening skills and the use of 'I' messages, aimed at encouraging ownership of what an individual says and how needs are expressed. The focus is on developing partnerships with health care providers when negotiating around health care needs, to enable the attainment of realistic choices.

---

promotion and health care needs of people with chronic, long term health conditions in the 21st century.

Limitations of the EPP

It has already been asserted that the EPP produces positive results (Barlow et al., 1998b). However, the EPP is not a panacea for addressing the needs of those with long term conditions and, as Wilson (2002) and Plews (2005) note, the programme is not unconditionally accepted by all. The evidence base that validates the EPP is not yet fully endorsed by individual clinicians or professional bodies. In particular, professional and philosophical concerns about the actual and potential impact of the EPP on matters of 'choice' and realistic expectations need to be explored, along with consideration of the practical and resource implications for local PCT policy-making (Farrell, 2004).

Concerns have been raised about the use of the term 'expert' (Kennedy et al., 2004; Shaw & Baker, 2004) and fears voiced that patients will challenge professionals' care decisions (Plews, 2005), particularly when patients' choices conflict with health professionals' recommendations (Wilson, 2002). Professional values and expectations influence attitudes towards patient involvement, and conflicts with professional ethics (such as non-maleficence) or a clear belief in the suitability of a particular option, interfere with professional engagement with, and acceptance of, the expert (involved) patient (Farrell, 2004). This potential source of conflict increases with the growing use of care pathways or protocols and the standardization of care implied by such guidelines (Farrell, 2004). Inevitably the lack of concordance between competing ethical (and practical) considerations can only be resolved through deliberation and discussion (Seedhouse, 1986, 1998). Reflecting upon difficult scenarios with peers may be helpful and, ultimately, compromise may be necessary to enable shared decision-making (Farrell, 2004).

Fitzpatrick (2007) suggests that the increasing focus on the 'expert patient' may shift the balance of responsibility for health management to the individual with the chronic condition, undermining traditional health care relationships and the importance of professional expertise in the provision and development of treatment and health care packages. Practitioners may feel their health care role is fundamentally undermined through the self-help ethos, and research published by the NPCRDC (2005) has indicated that GPs and other health care practitioners want to remain central to patients' treatment regimes. This, at least in part, reflected practitioners' apprehension (regarding liability and competency) when patients self-manage their conditions (Wilson, 2002), and there is some evidence that emphasizing self-management falsely implies to patients that the health condition is not serious (Lawton et al., 2005). Indeed, Hardy (2004) wonders if the focus on the expert patient may result in withdrawal of professional support. Iphofen (2003) notes that self-help requires a supportive partnership and that professional expertise should remain a core component of care and treatment for those with chronic health conditions. The importance of collaboration within consultation is emphasized. A good consultation is recognized as one characterized by mutuality, shared values and shared responsibility for treatment and care decisions (Farrell, 2004).

Practical and financial limitations have emerged too. Developing the scope and coverage of the EPP inevitably has resource implications for any health care services that are publicly funded. The EPP itself is a short intervention, lasting six weeks only, and benefits may be similarly short term (Riemsma et al., 2002). Therefore, the importance of continuing support is increasingly being recognized (Patient Liaison Group, 2005), with some PCTs providing review or reunion days (Wilson & Mayor, 2006). This inevitably impinges upon resources distribution. Moreover, the work of health professionals may be shaped by many different, often conflicting, agendas (different outcomes, different values/ideological focus) resulting in stress, conflict and inefficiency (Farrell, 2004). Conflicting policies and priorities at a local level (and the drive to meet national and regional targets) may mean that the development of bespoke delivery packages may be jeopardized. Indeed, Lee et al. (2006) indicated that there is an 'implementation gap' between national aspirations and the actual number of EPPs operating at a local level, with local priorities taking precedence within PCTs.

Choice and responsibility

Returning to the notion of 'choice' as it relates to health matters raises some problematic issues, despite its positive connotations. The notion of choice and health has considerable contemporary resonance.

'We are committed to ensuring that the fundamental mission of the NHS to promote physical and mental well-being and prevent illness is pursued effectively in the 21st century.' (DOH 2004a; p. 5)

'Our starting point is informed choice.' (DOH 2004a: p. 6)

The contribution of the EPP to promoting choice (autonomy and empowerment) and the elemental role of this in promoting health have already been discussed at some length.

While evidence suggests that the EPP provides participants with information and other prerequisite skills to facilitate informed choice (generally considered a 'good thing'), there may be a danger that it becomes prescriptive. The programme is criticized for being too rigid with no reference made to important socioeconomic factors and welfare issues that affect health such as benefit entitlements (NPCRDC, 2005). Moreover, enabling 'choice' may simply be a euphemism for 'individual responsibility' (Patient Liaison Group, 2005). The programme is seen by some as a way of reducing demand for mainstream services (NPCRDC, 2005; Taylor & Bury, 2007) and improving compliance and concordance through more active self-management (DOH, 2001). This broad objective may not be equally welcomed across the social spectrum. Personal responsibility appealed less to people living in deprived areas, where higher value may be placed on the relationship with GPs (NPCRDC, 2005) and the programme may well be unsuitable for some patients (Patient Liaison Group, 2005). Some minority ethnic groups, for instance, are unfamiliar with concepts of preventative medicine (Griffiths et al., 2001) and those who have reduced mobility and limited contact with social network groups may find access difficult.

More seriously, there is a growing tendency in the health arena for unarticulated assumptions to be made about what constitutes an informed or 'good' choice (Seedhouse, 1997, 2001), innocuously articulated on various pages in *Choosing Health: Making healthy choices easier* (DOH, 2004a: pp. 5–6) as follows:

'Health improvement depends upon people's motivation and their willingness to act on it. The Government will provide information and practical support to get people motivated and improve emotional wellbeing and access to services so that healthy choices are easier to make . . . achieving a balance between the healthy outcome we want to see and the equally valued freedom to determine our own way of life that is so important in a democratic society . . . so that it is easier to do the *right thing.*' [authors' emphasis]

While a balance between different aspirations is noted, the implication is that there is a right thing to do and a wrong thing to do. Concerns have already been raised about professional/patient conflicts around 'choice' (Wilson, 2002), but on a more fundamental level caution needs to be exerted when making exhortations about what represents the 'right' choice, particularly in relation to matters concerning health. The notion of 'right' or 'wrong' in this context has the potential for being misleading and pejorative as there are no universally prescribed goals or specified ways of living (Seedhouse, 2004). Definitive claims about what constitutes the 'right' thing to do are contestable. Indeed, assertions of this kind undermine the very basis of autonomy. Autonomy is a fundamental concept in Western ethical philosophy (Gillon, 1990; Beauchamp & Childress, 1994; Cribb & Duncan, 2002;

Seedhouse, 1988, 1997, 1998, 2001, 2004). John Stuart Mill (1806–1873), the 19th century philosopher and author of *On Liberty*, believed that autonomy was the central feature of being a person and that each person is the best judge of their own happiness such that the autonomous pursuit of goals is itself a major source of happiness. Essentially this implies that an individual must be allowed to choose his or her own life goals and these may legitimately be many and varied. John Stuart Mills asserted that:

> 'the only purpose for which power can rightfully be exercised over any member of a civilised society is to prevent harm to others. His own good, either physical or moral, is not a sufficient warrant.' (Seedhouse, 2001: p. 107)

Exercising choice, exercising our autonomy and pursuing the things we value in life must therefore also include the choice to smoke, drink, not exercise or, in point of fact, not attend an EPP or self-manage a chronic health condition. There may be a danger that attendance at an EPP becomes a mandatory component of a health care package for those with a long term health problem. While this may seem innocuous, it could fundamentally undermine the principle of choice (according to *Compatibilists*, philosophers such as Hume and Hobbes, free will, and therefore responsibility, only exists when an individual is not forced to make a certain choice). As Taylor and Bury (2007: pp. 32–33) note, the existence of the EPP could change:

> 'professional/patient relationships to the extent to which more aggressively managed systems of care may have an impact not only on clinical judgements but also . . . on health service users' freedoms and opportunities to cope with the challenges of chronic illness in ways that they find most effective and appropriate.'

Within the context of the EPP, subtle persuasion may also be exerted on an individual to conform to particular behavioural or treatment regimes (Taylor & Bury, 2007). The EPP can, however, provide firm foundations for health without falling into the trap of 'prescribing choice', as long as sanctions concerning what constitutes the 'right' choice are absent and alternative treatment and care options remain available.

Action Learning Point

- Consider the issues raised in the section above. In particular, have a discussion with your colleagues about what they think interferes with patient involvement.
- Identify if any of you have had any experiences when you felt a patient's request for care or treatment conflicted with what you, or a colleague, thought was best practice.
- Discuss any conflicts there are between the patient's autonomy, professional codes of conduct, the law and resource issues. How might these conflicts be resolved or managed?

Get hold of a copy of the DOH report compiled by Christine Farrell (2004). You can download a pdf copy of this report from www.dh.gov.uk. Type Farrell in the 'Search this site' box on the top right-hand side of the screen and look for the title *Patient and Public Involvement in Health: Evidence for policy implementation*. This report provides some useful ideas about practice and practical discussions for improving patient involvement.

Implications for practice

The existence and success of the EPP has consequences for professionals' work in several ways, necessitating philosophical and practical changes to traditional practice. The EPP requires a shift in health professional/patient relationships, changing the focus from normative values towards expressed needs and lay perceptions (Rowley, 2005). As Iphofen (2003: p. 39) notes:

'responsibility for health has to be shared between those who possess the knowledge, skills and access to the finite resources of health . . . There is a mutual responsibility between professionals and client.'

Additionally, our taken-for-granted perceptions of what constitutes 'health' and the 'promotion' of health need to be extended beyond limited notions of health as the absence of disease (Rowley, 2005). Instead, it is important to acknowledge that positive health outcomes should be based on what people value as life goals and not simply in terms of shifts in states of illness or disease (Cowley & Billings, 1999). We have suggested in this chapter that, particularly in the context of the EPP, the foundations concept of health (Seedhouse 1988, 1997, 2001, 2004) provides a sound theoretical and conceptual framework for health professionals to ponder such matters.

Finally, some other practical considerations concerning the EPP should be mentioned. Generally, programmes have run more frequently and extensively in PCT areas with a dedicated champion or leader (NPCRDC, 2005; Lee et al., 2006) as this enables more effective co-ordination of activities as well as offering the potential for developmental support for lay group leaders, for example, around group management skills (NPCRDC, 2005). Health professionals may therefore additionally have to engage with more active promotion, or at least endorsement of the EPP. While the EPP is based on the principle of self-referral, health professionals could act as an appropriate source of information or encouragement to patients who may be unaware or sceptical about the programme (Wilson & Mayor, 2006). It might ultimately be a more effective means of ensuring the EPP reaches the appropriate target groups (NPCRDC, 2005). This, in itself, requires the education of professionals regarding the purpose and process of the EPP, with better integration of the EPP within mainstream resources (NPCRDC, 2005). Lee et al. (2006) suggest that some programmes could be usefully led by professionals to enhance coverage and to complement more traditional, mainstream disease management provision, and that occupational health departments could be involved in the publicity, if not delivery, of EPPs (Patient Liaison Group, 2005). Flexible and innovative modes of delivery and culturally appropriate content are needed to effectively meet the needs of diverse communities and individuals still in employment (Patient Liaison Group, 2005).

Conclusions

In this chapter we have explored components of the EPP. In particular, we have attempted to reinforce the validity of this type of 'non-traditional' health care intervention by exploring a variety of theoretical and conceptual matters that underpin the 'taken-for-granted' claims about the contribution of the EPP to the promotion of health. What emerges from this is an extension of our understanding about the nature of work for health and deeper insights into what legitimately can be considered a 'health gain'. More importantly, we have attempted to illustrate how the existence of programmes such as the EPP should be supported because it enables individuals to become more autonomous and that this is a valuable outcome, regardless of shifts in disease status or health care costs. Notwithstanding these benefits, we have also introduced points of debate concerning some fundamental ethical and philosophical principles around notions of 'choice', which must be considered in the context of developing health care systems to meet needs if the basic principle of non-maleficience (do no harm) is to be upheld.

References

Altschuler, J. (1997) *Working with Chronic Illness*. Basingstoke, Macmillan.

Amos, M. (2002) Community development. In: L. Adams, M. Amos & J. Munro (eds) *Promoting Health – Politics and practice*. London, Sage Publications, pp. 63–71.

Baggott, R. (2004) *Health and Health Care in Britain*, 3rd edn. Basingstoke, Palgrave.

Bandura, A. (2000) Health promotion from the perspective of social cognition theory. In: P. Norman, C. Abraham & M. Conner (eds). *Understanding and Changing Health Behaviour: From Health Beliefs to Self-Regulation*. The Netherlands, Harwood Academic Publishers, pp. 299–339.

Bandura, A. (2002) Self-efficacy assessment. In: R. Fernandex-Ballesteros (ed.) *Encyclopedia of Psychological Assessment*. London, Sage Publications, pp. 848–852.

Barlow, J.H., Turner, A.P. & Wright, C.C. (1998a) Sharing, caring and learning to take control: self management training for people with arthritis. *Psychology, Health and Medicine* 3: 387–393.

Barlow, J.H., Turner, A.P. & Wright, C.C. (1998b) Long-term outcomes of an arthritis self-management programme. *British Journal of Rheumatology* 37 (12): 1315–1319.

Barlow, J.H., Williams, B. & Wright, C.C. (1999) Instilling the strength to fight the pain and get on with life: learning to become an arthritis self manager through an adult education programme. *Health Education Research* 14: 533–544.

Beauchamp, T.L. & Childress, J.F. (1994) *Principles of Biomedical Ethics*, 4th edn. Oxford, Oxford University Press.

Berger, P.L. & Luckmann, T. (1966) *The Social Construction of Reality: A treatise in the sociology of knowledge*. New York, Doubleday.

Conner, M. & Norman, P. (eds) (1996) *Predicting Health Behaviour*. Buckingham, Open University Press.

Cowley, C. & Billings, J.R. (1999) Resources revisited: salutogenesis from a lay perspective. *Journal of Advanced Nursing* 29 (4): 994–1004.

Cribb, A. & Duncan, P. (2002) *Health Promotion and Professional Ethics*. Oxford, Blackwell Publishing.

Crossley, M.L. (2000) *Rethinking Health Psychology*. Buckingham, Open University Press.

Damasio, A. (1994) *Descartes' Error*. New York, Grosset Putnam

Department of Health (1999a) *Saving Lives, Our Healthier Nation*. London, Stationery Office.

Department of Health (1999b) *The Health Act*. London, Department of Health.

Department of Health (2000) *The NHS Plan: A plan for investment, a plan for reform*. London, Department of Health.

Department of Health (2001) *The Expert Patient: A new approach to chronic disease management for the 21st century*. London, Department of Health.

Department of Health (2003) *Future Partnerships, Primary Care in 2020.* London, HMSO.

Department of Health (2004a) *Choosing Health: Making healthier choices easier.* London, Department of Health.

Department of Health (2004b) *Improving Chronic Disease Management.* London, Department of Health.

Department of Health (2004c) *The NHS Improvement Plan: Putting people at the heart of public services.* London, Department of Health.

Department of Health (2004d) *At Least Five a Week – Evidence on the impact of physical activity and its relationship to health.* Report from the Chief Medical Officer. London, Department of Health.

Department of Health (2005a) *Supporting People with Long Term Conditions: An NHS and social care model to support local innovation and integration.* London, Department of Health.

Department of Health (2005b) *National Service Framework for Long-term Conditions.* London, Department of Health.

Department of Health (2005c) *Creating a Patient-led NHS – Delivering the NHS improvement plan.* London, Department of Health.

Department of Health (2005d) *Self Care – A real choice: Self care support – A practical option.* London: Department of Health.

Department of Health (2006) *Our Health, Our Care, Our Say.* London, Department of Health.

Ewles, L. & Simnett, I. (1999) *Promoting Health – A practical guide*, 4th edn. Edinburgh, Bailliere Tindall in association with the Royal College of Nursing.

Farrell, C. (2004) *Patient and Public Involvement in Health: Evidence for policy implementation. A summary of the results of the Health in Partnership research programme.* London: Department of Health.

Fitzpatrick, M. (2007) Empowering Patients: New Labour's unhealthiest idea? www.spiked-online.com [accessed 24 May 2007].

Gastaldo, D. (1997) Is health education good for you? Re-thinking health education through the concept of bio-power. In: A. Petersen & R. Bunton (eds) *Foucault – Health and medicine.* London, Routledge, pp. 113–133.

Gillon, R. (1990) *Philosophical Medical Ethics.* Chichester, John Wiley.

Green, J. & South, J. (2006) *Evaluation.* Buckingham, Open University Press.

Griffiths, C., Kaur, G., Gantley, M. et al. (2001) Influences on hospital admission for asthma in south Asian and white adults: qualitative interview study. *British Medical Journal* 323: 962–966.

Hardy, P. (2004) The Expert Patient Programme: A critical review. MSc lifelong learning, policy and research – programme evaluation, quality assessment and learning processes. www.pilgrimprojects.co.uk/papers/epp_mc.pdf [accessed 9 November 2007].

Harris, J. (1985) *The Value of Life: An introduction to medical ethics.* Abingdon, UK, Routledge and Kegan Paul.

Hillsdon, M., Foster, C., Cavill, N., Crombie, H. & Naidoo, B. (2005) *The Effectiveness of Public Health Interventions for Increasing Physical Activity among Adults: A review of reviews – evidence briefing*, 2nd edn. Department of Epidemiology and Public Health, University College London/British Heart Foundation Health Promotion Research Group, University of Oxford/Health Development Agency. www.nice.org.uk/download.aspx?o=505281 [accessed 30 April 2007].

Illich, I. (1977) *Limits to Medicine. Medical nemesis: The expropriation of health.* London, Pelican Books.

Iphofen, R. (2003) Social and individual factors influencing public health. In: J. Costello & M. Haggart (eds) *Public Health and Society.* Basingstoke, Palgrave Macmillan, pp. 23–41.

Jones, F.R. (2003) Can Expert Patients Be Created? *Expert Patient Conference* May 2003. http://www.rpsgb.org/pdfs/exptpatsem6.pdf [accessed 18 May 2007].

Kagan, C. (2006) *Making a Difference – Participation and wellbeing.* RENEW Intelligence Report. www.RENEW.co.uk [accessed 18 May 2007].

Katz, J., Perbedy, A. & Douglas, J. (2000) *Promoting Health: Knowledge and practice,* 2nd edn. Basingstoke, Open University Press with Palgrave.

Kennedy, A., Gatley, C. & Rogers, A. (2004) *EPP Evaluation Team; Notional Evaluation of Expert Patients Programme. Assessing embedding EPP in the NHS preliminary survey of PCT pilot sites.* Manchester, Manchester National Centre for Primary Care Research and Development with Universities of York and Manchester.

Koelen, M.A. & van den Ban, A. (2004) *Health Education and Health Promotion.* Wageningen, Academic Publishers.

Lau, R.R., Hartman, K.A. & Ware, J.E. (1986) Health as value: methodological and theoretical considerations. *Health Psychology* 5: 25–43.

Lawton, J., Peel, E., Parry, O. et al. (2005) Lay perceptions of type 2 diabetes in Scotland: bringing health services back. *Social Science and Medicine* 60: 1423–1435.

Lee, V., Kennedy, A. & Rogers, A. (2006) Implementing and managing self-management skills training within primary care organisations: a national survey of the expert patients programme within its pilot phase. *Implementation Science* 1: 6. www.implementation-science.com/content/1/1/6 [accessed 25 April 2007].

Lenker, S., Lorig, K. & Gallagher, D. (1984) Reasons for the lack of association between changes in health behaviour and improved health status: an exploratory study. *Patient Education and Counselling* 6 (2): 69–72.

Liss, P.E. (1990) *Health Care Need: Meanings and measurement.* Sweden, Linkoping University.

Lorig, K., Gonzalez, V. & Laurent, D. (1997) *The Expert Patients Programme Chronic Disease Self-Management Course: Leader's Manual.* California, Stanford Patient Education Research Centre. (Copyrighted by the Board of Trustees of the Leland Stanford Junior University. Adapted for the UK by J. Phillips & J. Thompson.)

Lorig, K. & Holman, H. (2003) Self-management education: history, definition, outcomes, and mechanisms. *Annals of Behavioral Medicine* 26: 1–7.

Lorig, K., Holman, H., Sobel, D., Laurent, D., Gonzalez, V. & Minor, M. (2000) *Living a Healthy Life with Chronic Conditions – Self management of heart disease, arthritis, diabetes, asthma, bronchitis, emphysema and others,* 2nd edn. Boulder, Bull Publishing Company.

Lorig, K., Sobel, D., Stewart, A. et al (1999) Evidence suggesting that a chronic disease self-management program can improve health status while reducing hospitalization: a randomised trial. *Medical Care* 37: 5–14.

Mooney, G. (1998) Beyond health outcomes: the benefits of health care. *Health Care Analysis* 6: 99–105.

Naidoo, J. & Wills, J. (1994) *Health Promotion – Foundations for practice.* London, Bailliere Tindall.

Naidoo, J. & Wills, J. (2000) *Health Promotion – Foundations for practice,* 2nd edn. London, Bailliere Tindall with the Royal College of Nursing.

National Assembly for Wales (2001) *Expert Group on Indicators of Health Inequality: Report on phase 1, Health indicators – better health, better Wales.* Wales, Health Promotion Division.

National Primary Care Research and Development Centre (NPCRDC) (2005) *Executive Summary 36: How has the EPP been delivered and accepted in the NHS during the pilot phase.* www.npcrdc.ac.uk [accessed 26 April 2007].

National Primary Care Research and Development Centre (NPCRDC) (2007) *Executive Summary 44: National evaluation of the Expert Patient Programme – key findings (research into expert patients – outcomes in a randomised trial)*. www.npcrdc.ac.uk [accessed 26 April 2007].

Norman, P. & Bennett, P. (1996) Health locus of control. In: M. Conner & P. Norman (eds) *Predicting Health Behaviour*. Buckingham, Open University Press, pp. 62–94.

Ogden, J. (2002) *Health and the Construction of the Individual*. New York, Routledge with Taylor Francis.

Patient Liaison Group (2005) *The Expert Patients Programme – A discussion paper*. London: British Medical Association.

Perbedy, A. (2002) Evaluating Community Action. In: L. Jones, M. Sidell & J. Douglas (eds) *The Challenge of Promoting Health – Exploration and Action*, 2nd edn. Buckingham, Open University Press, pp. 85–102.

Pitts, M. (1996) *The Psychology of Preventive Health*. London, Routledge.

Plews, C. (2005) Expert Patient Programme: managing patients with long-term conditions. *British Journal of Nursing* 14 (20): 1086–1089.

Pomerleau, J. & McKee, M. (eds) (2005) *Issues in Public Health*. Berkshire, Open University Press.

Raeburn, J. & Rootman, I. (1998) *People Centred Health Promotion*. Chichester, John Wiley.

Raphael, D. (2000) The question of evidence in health promotion. *Health Promotion International* 15 (4): 355–367.

Riemsma, R.P., Kirwan, J.R., Taal, E. & Rasker, J.J. (2002) Patient education for adults with rheumatoid arthritis. *Cochrane Database Systematic Review* 3: CD003688.

Rogers, A., Bower, P., Gardner, C. et al. (2006) *The National Evaluation of the Pilot Phase of the Expert Patient Programme – Final report*. Manchester and York, National Primary Care Research and Development Centre.

Rowley, C. (2005) Health needs assessment. *Journal of Community Nursing* 19 (6): 11–14. www.jcn.co.uk/journal.asp?MonthNum=06&YearNum=2005&Type=backissue&ArticleID=808 [accessed 12 April 2006].

Salkeld, G. (1998) What are the benefits of preventive health care? *Health Care Analysis* 6: 106–112.

Schwarzer, R. (1992) Self-efficacy in the adoption and maintenance of health behaviour: theoretical approaches and a new model. In: R. Schwarzer (ed.) *Self-Efficacy: Thought control of action*. Washington DC, Hemisphere, pp. 217–243.

Seedhouse, D. (1986) *Health. The foundations for achievement*. Chichester, John Wiley.

Seedhouse, D. (1988) *Ethics – The heart of health care*. Chichester, John Wiley.

Seedhouse, D. & Buchanan, I. (1997) *Health Promotion. Philosophy, prejudice and practice*. Chichester, John Wiley.

Seedhouse, D. (1998) *Ethics – The heart of health care*, 2nd edn. Chichester, John Wiley.

Seedhouse, D. (2000) *Practical Nursing Philosophy*. Chichester, John Wiley.

Seedhouse, D. (2001) *Health. The foundations for achievement*, 2nd edn. Chichester, John Wiley and Sons.

Seedhouse, D. (2004) *Health Promotion. Philosophy, prejudice and practice*, 2nd edn. Chichester, John Wiley.

Shaw, J. & Baker, M. (2004) Expert patient – dream or nightmare? *British Medical Journal* 328: 723–724.

Taylor, D. & Bury, M. (2007) Chronic illness, expert patients and care transition. *Sociology of Health and Illness* 29 (1): 27–45.

Tones, K. & Green, J. (2004) *Health Promotion: Planning and strategy*. London, Sage Publications.

Tudor, K. (1996) *Mental Health Promotion – Paradigms of practice*. London, Routledge.

Unwin, N., Carr, S., Leeson, J. & Pless-Mulloli, T. (1997) *An Introductory Study Guide to Public Health and Epidemiology*. Buckingham, Open University Press.

Wallcraft, J. (1996) Becoming fully ourselves. In: J. Read and J. Reynolds (eds) *Speaking our Minds – An anthology of personal experiences of mental distress and its consequences*. Basingstoke, Macmillan.

Wanless, D. (2004) *Securing Good Health for the Whole Population (Wanless Report)*. London, HM Treasury.

Warnock, M. (1998) *An Intelligent Person's Guide to Ethics*. London, Duckworth,

Williams, R. (1983) Concepts of health: an analysis of lay logic. *Sociology* **17** (2): 185–205.

Wilson, P.M. (2002) The expert patient: issues and implications for community nurses. *British Journal of Community Nursing* **7** (10): 514–519.

Wilson, P.M. & Mayor, V. (2006) Long-term conditions: 2. Supporting and enabling self-care. *British Journal of Community Nursing* **11** (1): 6–10.

Chapter 4

Informal carers: valuing our assets

Maureen Deacon, Marilyn Fitzpatrick and Margaret Presho

Key points

- Presenting a profile of the informal caring population
- Examining the cultural influences on the experiences of carers
- Discussing policies that affect carers and those in receipt of care
- Presenting a problem-solving approach for practitioners who have responsibility for supporting informal carers

In this chapter we aim to carefully consider the needs of informal carers and how practitioners can enable them to gain access to more effective, person-centred support. Initially we unpack ideas about this group of people and consider the impact of these ideas on how carers may be perceived. We argue that these perceptions need to be confronted and challenged if we are to value the experiences of individuals and the unique context in which they care. Having examined the social context of caring, we then move on to discuss policy and what is known about carers as a population group. This leads to the observation that carers may suffer from 'multilayered disadvantage' (Carers UK, 2007a). Finally, we discuss some contemporary potential solutions to the well-established problems and offer practical tips to the individual practitioner.

The context of informal care

Kinship obligations

The activity of informal caring is both an ordinary and extraordinary feature of social life. Ordinary in the sense that caring is taken for granted as being completely normal and natural in many social circumstances, but extraordinary in other senses. For example, we expect parents to care for their children and consider it entirely unremarkable when parents devote a great deal of their resources to this activity. However, if a child has a long term condition demanding complex medical regimes, we perceive this as extraordinary. Stalker (2003) observes that it was only in the latter part of the 20th century that the 'carer' became a category of social concern and it was not until the 1970s that any official financial support was available for this work in the form of the invalid care allowance. The decision to bar married women from claiming this benefit added to a strong feminist appraisal of community care (Twigg & Atkin, 1994). This argued that the cross-cutting policy of community care relied mainly on women to do informal caring. Tracing the historical emergence of social and policy concern for carers in detail is not our task here but it is useful for current purposes to note the relationships between informal caring, changing patterns of employment, an ageing population, the deinstitutionalization of people with long term conditions and the reduced mortality of people with particular health problems. These macro social issues impact on the ways in which we think about caring and this has practical ramifications for the services that carers receive. Practitioners may be tempted to skip this discussion but we argue that it is this taken-for-granted thinking that provides an interpretive background for practice that can get in the way of enabling effective carer support.

Twigg and Atkin (1994: p. 2) and Stalker (2003) provide interesting analyses of scholarly interest in carers. The former note how an important debate has been that of our understanding of 'kinship obligation' – that is, in this case, who we as a society regard it as normal and natural to take responsibility for caring for. There has been academic interest in unpacking these assumptions about relationships within real life settings, and the idea that contemporary families do not provide care has been definitively challenged. Chamberlayne and King (2000) argue that these assumptions are culturally produced rather than arising as a consequence of welfare provision. Feminists challenged these assumptions about the family. Their work, by the 1980s, allowed a more complex understanding of caring relationships to emerge (Twigg & Atkin, 1994). For example, empirical data allowed the relationships between gender and caring to be more closely examined. Another important theme of scholarly work has concerned carer burden and this has illuminated the sometimes tough, unremitting work that caring involves. Howard (2001) argues that caring can result in social exclusion through poverty and restricted access to resources connected to social status and to poorer health. These issues have been politicized through organizations that lobby on the carers' behalf, for example Carers UK. The literature regarding the feminist analysis and that concerning the burden of care shares the observation that carers are often regarded non-problematically as resources by policy-makers and formal care providers.

More recently, disabled people have lobbied for the idea that disability is a socially constructed phenomenon and this has had implications for the debates concerning informal caring (Stalker, 2003). The 'cared for' have argued for the right to employ their own carers and for an awareness that there is interdependence and mutual benefit between the different parties involved (Stalker, 2003). Stalker notes too how these relationships have their own history and interpersonal features and that together these have an enormous influence on intersubjective experiences.

Twigg and Atkin (1994) discuss the pros and cons of categorizing carers in a generic fashion and they point out that whilst carers hold much in common, there are important differences too. Eley (2003) comments that we have failed to fully appreciate the diversity of carers, including how some people are carers more than once and for more than one person at a time. She sets out the different categories that have been examined, for example ethnicity and household type, but shows how limited our understanding of diversity is overall. Moreover, she draws attention to the issue of stigma, noting how carers of persons with stigmatized conditions may be stigmatized in turn: a phenomenon Goffman (1963) referred to as *courtesy* stigma.

We argued above that our mundane, unexamined perceptions of carers provide an interpretive backcloth for practice. To summarize, we may make assumptions about the 'rightness' of who is doing the caring and exactly what kind of work that might involve; we may fail to see the complex present and future consequences for a person undertaking the caring role; we may assume that the 'cared for' want to be engaged in this relationship and that there is little reciprocity in the arrangement; and we may fail to understand the impact of the features of the unique relationship in front of us. The following case study illustrates some of these matters.

Case study 1

One woman in her late fifties who cared for her elderly mother, who had dementia, contacted emergency services when her mother continually kept the family up all night running baths, leaving electrical appliances on and shouting that her grandson was an intruder trying to molest her. Furthermore the elderly mother was also refusing to take food or fluids, insisting that someone was trying to poison her, thus rapidly becoming dehydrated. When the ambulance service arrived, the carer herself had such a haggard appearance that the ambulance service thought that she was the patient until her family intervened. The carer had been unable to secure any support from health and social care providers, not even respite care, despite having cared for her elderly mother since the death of her father four years previously. On consulting her mother's GP, she had been told that she should be able to manage as her mother would not be alive for very long and that she would not like her mother to die alone in hospital.

There are two cross-cutting social categories that are considered when we define caring as either routinely normal or as remarkable: the type of relationship between the carer and the cared for (assuming that this is always straightforward) and the degree of caring activity involved. Within this overall scheme, the point at which we conceptualize caring as either ordinary or extraordinary is contingent reflexively on both cultural and personal mores.

The consequences of this discussion about kinship obligations for practice development are outlined below but now we turn to the bigger picture of policy and what is known about the informal carers of people with a long term condition as a population group.

The bigger picture

The NHS is currently considered to be in financial crisis (Royal College of Nursing, 2007) but it has been argued that it would have slipped into financial meltdown long ago if it were not for the 6.8 million adults who act as carers for family, friends and neighbours who would otherwise, temporarily or permanently, be unable to care for themselves. According to Andersen et al. (2007), 2 million referrals to Councils with Responsibility for Social Services were made in 2005/6 for people with newly identified needs, with a further 1.2 million reviews of existing social services clients, but there are an estimated 34 million people living with long term health problems. A quarter of those with long term health problems will have three or more concomitant conditions and that figure rises to almost 70% of people with concomitant long term conditions in those aged 65 years or more (Department of Health (DOH), 2004). These statistics indicate that the potential pool of those requiring some degree of informal care is vast and that those with long term conditions who are self-caring represent a large proportion of the population, with the less affluent population being most greatly disadvantaged (Wanless, 2004). Those experiencing multiple and complex health problems are much more likely than the general populace to require formal or informal care at some point in their lives. The greater the number of long term conditions simultaneously experienced, the greater the potential requirement for formal health and social care contact, GP consultations and hospital admission, with hospital inpatient stays being of a longer duration for this group (DOH, 2004: p. 15).

The management of people with long term conditions is central to current health policy and focuses on obtaining a reduction in the number of hospital bed days associated with acute admissions (DOH, 2006a). Subsequently, even greater demands will be placed on health and social services and, importantly, on patients and informal carers. The latter save the UK economy an estimated £57 billion each year, which, as Carers UK (2002) point out, was roughly the same as the annual cost of the whole NHS at that time. The assertion that carers 'save' us a large amount of national spending rests on the fragile territory of kinship obligations, that is, if we were certain that it was morally right for people to 'look after their own' then this claim would not arise.

As the government have acknowledged, older people (who are most likely to experience long term conditions) have often been discriminated against with organizational barriers put in place to prevent them accessing services that would enable greater independence for a longer duration (DOH, 2001a). Howard (2001) suggested that access to health and social care services remained a lottery despite the Carer's Act 1995 and government acknowledgement that carers should be valued as a resource and treated as collaborative partners by professionals (DOH, 2001b). Howard's suggestion is clearly rooted in reality given that the government have passed further legislation in the form of the Carer's (Equal Opportunities) Act 2004, which came into force in April 2005. This Act places a duty on Councils with Responsibility for Social Services to inform carers of their right to an assessment, and to ensure that any assessment undertaken takes into consideration the carer's rights to work, education and leisure time and also that any other authorities requested to support the carer (such as housing and education) should take that request into due consideration. However, in the 'real world' of caring, policy is often not synonymous with practice and despite legislation, carers continue to experience barriers to obtaining the support that they require when it is most needed.

Many informal carers are not paid for their caring work; others are in receipt of benefits associated with caring such as the 'carer's allowance'. Keeley and Clarke

(2002, 2003) note that 1.7 million people are the sole carers of those in need, each providing at least 20 hours of care per week; with more than 1 million giving more than 50 hours of their time each week. These figures relate to adults and do not take into account the number of children playing a role in caring for family members, some of whom are sole carers and may well be invisible to health and social care service providers (see Chapter 7).

Although a number of large-scale studies have been conducted to collect data on carers and their experiences, it was only recently that the topic was considered to be of sufficient significance to merit inclusion in the national census. The national census is used to survey the UK population once every ten years. The census collects a range of socioeconomic data but, although established in 1801, it was not until 2001 that a question was included to identify the prevalence of informal carers and the amount of time that they spent each week on caring activities (Office for National Statistics, 2007). The 2001 findings indicate that 6 million people are carers: just under a million less than the number projected from the findings of the 2000/1 general household survey (GHS). This discrepancy is not surprising as, compared with the census, which includes all addresses, the 2000/1 GHS sample comprised 12 393 eligible addresses, resulting in 8221 interviews (Maher & Green, 2002) and there is bound to be a margin of error when extrapolating findings to the population as a whole. However, demographic monitoring via the GHS indicates that the prevalence of (adult) informal carers remained more or less constant in the decade preceding the 2000/1 survey (Maher & Green, 2002). This is likely to change as the proportion of people over the age of 75 is anticipated to increase by 3 million over the next 30 years and this will necessitate a simultaneous increase in informal carer support (George, 2001).

Action Learning Point

- Do the GPs with whom you have professional contact keep a register of carers as advocated by the General Medical Services contract (British Medical Assocation/NHS Employers, 2006)?
- How are patients and their carers referred for formal assessment as determined by the Health and Social Care Act 2001?
- Where is the nearest local Carers' Centre and how do patients and their carers find out about the service or access it?

The GHS was first implemented in 1971 and, with two exceptions, it has been administered every five years (Office for National Statistics, 2007). Since 2000, the GHS has comprised two elements: a continuous survey and trailers. One of the 2000/1 trailers focused on informal carers and the resulting publication *Carers 2000* (Maher & Green, 2002) presents a comprehensive range of sociodemographic information. This is particularly useful for policy-makers but less so for practitioners because, as discussed above, carers are not a homogeneous group and cannot be treated as such in practice.

The 2001 census question, which elicited statistics on the number of carers and the time spent caring, was not formulated to distinguish between carers who share a home with their dependent and those who provide care elsewhere. Conversely, the GHS was designed to collect information on not only the prevalence of carers and the site of caring, but a wide range of other issues related to the caring experience. The GHS collected data on all carers in the households sampled but, where caring was an activity shared by more than one person, the questions focused on the main carer (the person self-identified as providing the most care). Likewise, where there was more than one person in receipt of care in the household, questions centred on the person who was most dependent.

In the Office for National Statistics' 'Focus on health' series, Wheller (2006) provides a useful summary of available data on carers and their dependents. He highlights that the 2000/1 GHS revealed the provision of practical help as the dominant form of caring, although monitoring the person's well-being and care aimed at promoting social interaction (for example, keeping the person company or taking them out) also scored highly. Help with personal care and physical activities appeared less frequently when care was provided for someone in another household. In this situation, the main care recipients were parents (46%). Friends or neighbours (29%) were the second most common group to receive care from someone outside their household, closely followed by other relatives (27%).

Where care was carried out in the same household, 55% were providing care for their spouse or partner, 27% for a parent or parent-in-law, and 20% for a child. The provision of help with personal hygiene and physical care (for example, assisting with mobility) featured highly in the range of caring activities (Maher & Green, 2002). Unsurprisingly, caring input was much higher when carers and dependents shared a home. In terms of weekly commitment to caring activities, 32% spent 20–49 hours per week and 31% spent over 50 hours, compared with 9% and 1%, respectively, for carers who looked after someone in a different household (Maher & Green, 2002).

The risks of caring

The self-reports of ill health amongst informal carers increase according to the number of hours spent caring (Dahlberg et al., 2007). The 2000/1 GHS found that 61% of carers providing 20–49 hours of care and 72% of those providing 50 hours or more reported that their health had been affected by caring. Furthermore, ill health was more frequently reported by carers who shared a home with the looked after person (59% compared with 29% of those who provided care elsewhere). In this group, 51% had suffered a physical injury as a direct result of performing a physical care activity (DOH, 1999a). However, injuries (physical and psychological) are sometimes sustained as a result of aggression by the care recipient (Ayres & Woodtli, 2001; Princess Royal Trust for Carers, 2004). This may be due to mental health difficulties or a poor relationship between the carer and the looked after person. Despite this, carers do not meet the Department of Health (2000) definition of a 'vulnerable person' – a category that brings protection entitlements. This is problematic, especially for older people who comprise the main carer population, because the act of caring may itself render carers vulnerable to abuse and this needs to be further investigated if government policies on carer support are to be successful.

Although there is a growing body of literature on the health of carers (for example, see Carers UK, 2004; Hare, 2004; Hirst, 2004), comparatively little is written from the perspective of the person cared for. McCann and Evans (2002) conducted interviews with 55 older people who were recipients of informal care, to ascertain their views on their experiences of being looked after. Whilst the vast majority were highly satisfied with the care that they received, over half of the respondents expressed concerns about the health of their carer and what might happen to them if the carer was not there. They were sensitive to the potential fragility of the arrangements they encountered. Respondents were asked whether their carer had ever been violent, angry or frustrated with them. The majority denied that they had been abused in any way but over a third reported that their carers sometimes got angry: one in ten had been shouted at, nine reported that their carer had lost their temper and one stated that they had been slapped or hit. These findings support those of previous studies (Ogg and Bennett, 1992; Action on Elder Abuse, 2000), which highlight 'carer stress' as a risk factor in elder abuse. Physical violence by carers may be under-reported due to a number of factors but self-reported feelings of frustration and anger on the part of the carer are not uncommon and may often be accompanied by guilt (Brewin, 2004; Princess Royal Trust for Carers, 2004). However, it is important to remember that such feelings do not necessarily result in abuse: on the contrary, the vast majority of carers provide high quality care for their dependents (McCann & Evans 2002) and commonly find satisfaction in their caring relationships (Carers UK, 2007b; DOH, 1999a). Brechin et al. (2003) found that carers had good and bad times and they argue that polarizing carers as either 'good' or 'bad' risks ignoring the complexity of their experiences of caring.

In relation to carer characteristics, the 2000/1 GHS findings generally mirror those of the 2001 census. Both surveys found that the majority of carers for people under the age of 65 years are women, whereas the reverse is true in relation to those caring for people aged 65 plus. It is postulated that the reason for the slightly greater number of male carers for the over 65s is that very elderly women are more likely to be in need of carer support (so, for example, a son may take on the caring role for his aged mother) and, when both sexes are of a comparable age, women are more inclined to suffer a disability (Maher & Green, 2002). Where the care recipient has a high level of disability, care is more likely to be provided by a carer sharing the same household (Wheller, 2006).

Just as the population of those with long term conditions is ageing, so are their informal carers. This does not auger well for the future of lay care for two key reasons. Firstly, unless there is a rapid rise in the birth rate, there will not be a new population of informal carers to replace existing carers as time progresses. Secondly, the greater number of hours that are spent in providing informal care, the less likelihood there is of being able to hold down a full-time job, thus the greater the potential for people acting in a caring role to claim benefits rather than contributing to the economy. Keeley and Clarke (2002) found that only 21% of the 2800 carers they surveyed were in employment, with only 7% of those being in full-time employment; 68% of those surveyed were under 65 years of age. Unemployment may ultimately lead to poverty, social exclusion and a greater potential for health problems in the lay care population.

It is important to consider gender issues in relation to the context of care provision. The GHS findings reveal that most carers (approximately two-thirds) look after someone who is not living with them. Furthermore, 60% of these carers are female; in the main, they are women who are either married or cohabiting and 28% have dependent children. For those providing care in the same household, gender differences are less marked (54% of women carers compared to 46% of men) (Maher & Green, 2002).

The GHS data fail to distinguish between the gender of the carer and the nature of the caring tasks performed. However, it has been found that where household chores are part of caring activities, men appear to be more inclined than female carers to accept help (Parker, 1993). Additionally, Twigg and Atkin (1994) suggest that male carers are less willing to perform intimate care for a female dependent. These differences may result from gender socialization or, in the latter case, arise from a fear of being vulnerable to accusations of sexual abuse. It is essential to remember that carers are individuals and stereotyping on grounds of gender creates the potential for numerous problems. However, it would appear that the role of the carer lies predominantly with women. Carmichael and Charles (2003) suggest that life expectancy and tradition are not the only reasons for this. They argue that the whole wage-earning and job market infrastructure is so organized that paid male job roles are less likely to offer part-time positions or flexible working practices that take into consideration the potential impact of being a carer; whereas the female job market has traditionally been structured to encourage part-time labour opportunities and consequently lower wage-earning capacity. Thus for men to become sole carers, their likelihood of being able to simultaneously earn and care is much lower than that for women unless their caring hours are very limited. Additionally, as women live longer than men, despite the current disparity in retirement age, men in the older population are also more likely to have been accruing a pension. Abandoning paid work results in the loss of pension income.

Cultural mores may also play a part in gender roles but, again, care must be taken not to make generalizations. Katbamna et al. (2004) investigated informal caring amongst South Asian families in the UK. They describe how touch is prohibited between adult family members who are not married. They explain that a woman providing intimate care for her husband cannot rely on help from her female relatives as they would be prohibited from contributing caring activities other than those of a non-physical nature. Furthermore, assistance from male relatives was found to be unreliable, thus resulting in an overall lack of support. Contrary to this, male carers with a female dependent received greater support from female relatives, who tended to take on both intimate and household tasks. The role of female relatives diminished only in situations where a male carer had responsibility for a dependent of the same sex. In this instance, intimate care activities were shared with other male relatives.

Hence, in South Asian families, caring roles are largely dictated by the gender of the looked after person and Katbamna et al. (2004: p. 404) assert that their findings:

'challenge the pervasive assumption and stereotype that South Asian people live in self-supporting extended families, and therefore, that the support of the social services is largely unnecessary.'

Moreover they point out that obtaining statutory services may be particularly difficult for South Asian women due to language and communication difficulties: an issue that also holds true for many people from other minority ethnic groups (Carers UK, 1998; Arksey et al., 2003; Arksey & Hirst, 2005).

Caring for the carers

In 2006, the Department of Health in the White Paper *Our Health, Our Care, Our Say* (DOH, 2006b) revealed its plan to review the 1999 National Strategy for Carers. With the intention of informing government policy, Carers UK conducted a survey of carers to ascertain their priorities. Analysis of nearly 3000 responses identified 'recognition by professionals' as the main priority (Carers UK, 2007b: p. 1). The vast majority of respondents in this survey provided over 50 hours of care per week and therefore are not representative of carers as a whole. None the less, it draws attention to the plight of those providing the most intensive caring input and given that this group suffer the poorest health (Maher & Green, 2002), merits urgent attention.

The 2007 Carers UK report provides only minimal information on the methods used in its survey and insufficient detail to determine the finer characteristics of its sample, so it is a matter of conjecture whether carers from black and minority ethnic groups were adequately represented. At present, the relatively small proportion of older people who belong to a minority ethnic group are likely to have come to Britain in the 1950s and 1960s as young adults (Murray & Brown, 1998). As with dependent people from the indigenous population, care is most likely to be provided by relatives and these carers are among those providing the largest amount of care (Wheller, 2006).

Drawing on government surveys highlights findings that classify carers into the following ethnic groups: 'white', 'mixed (race)', 'Asian', 'black' and 'Chinese and other'. In all black and minority ethnic groups there were more female than male carers. Approximately 20% of these carers provided high intensity care (defined as 50 hours or more per week). Across all groups, more women than men were acting as the main carers. This difference was particularly marked in the Asian population as almost 30% of female carers, compared to 18% of male carers, were providing high intensity care. These findings add substance to the work of Katbamna et al. (2004) who found that South Asian women were not only the main carers but were often isolated in terms of support from other family members.

The dependents of the majority of carers receive no health or social care services (DOH, 1999a). This may be because they are not known to the services or they require no external help. Additionally, they may be reluctant to accept formal care, preferring to rely on relatives and friends or, as Case study 2 illustrates, be unable to effectively articulate their situation.

Case study 2

Rani has cared for her husband, Amir, for the past 18 months since he suffered a stroke that left him with a right hemiparesis. They have a married daughter who lives many miles away and they share their home with their son and pregnant daughter-in-law who both work full time. Rani's daughter-in-law does the shopping and helps clean the house; her son gets his father up in the mornings and puts him to bed. Rani spends most of the day alone with her husband. In addition to cooking and cleaning for her family, Rani helps her husband to eat and takes care of his personal hygiene needs. Although only 65 years old, Rani is a frail lady and she recently sustained a back injury when trying to reposition her husband in bed. She was given pain killers by her English GP who, being aware of Amir's ill health, enquired how she was coping. Unfortunately, due to her poor mastery of spoken English, Rani was unable to effectively express her needs. As a consequence, the situation continued, leaving Rani vulnerable to ill health.

Carers may request an assessment under the Carers and Disabled Children Act 2000 but this relies on knowing their rights and, again, an ability to effectively communicate with health and social care workers. It should also be noted that even if an assessment has been undertaken and needs are identified, no services can be forced on the person cared for (DOH, 2006a) and so the burden of care may not be alleviated.

Pickard and Glendinning (2002) assert that, despite a range of policies to support carers, the intended results are not always being achieved. In 1998, Arber et al. found that health and social care workers were more sympathetic and more responsive to the needs of male carers. A more recent study by Bywaters and Harris (2001) suggests that, to some extent, this situation remains as they found that care managers had higher expectations in terms of caring contributions when the carer was female. Furthermore, gender differences were apparent also in the use of respite and day care services as there is a greater uptake by the dependents of male carers. However, when considering gender issues in caring, it is important to remember that, for some, gender boundaries are becoming more blurred and previous findings may not hold true in contemporary society.

Having examined some of the data available about carers as a group, we now turn to the highly skilled and complex work of caring and some of its ramifications for the carer's own life.

What do carers do?

Twigg and Atkin (1994) identified how caring can fall into several categories including work requiring immediate attention and that which can be deferred. The former includes activities such as toileting, dressing, nursing and personal care whilst the latter includes shopping and housekeeping (although clearly these can only be delayed temporarily). Attending and financial support are equally important elements of caring for someone with a long term condition. For example, in practice, it has been observed that some patients who experience dyspnoea as a result of chronic obstructive pulmonary disease will complain of exacerbation when their usual carer leaves the house to shop, visit friends or engage in other leisure pursuits. Contact with emergency services may be instigated at such times. Health care professionals and carers may regard this as a form of 'attention seeking' but in reality, as Bailey (2004) reports, there is an inextricable link between anxiety and breathlessness that is not fully understood. Thus just being physically and psychologically present is an important aspect of care provision and this can be emotionally draining. Goldstein et al. (2000), in their research of carers looking after people with motor neurone disease, demonstrated how the impact of caring for someone on an informal basis is much greater when they feel less able to control the situation and have no additional network of informal or formal support mechanisms to fall back on. In some ways this mirrors the impact of having a long term condition, in that the more control a person has over their lives, the greater their ability to cope with and make sense of what is happening to them. That control for patients may take the form of self-managing medication, being able to engage in the normal activities of daily living, or relating to activities outside of the sphere of their illness and its associated links. Carers who have additional support that they may if necessary call upon, confidence in the care and management that they can provide for the person being cared for, and engagement in activities or pursuits beyond their role as carer may well fare much better in terms of quality of their own lives.

We have shown that carers are not a homogeneous group and nor is the detail of their caring work. We should beware of making ill-informed judgements about the kinds of work and its local context, especially in relation to how we perceive the level of associated burden. For example, the carer of a person with schizophrenia could give the superficial impression of doing very little because the care recipient is able to care for himself physically. However, closer investigation could reveal that the carer is exhausted and low in mood following sleepless nights caused by constant talking and reassurance giving. Moreover, there may well be more than the carer/care recipient relationship to consider. A carer, for example, may also be a victim of domestic abuse from another party within the household.

As discussed above, a negative consequence of caring is financial insecurity and poverty. Carers Northern Ireland (2007) reports how many carers miss out on holidays, are unable to pay utility bills, can not afford essential home repairs and even cut back on food purchase and consumption. Howard (2001: p. 124) argues that many carers live 'on the breadline' and she discusses the social and financial impact of transitions in caring. For example, those no longer required to care may find it difficult to get back into the job market and those whose caring work is interrupted may fall foul of an inflexible welfare benefit system. Moreover, whilst many carers are unable to secure employment due to their caring duties, unlike in the general population, there is no recognized retirement age as they continue to care until the person that they care for is taken into formal care or dies or until the carers themselves become too ill to care. Carers UK (2007a: p. 34) argues that carers experience 'multilayered disadvantage'.

Action Learning Point

- If you have formal or informal contact with carers (possibly family or friends), discuss with them how caring affects their lives both in a positive and negative context. If your contact is on a professional level, you could conduct an audit of the levels of support that your identified group of carers are aware of, have access to, or would most want if available.
- Is there any mechanism that you, as a practitioner, are able to put in place to support them?
- What are the barriers to implementation?

We have painted a bleak picture and a lot of the literature about informal caring is of the 'ain't it awful' genre, yet as a society we consider it normal and natural to care for our kin. Indeed most of us would probably prefer to be cared for by our loved ones, rather than within or from a faceless organization (Parker, 1998). Hollinghurst (1998: p. 36) refers to 'a tangled web of emotions . . . love, fear, resentment, guilt' as she narrates her experience of caring for her mother. This is a useful insight into the lived experience of caring and it teaches us that we should avoid making assumptions that situations are all good or all bad, all wanted or all resented, always tender and loving or always vicious and abusive. It may, in reality, be all or none of these things and we now move on to discuss some potential solutions to the problems identified.

Potential solutions

Campaigns by carer organizations, research and recent government legislation should, in theory, be improving the prospects for carers in relation to the difficulties outlined above. Indeed the latest report from Carers UK (2007a) shows some small but positive indications that financial hardship amongst carers has reduced since 2000. This report concentrates its fire predominantly on financial issues, analysing the practices involved in the welfare benefit system and proposing solutions in this light. The report's publication may be timely given the current government's pledge 'to listen'.

The advent of Carers' Centres supported by the Princess Royal Trust has enabled direct access to practical support by carers regardless of the nature of those being cared for. Additionally, GPs are being encouraged by the Princess Royal Trust to keep a register of carers for various purposes, such as targeting those carers who are most likely to require support because of the intensive nature of their caring role, signposting carers to resources that would best support them, or initiating an assessment of their needs, as advocated by the national carers' strategy (DOH, 1999a), and legal rights (as discussed above). Where carers are registered with the same GP as those that they care for, this makes administration of this system much easier for health care professionals to handle. However, often this may not be the case and collaboration between primary care service providers may be necessary for the system to operate more effectively. Identifying carers is a primary concern in establishing a network of support for those providing informal care in the community.

Communication between all members of the primary health care team as well as referrals from secondary care may provide the information necessary to set up the register of carers, although the register will be a 'live' document given that its detail will change frequently. Policy-makers have added an incentive for such registers to be developed: GPs now have a vested interest in establishing a register of carers given that this activity attracts three quality points under the practice management domain of the General Medical Services contract (British Medical Association/NHS Employers, 2006). This is an important and strategic addition to the contract and raises the profile of carers within the domain of general practice and primary care. One outcome of identifying carers is that the practice may be able to better take their needs into consideration, such as organizing appointments to fit in with the caring schedule, arranging fast track prescriptions and alerting out of hours services to the specific problems that the carer and the person being cared for may experience, thus expediting responses from those services. A further aspect of the same practice management domain, within the context of points acquisition in the Quality Outcomes Framework, is that practices should have a mechanism of referral for social services assessment. This may be by direct referral to social services or via referral to a Carers' Centre. In making those referrals, carers will potentially benefit from access to advocacy services, benefits advice and have a greater probability of support from carer organizations or specialist health professionals with interest in specific long term conditions. The latter may range from access to Sapphire Nurses providing support for those with epilepsy, to encouragement to become a member of the Parkinson's Disease Society. Engagement with such resources may help carers to better understand the issues of import to themselves and those they care for and enable a range of coping strategies by drawing upon the experiences of others in similar situations. These support mechanisms are also possible outcomes of referral to Expert Patient Programmes (DOH, 2001c) although, in practice, some carers and people with long term conditions state that attendance at Expert Patient events is difficult for those who are non-ambulatory or have a range of long term conditions that restrict their mobility. Wilson (2001) argues that Expert Patient initiatives are a means of taking responsibility away from the state for those who require care resources by putting the onus on individuals to take responsibility for their own care. She also argues that these initiatives do not challenge the professional perception of those with chronic health problems, whereas health professionals may contest this notion and consider such initiatives as a means of patient empowerment (see Chapter 3).

The development of active case manager and community matron roles in the care of people with complex long term conditions includes responsibility for the co-ordination of carer support. However, the onus is on all health and social care practitioners to be alert to cues from carers and those being cared for. As one male carer commented in Keeley and Clarke (2003) *Primary Carers – Identifying and providing support to carers in primary care*, he just felt like the person who opened the door to let in health care professionals visiting his mother. Clearly, acknowledging that someone performs a valuable caring role can make a huge difference to that individual regardless of any practical support that may be offered, and paying this essential respect is the cornerstone of person-centred initiatives. Keeley and Clarke (2003) have also provided a range of practical recommendations for those working in primary care (particularly in general practice) on how to support carers and Carers' Centres are charged with making that practical support a reality.

Our discussion so far has indicated a number of important matters that will require assessment and subsequent action by practitioners. Methods for systematically and accountably assessing carers' needs have been published (see, for example, Nolan et al., 1998) and care organizations have devised their own carer assessment tools. These will differ in their fine detail and in their relationships to other relevant policies. For example, within secondary mental health services, carer assessment tools will be integrated through the care programme approach (DOH, 1999b) and where appropriate, with section 117 of the Mental Health Act 1983. However, they are likely to share much in common too.

Whatever specific tool a practitioner is organizationally equipped with, there will remain a relationship between their enthusiasm and sensitivity in conducting a carer assessment and the resources available to meet the needs established through the process. Consequently, practitioners need a confident grasp on what is available and on how to go about enabling carers to get it. This is undoubtedly a challenge because what specific services (particularly those with fragile incomes) can and cannot offer may frequently change. The development of a network of Carers' Centres promises to ease these difficulties of having accessible, local and up-to-date information.

At the level of individual practice, establishing and attending to the needs of a carer requires an advanced level of interpersonal communication skills throughout the course of professional involvement. Caring is a dynamic, complex process that takes place in an equally complex social context and nobody understands this better than the carer themselves. What a carer needs today may be very different from what they need tomorrow and sensitivity to this changing landscape is essential. This potential level of complexity can lead to the oft-heard proverbial practitioner's fear of 'opening a can of worms'. This fear can be solved by engaging in a person-centred problem-solving partnership and by respecting that carers well know that there are no magical solutions to the 'tangled web' (Hollinghurst, 1998) of their caring world. A useful way into this type of therapeutic engagement is to ask focusing questions. For example:

- Is there anything that you find rewarding about your caring role?
- What are you struggling with the most at the moment?
- What kind of help would be most useful to you?
- What would be the smallest thing that would make a difference to how you are feeling?

An important consideration when working this way is to consider the therapeutic context. For example, it might be very hard for a particular carer to 'think straight' or to talk freely when the person they are caring for is present. Alternatively, they might have an extremely intimate relationship and want to take the opportunity to review things together.

This interpersonal strategy may well open up challenges to the professional and organizational network, be at odds with current policy drivers and upset the care recipient. The carer may say that they no longer want to care or that they need regular respite. Problems can only be systematically solved when we know what they are, and getting to grips with solving specific difficulties is the only way to enable a carer to be effectively supported. Practitioners need to be willing to act as advocates and sometimes this may place them at odds with their managers and policy-makers. This takes moral courage, determination and tenacity; the hallmarks of the best health and social care practitioners.

In conclusion, if we are to 'value our assets' we should form respectful, collaborative relationships with carers and be bold in attending to their unique strengths and difficulties. Practitioners need to reflect on their own perceptions of kinship obligations and learn to deliberately put these to one side when collaborating with carers, lest they make unhelpful assumptions about what they require. The priority is to focus on the carer and to do this with the full understanding that their caring work is but one part of a whole life.

References

Action on Elder Abuse (2000) *Listening is Not Enough. An analysis of calls to Elder Abuse Response – Action on Elder Abuse's national helpline.* London, Action on Elder Abuse.

Andersen, K., Sylvester, K., Archer, S. & Alamdri, A. (eds) (2007) *Community Care Statistics 2005–06: Referrals, assessments and packages of care for adults, England.* London, Information Centre, Government Statistical Service.

Arber, S., Gilbert, N. & Evandrous, M. (1998) Gender, household composition and receipt of domiciliary services by elderly disabled people. *Journal of Social Policy* **17** (2): 153–175.

Arksey, H. & Hirst, M. (2005) Unpaid carers' access to and use of primary care services. *Primary Health Care Research and Development* **6** (2): 1011–1016.

Arksey, H., Jackson, K., Wallace, A., Baldwin, S., Goldner, S., Newbronner, E. & Hare, P. (2003) *Access to Health Care for Carers: Barriers and interventions.* London, National Co-ordinating Centre for NHS Service Delivery and Organisation.

Ayres, M. & Woodtli, A. (2001) Concept analysis: abuse of ageing caregivers by elderly care recipients. *Journal of Advanced Nursing* **35** (3): 326–334.

Bailey, P.H. (2004) The dyspnea–anxiety–dyspnea cycle – COPD patients' stories of breathlessness: 'it's scary when you can't breathe'. *Qualitative Health Research* **14** (6): 760–778.

Brechin, A., Barton, R. & Stein, J. (2003) Getting to grips with poor care. In: K. Stalker, (ed.) *Reconceptualising Work with 'Carers'. New directions in policy and practice.* Research Highlights in Social Work No. 43. London, Jessica Kingsley Publishers.

Brewin, A. (2004) The quality of life of carers of patients with severe lung disease. *British Journal of Nursing* **13** (15): 906–912.

British Medical Association/NHS Employers (2006) *Revisions to the GMS Contract 2006/07: Delivering investment to general practice.* London, British Medical Association/NHS Employers.

Bywaters, P. & Harris, A. (2001) Supporting carers: is practice still sexist? *Health and Social Care in the Community* **6** (6): 458–463.

Carers Northern Ireland (2007) Paying the Price: Caring on the breadline. http://www.carersni.org/Newsandcampaigns/Fairdeal/Payingtheprice [accessed 19 April 2007].

Carers UK (1998) Policy Briefing: Black and minority ethnic carers. http://www.carersuk.org/Policyandpractice/PolicyResources/Policybriefings/blackminethniccarers.pdf [accessed 19 April 2007].

Carers UK (2002) *Without Us . . . ? Calculating the value of carers' support.* London, Carers UK.

Carers UK (2004) *In Poor Health. The impact of caring on health.* London, Carers UK.

Carers UK (2007a) *Real Change not Short Change. Time to deliver for carers.* London, Carers UK.

Carers UK (2007b) *Our Health, Our Care, Our Say for our Caring Future. Carers' priorities for a new National Strategy for Carers.* London, Carers UK.

Carmichael, F. & Charles, S. (2003) The opportunity costs of informal care: does gender matter? *Journal of Health Economics* **22**: 781–803.

Chamberlayne, P. & King, A. (2000) *Cultures of Care. Biographies of carers in Britain and the two Germanies.* Bristol, Policy Press.

Dahlberg, L., Demack, S. & Bambra, C. (2007) Age and gender of informal carers: a population-based study in the UK. *Health and Social Care in the Community* **15** (5): 439–445. http://www.blackwell-synergy.com/toc/hsc/0/0 [accessed 19 April 2007].

Department of Health (1999a) *National Strategy for Carers.* London, Department of Health.

Department of Health (1999b) *Effective Care Co-ordination.* London, Department of Health.

Department of Health (2000) *No Secrets: Guidance on developing and implementing multiagency policies and procedures to protect vulnerable adults from abuse.* London, Department of Health.

Department of Health (2001a) *National Service Framework for Older People: Modern standards and service models.* London, Department of Health.

Department of Health (2001b) *Valuing People: A new strategy for learning disability in the 21st century.* London, Department of Health.

Department of Health (2001c) *The Expert Patient: A new approach to chronic disease management for the 21st century.* London, Department of Health.

Department of Health (2004) *Chronic Disease Management: A compendium of information.* London, Department of Health.

Department of Health (2006a) Caring about Carers: Frequently asked questions. http://www.carers.gov.uk/elearningfaqs.htm [accessed 19 April 2007].

Department of Health (2006b) *Our Health, Our Care, Our Say: Investing in the future of community hospitals and services.* London, Department of Health.

Eley, S. (2003) Diversity among carers. In: K. Stalker (ed.) *Reconceptualising Work with 'Carers'. New directions in policy and practice*. Research Highlights in Social Work No. 43. London, Jessica Kingsley Publishers.

George, M. (2001) *It Could Be You: A report on the chances of becoming a carer*. London, Carers UK.

Goffman, E. (1963) *Stigma. Notes on the management of spoiled identity*. London, Penguin Books.

Goldstein, L.H., Adamson, M., Barby, T., Down, K. & Leigh, P.N. (2000) Attributions, strain and depression in carers of partners with MND: a preliminary investigation. *Journal of the Neurological Sciences* **180**: 101–106.

Hare, P. (2004) Keeping carers healthy: the role of community nurses and colleagues. *British Journal of Community Nursing* **9** (4): 155–159.

Hirst, M. (2004) *Hearts and Minds: The health effects of caring*. York, University of York Social Policy Research Unit.

Hollinghurst, V. (1998) A 'tangled web' of emotions. In: M. Allott & M. Robb (eds) *Understanding Health and Social Care. An introductory reader*. London, Open University Press.

Howard, M. (2001) *Paying the Price: Carers, poverty and social exclusion*. London, Child Poverty Action Group and Carers UK.

Katbamna, S., Ahmed, W., Bhakta, P., Baker, R. & Parker, G. (2004) Do they look after their own? Informal support for South Asian carers. *Health and Social Care in the Community* **12** (5): 398–406.

Keeley, B. & Clarke, M. (2002) *Carers Speak Out. Project report on findings and recommendations*. London, Princess Royal Trust.

Keeley, B. & Clarke, M. (2003) *Primary Carers – Identifying and providing support to carers in primary care*. London, Princess Royal Trust.

Maher, J. & Green, H. (2002) *Carers 2000*. London, HMSO.

McCann, S. & Evans, D. (2002) Informal care: the views of people receiving care. *Health and Social Care in the Community* **10** (4): 221–228.

Murray, U., & Brown, D. (1998) *Great Britain. They look after their own, don't they? Inspection of community care services for black and ethnic minority older people*. London, Department of Health Social Services Inspectorate.

Nolan, M., Grant, G. & Keady, J. (1998) *Assessing the Needs of Family Carers. A guide for practitioners*. Brighton, Pavillion Publishing.

Office for National Statistics (2007) General Household Survey. Social Survey Division of the Office for National Statistics. http://www.statistics.gov.uk/ssd/surveys/general_household_survey.asp [accessed 12 April 2007].

Ogg, J. & Bennett, G. (1992) Elder abuse: a national survey. *British Medical Journal* **305**: 998–999.

Parker, G. (1993) *With this Body: Caring and disability in marriage*. Buckingham, Open University Press.

Parker, R.A. (1998) The persistent image. In: M. Allott & M. Robb (eds) *Understanding Health and Social Care. An introductory reader*. London, Open University Press.

Pickard, S. & Glendinning, C. (2002) Comparing and contrasting the role of family carers and nurses in the domestic health care of frail older people. *Health and Social Care in the Community* **10** (3): 144–150.

Princess Royal Trust for Carers (2004) *Carers Health Survey: Main findings*. London, Princess Royal Trust for Carers http://www.carers.org/data/files/carershealthsurvey-12.pdf [accessed 12 April 2007].

Royal College of Nursing (2007) *Our NHS – Today and Tomorrow: A Royal College of Nursing commentary on the current state of the National Health Service and the steps needed to secure its future*. London, Royal College of Nursing.

Stalker, K. (2003) (ed.) *Reconceptualising Work with 'Carers'. New directions in policy and practice*. Research Highlights in Social Work No. 43. London, Jessica Kingsley Publishers.

Twigg, J. & Atkin, K. (1994) *Carers Perceived: Policy and practice in informal care*. Buckingham, Open University Press.

Wanless, D. (2004) *Securing Good Health for the Whole Population: Final report*. London, HMSO.

Wheller, L. (2006) Caring and carers. In: M. Bajekal, V. Osbourne, M. Yar & H. Meltzer, (eds) *Focus on Health*. Basingstoke, Palgrave Macmillan.

Wilson, P.M. (2001) A policy analysis of the expert patient in the United Kingdom: self care as an expression of pastoral power? *Health and Social Care in the Community* **9** (3): 134–142.

Chapter 5

The National Service Framework for Long Term Conditions: towards the integration of a learning disability perspective

Garry Diack

Key points

- Outlining the history and development of the National Service Frameworks
- Identifying the areas that are of particular relevance to the learning disability nurse
- Suggesting ways of working within the frameworks that facilitate the achievement of improvements in the quality of service that is delivered to people with learning disabilities

---

This chapter will have a duality of purpose in that it will serve to highlight the issues pertaining to people with learning disabilities for a general nursing audience and will also clarify ways forward for those working in learning disability (LD) services. There has been a historic lack of engagement with primary health care strategic planning, in part due to the integrated nature of LD services that arose from the lead commissioning arrangements detailed in section S.31 of the Health Act 1990. The other compelling aspect of the lack of engagement has been the competing priorities experienced within integrated services combined with a lack of awareness of LD issues. It is hoped that this chapter will offer suggestions on how to influence the agenda and ensure that people with learning disabilities are properly represented within National Service Framework (NSF) strategic forums.

Health needs of people with a learning disability

The health needs of the LD population in comparison to those of the non-learning disabled population are better understood following the research that accompanied *Valuing People* (Department of Health (DOH), 2001a). People with learning disabilities have more significant experience of health-related problems; they also have difficulty in accessing secondary health care because of a lack of knowledge on the part of secondary health care staff, communication difficulties and 'diagnostic overshadowing'. This issue has challenged LD services for many years as other professionals have tended to view any presentation in the context of learning disability rather than specific ill health.

The health status of people with a learning disability is improving, albeit slowly; one significant area is in terms of mortality and morbidity. Life expectancy continues to increase and is now comparable to life expectancy in the general population (Linehan et al., 2004). Wanless (2002: pp. 38–39) identified that people are living much longer and as a consequence perhaps experiencing more ill health. The scenario of 'slow uptake' is described and there are many parallels with the experiences of people with a learning disability, who can be said to experience inequalities in health and an increased likelihood of chronic ill health. The increasingly technologically sophisticated nature of modern health care has resulted in increases in survivability and longevity. People with learning disabilities have also experienced the benefits and are now able to enjoy a lifespan approaching that of the non-LD population.

The White Paper *Valuing People* (DOH, 2001a) was a bold attempt to delineate a clear national agenda for addressing the various and complex needs of people with learning disabilities. Six years on from its publication it is not without its detractors; one of the principal issues being that whilst its recommendations and ideas are revolutionary it is constrained by not being legislative. One only has to consider the number of targets that have been set that have not been achieved, such as 'everyone should have a health action plan by 2005', for example, to appreciate the potential failings and to understand the criticisms of *Valuing People*.

Fyson and Simons (2003) comment that *Valuing People* was not created in response to a particular concern about standards in the same way as *Better Services for Mentally Handicapped People* (Department of Health and Social Services, 1971), the latter having been written in response to the alarming findings from long-stay hospitals of that time. However, it is worth commenting that in the light of the Budock and Sutton and Merton Primary Care Trust (PCT) enquiries, there will once again be a renewed concern about, and scrutiny of, LD services. It is perhaps incumbent upon services to attempt to capitalize on some of the progress that has been made by *Valuing People* and attempt to set in stone its achievements. The NSFs offer a coherent model in order to try to deliver against targets. In their critique of *Valuing People*, Fyson and Simons (2003) call for the translation of *Valuing People* as a national plan into effective local action. Arguably the NSF quality requirement groups will provide a means to facilitate that translation from national plan into local action. There will need to be some creative thinking and interpretation of the quality requirements but it would be possible to couch many of the goals, aspirations and targets of *Valuing People* (DOH, 2001a) in terms of NSF quality requirements. This would seem to be particularly relevant if one considers the long term conditions quality requirements. It is essential not to downplay the importance of the other NSFs and, arguably, learning disabled people should have been adequately and appropriately represented in all the NSF subgroups thus far. There are, however, rather too many indicators that this is not the case and people with learning disabilities are not receiving the level of care that is necessary.

The Disability Rights Commission (2006) commissioned research into the health inequalities of people with learning disabilities and mental health needs; the findings were alarming and made uncomfortable reading for many. People with a learning disability were less likely to be offered appropriate health screenings and investigations, were more likely to die young and more likely to live with preventable (long term) conditions. Mencap produced a disturbing report *Death by Indifference* (2007) that highlighted how six people with learning disabilities had died unnecessarily as a consequence, in part, of insufficient knowledge on the part of the health professionals. The report followed *Treat Me Right!* (Mencap, 2004) that highlighted the inequalities in care that were experienced by people with a learning disability. These reports demonstrate how all practitioners have a duty of care to those with a learning disability.

The National Service Framework for Long Term Conditions

The NSF for Long Term Conditions describes a number of conditions that are considered to be within the domain of 'long term conditions'. Epilepsy is one such condition and is particularly significant in the context of LD services. Prevalence and incidence figures are difficult to ascertain with any veracity, although it is widely accepted that for people with a mild to moderate learning disability, the incidence of epilepsy may be 1:3, and for people with a severe to profound disability, the incidence may be as high as 1:2. Given the degree of brain damage that has, in all probability, been a causative factor in the learning disability it is reasonable to predict that the epilepsy will often be difficult to treat. In such instances the use of adjunctive therapy may be required and there are stringent requirements around monitoring of the condition. For many people with a learning disability their experience within health care settings has been unsatisfactory, although precise qualitative data are not readily available.

> 'Epilepsy is one of the most prevalent neurological disorders that can be effectively prevented and treated at an affordable cost. It is the most common serious brain disorder worldwide with no age, race, social class, national nor geographic boundaries.'
> (World Health Organization, 2007)

Buck et al. (2006) describe the use of the ELDQOL (Epilepsy and Learning Disabilities Quality of Life) scale which, based on current research, presents as a tool with good evidence of reliability and validity. It is potentially an effective instrument to assess the quality of life of children and young adults with epilepsy and learning disabilities.

Despite the well-documented evidence that has emerged in the wake of *Valuing People* (DOH, 2001a) and specific research within the LD field, there is still a lack of participation in NSF strategic planning. *Valuing People* itself heralded a significant step forward for LD services although it was to some degree fettered by its status as guidance rather than legislation. A consequence of this was that services may have had the volition but not necessarily the motivation to address all the issues identified within the scope of the document. Resources that could have usefully been targeted towards significant improvements in health status were perhaps utilized in domains requiring specific feedback to government.

The publication of NSFs from the *NHS Cancer Plan: A plan for investment, a plan for reform* (DOH, 2000) onwards were potentially significant in helping to improve the situation. A long history of difficulties in accessing services has been acknowledged:

> 'People with LD have the same rights of access to NHS services as everyone else but may require assistance to use them.

Notwithstanding the above sentiment there have been continuing difficulties with regard to the NSFs in a LD context. An example of this is the NSF for Older People (DOH, 2002) that initially seemed to be the ideal vehicle with which to address the needs of an ageing LD population. Block and Justham (2004) under-took a study to try to ascertain nurses' understanding and awareness of the NSFs. There are acknowledged shortcomings in the research process in terms of the ability to discriminate between awareness and knowledge, for example. The overall findings were of concern in that levels of awareness of the different NSFs were found to be low to moderate. Furthermore, a proportion of the nurses who responded to the research had not attempted to discover any more about NSF documentation. This is a potentially worrying situation and goes part way to explaining the lack of interest and response to NSFs. It is therefore incumbent upon LD nurses to attempt to become more politically aware and conversant with the NSFs in order to be able to deliver against targets.

Action Learning Point

Try to complete the following without recourse to any reference material.

- List the NSFs currently published.
- What is a quality requirement?
- How is the success of each quality requirement reported, and to whom?
- What is an external reference group?

The publication of an NSF is not in itself a panacea for all ills. Thompson and Crome (2002) point out that the NSF for Older People (DOH, 2002), whilst generally accepted, was subject to some re-presentation. In order to satisfy the meeting of a particular standard, parts of a hospital's admission criteria were rewritten in order not to fall foul of accusations of discrimination. The case in point involved the substitution of a term that referred to age being replaced with another, apparently innocuous, term that in essence meant the same thing. What may be regarded as a somewhat cynical move is understandable, though not defensible, in the light of the audit culture that prevails within the NHS and the litigious society in which we live.

Palliative care as an issue is important and the NSF quality requirement 10 (QR10) adds weight to the considerations already raised in the Carer's Act 2000. This is particularly relevant as research now confirms that people with a learning disability are living much longer even with complex medical conditions (DOH, 2001b).

It is now widely understood that people with a learning disability experience much more ill health than the general population, some examples of which are listed here (Institute of Health Research, 2003):

- *Epilepsy*: up to one person in three with a learning disability may have epilepsy and one person in two with severe learning disabilities may have epilepsy.
- *Gastro-oesophageal reflux disorder* (GORD): up to 40% of people with a learning disability may have this condition. The risk of developing pneumonia as a consequence of aspirating food and/or stomach contents is high and represents a serious risk to health that often results in death. GORD-related complications are a leading cause of death in the LD population.
- *Gastrointestinal cancers*: there are much higher rates of incidence of gastrointestinal cancers in all people with LD.
- *Dementia*: people with Down's syndrome can begin to develop dementia in their late thirties/early forties.
- *Obesity*: this is on the increase, as in the general population, but poor economic status and education levels increases the likelihood for people with learning disabilities to be obese.
- *Complex health needs*: The conditions described often present as a multiple presentation, i.e. the person with learning disability is affected by more than one condition at one time and often by several.
- *Inequity of access*: Due to the complex health needs that may present, more intensive health interventions are required but, paradoxically, people with learning disabilities are often excluded from access to primary and secondary health care by a variety of means.
- *Dysphagia*: an increased rate of swallowing problems amongst people with learning disabilities contributes to lower body weight, poor nutritional status and a higher risk of premature death.
- *Cerebral palsy*: there are posture and mobility problems.
- *Respiratory problems*: these are common, particularly in people with Down's syndrome and people with compromised mobility and posture.
- *Sensory impairments*: people with learning disabilities have a greater incidence of sensory impairment. They may be 200 times more likely to have visual impairment; 40–60% have hearing impairment.
- *Cervical smears*: women with learning disabilities are less likely to be screened – 19% compared to 77%.
- *Mental health*: the prevalence of schizophrenia is three times higher; 40% of people with learning disabilities have additional mental health needs.
- *Coronary heart disease* (CHD): this is the second most common cause of death in this population.
- *Respiratory disease*: the leading cause of death in this population; 46–52% compared with 15–17% in the non-LD population.
- *Bone density*: people with learning disabilities have substantially lower bone density, which can lead to a high risk of osteoporosis. Perhaps in many cases

this is caused by the lack of exercise over a long period of time, in addition to poor level of nutrition.

- *Dental health*: one-third of people with learning difficulties have unhealthy teeth and gums (80% in people with Down's syndrome). There is for some people a historical context for this, in that daily dental care in long-stay hospitals was limited and for some people the main intervention was extraction because teeth had decayed so badly. An additional complication was gum disease caused by the use of some medications for epilepsy.
- *Nutrition*: less than 10% of people with learning disabilities eat a healthy diet; the potential consequences of this are obesity, diabetes, heart disease, gastrointestinal cancers and bowel cancers.

National Service Frameworks entered the health care lexicon in the wake of the Calman Hine Report (Expert Advisory Group on Cancer, 1995). The need to address the increasing problem of cancer had precipitated the development of a new approach. New Labour's 'Third way' was typified at the time by the White Paper *The New NHS: Modern, dependable* (DOH, 1997) and the establishment of the National Institute for Clinical Excellence (NICE) and the NSFs as the blueprints for a national standard approach. The precursor to the NSFs was the development of a national cancer plan by Kenneth Calman and Deirdre Hine. The plan was predicated on the use of an evidence base to inform planning that was not constrained by individual service approaches.

The NSFs have provided a specification for the services that would be provided as well as detailed quality standards. In addition, external reference groups were put in place for each NSF and their remit was to report on emerging issues. It has been suggested by Baker (2000) that the apparent dichotomy between the medical model, as represented by medical academics on the reference groups, and a more inclusive holistic model, as represented by health and social care professionals, carers and service users, resulted in significant bureaucratic problems. This was typified in the early days of the Mental Health NSF where intervention by the Health Secretary Frank Dobson was required to pre-empt resignations.

NSFs are characterized by four main features:

1 Specific nationally agreed standards.
2 Service models with clear parameters.
3 A clear implementation plan.
4 Performance indicators (PIs).

The NSF for Long Term Conditions (DOH, 2005) is specifically aimed at people with a long term neurological condition, although it is stated in the foreword by John Reid that anyone with a long term condition ought to be able to benefit from the findings. Specific mention is made of the importance of a person-centred approach and this is particularly pertinent to LD services. The NSF takes into account two other NSFs, the NSF for Children, Young People and Maternity Services (DOH, 2004a) and the NSF for Older People (DOH, 2002), and this is particularly relevant to LD services in view of the challenges that are encountered at transition. There are many complex issues centred on finance and logistics in the transition from children's services to adult services, or from adult services to older people's services. Transition is often unsatisfactory and is interpreted differently by different services. However, government intent was that the service be based on need rather than age.

In view of this it is perhaps useful to consider the NSFs as a matrix that is individual to each person. The quality requirements for each NSF may have some degree of overlap and a 'mapping' of the different elements could conceivably be incorporated into the person's needs-led assessment.

Davis (2005), in his editorial discusses the NSF for Long Term Conditions in relation to orthopaedic nursing and notes the philosophical changes engendered by the new NSF. Davis envisages a future where pre-emptive and proactive responses by health care professionals will avert costly reactive models of intervention. These initiatives will be led by specialist orthopaedic nurses who will work collaboratively with other health professionals to effect change and improvements in the experience of people with long term conditions. The demands addressed by the orthopaedic nursing profession are ones that will challenge LD nurses and perhaps add further weight to the health agenda of the LD nurse. The LD nurse is a specialist in the field of learning disability and is possessed of the clinical knowledge to operate effectively at both the interface between health and social care and the interface between LD services and secondary care.

The Better Metrics Project (Healthcare Commission, 2006) was developed in response to concerns that clinicians did not always engage with the targets and performance indicators used in the NHS. The intention of producing better metrics was to enable clinicians to work with clinically relevant measures of performance. The term is intentionally different to 'targets', 'indicators' and 'benchmarks' and is designed to encourage the achievement of factors that are important from a clinical perspective. Themes 8.09 and 8.10 in particular are relevant to the NSF for Long Term Conditions.

Public service agreements were instituted by the government in a series of White Papers from 2000 to 2004. This change in priorities for public spending is intended to channel investment towards education and health with a clear link to modernization. Objective II from the 2004 Spending Review identifies the need to offer personalized care plans for those deemed to be most at risk.

Standards for Better Health (2004b) established four national priorities; one of which is improved self-care in the community as a means to prevent hospitalization. For those people with a learning disability who live in the community and who receive a service from the LD team, there is an ideal opportunity here. The LD nurse can capitalize on the need to achieve outcomes in terms of quality requirements within the NSF for Long Term Conditions. Specific plans are required to be developed that take account of health priorities and this links very clearly with the health action planning agenda that has so dominated the work of LD services in the last few years.

Action Learning Point

Within your PCT or Acute Trust try to establish the membership of each of the quality requirement working groups for each NSF (use Table 1 as a basis for setting out the information gathered).

- What is the level of representation from learning disability services?
- Which of the NSFs are prioritized?
- Are NSF targets reflected in local plans?
- How is the information fed in to the PCT strategy?

Table 1 Use the table as a template to investigate local service provision of quality standards concerning National Service Frameworks.

National Service Framework	Number of quality requirements	Membership of quality requirement groups	Position of member	Feedback mechanism clear?	Links to local plans	Clear progress?
Cancer						
Coronary Heart Disease						
Paediatric Intensive Care						
Mental Health						
Older People						
Diabetes						
Renal						
Children						
COPD						
Long-term Conditions						

Quality requirements

The 'Good Practice Guide' (DoH, 2007) has been written at the request of service providers to assist them in implementing the National Service Framework for Long Term Conditions (DoH, 2005). The quality requirements that follow are addressed in the above framework and intended as a practical means of implementing quality within service provision.

Quality requirement 1: a person-centred service

The aim of this is to support people to manage their condition, maintain their independence and achieve the best possible quality of life through the integration of education, assessment, care planning, service delivery and information sharing. (DOH, 2005). The language used here has echoes in the ethos of LD services across the UK. Person-centred planning is a theme central to current philosophies in LD services and services are striving to make their services person-centred. There is a real opportunity offered with quality requirement 1 to actually set the concept of person-centred planning in stone. The quality requirement states that people with long term conditions are offered an integrated assessment or a plan of their health and social care needs. They are to be given possession of the information that they will need in order to make an informed decision about care and treatment. The aim would be that they will be able to manage their condition to whatever degree possible themselves. There is a particular challenge here in giving people with learning disabilities information to facilitate an informed decision about care and it will be very much incumbent upon the carer to make that information as accessible and understandable as possible. Learning disability services are experienced at providing user-friendly information in easy-read formats. Examples such as the White Paper *Valuing People* (DOH, 2001a) and the annual updates, which are available in easy-read format, are illustrative of this resource availability and there is significant expertise in this area amongst LD services. The challenge now becomes how to make information relevant to the particular long term conditions and accessible to people. The issue of 'asking the experts' (Rodgers & Namaganda, 2005) needs to be taken forward and services need to find ways of feeding information from NSF strategy groups into partnership boards.

Quality requirement 1 clearly describes the effectiveness of support, which involves multidisciplinary teams who have access to all the required information and who are able to work together in an effective and efficient way. Within this it is important that there is an integrated assessment process, a care planning process and a broad-based holistic assessment. If all these things are in place then it is suggested that there will be successful intervention.

Section 3d of the above rationale describes people who have long term neurological conditions experiencing improved quality of life if they are able to get appropriate support and advice and it specifically mentions specialist nurses. Arguably the LD nurse is such a specialist nurse and can adopt an important role within the context of the NSF. Implicit within the care planning process is the fact that the multidisciplinary team has to work as a cohesive unit. It has to be able to effectively consider the issues and act appropriately; as is stated in the NSF, care planning, if it is to be successful, must be person-centred and must also have a fluid component to it. The lack of engagement with NSFs is by no means unique to the LD format or forum. There are examples from secondary care and from primary health care where NSFs have also not been engaged with at the level that might have been expected. There have been numerous studies undertaken to examine where NSFs are now and to explore why there has not been the impact that was expected. One example comes from a sociological study undertaken by Checkland (2004) that highlights the dichotomy between the uptake of NSFs against the uptake of explicit clinical guidelines offered to GPs. In the main these clinical guidelines have been found to be more readily accepted and acted upon than the NSFs – the question is 'Why has this happened?'

Pickard and White (2006), in their editorial, summarized the position of the *National Service Framework for Long Term Conditions* (DOH, 2005) one year on from its publication and offered the *British Journal of Neurosurgery* as a forum for the publication of papers that would assist in the furtherance of the original ambitions of the NSF's architects. The editorial cites examples of apparent failings in the scope of the NSF that hinge upon the lack of financial support coupled with the changing demographic, which is arguably a testament to the success of modern medicine. The technological and pharmaceutical advances in acute care have reduced mortality rates at the same time as allowing increasing numbers of people to live much longer; albeit in some cases with a long term condition and possibly a reduced quality of life.

One particularly interesting aspect of Checkland's (2004) work is her survey of GPs in terms of their attitudes to NSFs. Once again there was a principal difference between their attitudes before the publication compared to their attitudes when they actually saw the NSF documentation. Commentary made by the GPs was essentially negative and focused around the idea that the NSFs did not actually offer practical help or practical direction. If one considers the phraseology used within the framework documents they are somewhat ambiguous and open to interpretation. This may account for some of the reasons why they are not taken on board to the extent that one would hope, although more ambiguity means less prescription and consequently greater clinical freedom.

There is a developing recognition of the requirement to address the needs of people with a learning disability and this has been reinforced by the publication of *Death by Indifference*, a report by Mencap (2007) that highlights six cases of people with a learning disability who died whilst receiving care that was not of the quality it should have been because of health and social care staff ignorance of the specific needs of people with a learning disability. The Disability Rights Commission (2006) findings and the disturbing findings from the Commission for Social Care Inspection (CSCI) investigations into Budock Hospital (Commission for Social Care Inspection & Healthcare Commission, 2006) and Sutton and Merton PCT (Commission for Healthcare Audit and Inspection, 2007) have all served to bring into sharp focus the experiences of inequality that people with a learning disability endure in the health service.

The *Lancet* published an editorial that cautioned all health professionals 'from undergraduates up' (Lancet, 2007) against complacency about the health needs and expectations of people with a learning disability. The need to prioritize training and education will hopefully serve as a clarion call that the LD nurse can respond to in a proactive manner. There are undoubtedly many examples of good practice around the country in terms of provision of training and awareness raising. The challenge for services is perhaps to take note of examples of good practice and adapt them for use in their own areas.

It would be cynical to assume that because of the payment by results system (British Medical Association/NHS Employers, 2006), GPs are more inclined to work within clinical guidelines produced by bodies such as the British Medical Association; however, one cannot ignore the issue of payment as one of the drivers for change. It also must be remembered that NSFs do not come with extra funding streams attached. The expectation is clearly stated that funding will come from within existing resources in order to facilitate the improvements required. The continuing focus on spiralling costs and increasing demand for services has meant that services must justify their performance and their expenditure; the acquisition and analysis of data has therefore assumed great importance. This pressure, in tandem with the continuing financial crisis that year (2006), which saw the ring-fencing around training budgets removed by the Department of Health, will likely further complicate the process of achieving the NSF targets.

Oliver (2005) comments that the NSFs have actually been increasing costs and yet at the same time there is no advice from NICE on how these extra costs can be met. This generates a potential dilemma in terms of how the NSFs can be implemented effectively. It would be reasonable to assume that costs will continue to increase as services meet more of the targets; a clear strategy for absorbing these costs and identifying appropriate funding streams therefore needs to be developed.

Perusal of the evidence-based markers for the quality requirements will tend to support this point – for example, p. 23 of the *National Service Framework for Long Term Conditions* (DOH, 2005), evidence-based marker number 4.

Local arrangements for providing information ensure that people receive timely, quality assured, culturally appropriate information in a range of formats. One only has to consider the potential ambiguities inherent in phrases such as 'timely', 'quality assured' and 'culturally appropriate' to realize that interpretation might be difficult. Consider for example the first phrase – timely. In order for something to be timely, one has to assume that there will be a specific timeframe apportioned to it. There is potential here for confusion and dissatisfaction if the detail of the timeframe within which the information is to be received is not clearly stated.

There is a significant amount of information required in terms of ensuring quality. There are quality action teams, quality groups, quality improvement frameworks and quality outcome frameworks – there are numerous mechanisms but what are the implications in practice of trying to achieve these quality directives?

The issue of cultural appropriateness is a specific problem. We live in a multicultural society and, arguably, LD services have a history of lack of engagement with specific cultures. In terms of the range of formats in which information is provided one only has to look at people who are deaf, people who are blind, people who are deaf/blind, and people whose first language is not English to realize that the range of formats available is indeed limited and will often come with a significant cost implication for which services are not adequately financed.

Another interesting issue is considered within a sociological study in terms of nurses' responses to the Expert Patient Programme (DOH, 2001c). The notion of the expert patient is one of the central concepts of the NSF for Long Term Conditions, the idea being that the patient is at the centre and in control of their own care, or is in receipt of a person-centred service. How to adequately represent the views of the learning disabled expert is a particular challenge to advocacy services.

Another intriguing concept or possibility offered by the NSF for Long Term Conditions is that a lot of the focus is on long term neurological conditions and the development of people who have expertise. Arguably, once again, the LD nurses – given their expertise in dealing with communication problems, psychosocial and emotional effects, cognitive behavioural problems, sensory difficulties and physical and motor problems – could be potentially regarded as having such expertise. Case examples such as this are all grist to the mill of the LD nurse given the presentation of people with learning disabilities who may have an attendant physical disability. Perhaps nurses who qualify in LD nursing are in a position to become experts and offer advice and guidance to other nursing colleagues and/or health and social care colleagues about the particular needs of their client group.

An interesting aspect of the introduction to the *National Service Framework for Long Term Conditions* (DOH, 2005) is the issue of addressing who will benefit from the NSF. A clear statement is made that this NSF is offered or delivered in the context of the government's overall strategy to improve health and social care support. It states in the policy document that all people living with long term conditions should benefit and it also states that whilst the quality requirements listed are derived from specific research that has been undertaken in the field of long term neurological conditions, elements of the quality requirements can be applied to people with other long term conditions. The list is indeed compelling:

- Prompt diagnosis.
- Person-centred care.
- Planning and liaison when people make transitions between services.
- Equitable assessment for fully funded NHS continuing care and adult social care with fair access to care services.
- Facts guidance.
- Providing palliative care to people who have conditions other than cancer.
- Supporting carers.

These are all issues that have particular pertinence to LD services because they often have difficulty in meeting the challenges of providing these aspects to their clients. Consider, for example, planning and liaison when people make transitions between services. Transition is an extremely complicated issue in services. There are two types of transition within LD services, that which occurs between children's and adult services and that which notionally occurs between adult services and older people's services. In the former case the transition happens on a sliding scale beginning notionally at the age of 14 when transition joint working begins. Different services have different approaches to this – there is no unified national approach to transition – and as a consequence the experience of transition in different services and in different parts of the UK is variable. What is more contentious perhaps is the nature of transition from adult services into older people's services when a person reaches 65.

Notionally, people are in adult services from the age of 18 to 65 years, but large numbers of people over the age of 65 continue to receive their services and more crucially their funding from adult services. There is a confused picture with regard to issues of charging from older people's services and a lack of a formalized transition process at the age of 65 years. Perhaps the NSF in attempting to set in stone these quality requirements will help to address this issue and maybe LD services will be able to couch their formalized transition process in terms of NSF quality requirements and standards.

A further issue that is worthy of consideration is the notion of equitable assessment for fully funded continuing care and adult social care under *Fair Access to Care Services* (DOH, 2003). The most notable case example would be that of early-onset dementia in people with Down's syndrome. There has been a significant amount of research regarding the early onset of dementia and organic changes are being detected as early as the second to third decade. Potentially, by the time people with Down's syndrome are in their fifth decade they will either have the condition or it will be developing. A difficult issue in this regard is that people are being referred to dementia services that traditionally deal with people who are older, as a consequence they are deemed ineligible in terms of age, irrespective of their clinical presentation. Furthermore, the issue of having a learning disability is considered to be critical as such people with dementia do not readily fit into a particular service. The person with a learning disability will be redirected back to the LD service as the most appropriate service to meet their needs. This is one of the many examples of so-called inappropriate referrals that can constrain and frustrate services, let alone not meet the needs of the client group.

Diagnostic overshadowing (Reiss et al., 1982) is a problem encountered frequently in psychiatric services, where the diagnostic significance of a person's mental health presentation assumes a lesser significance if a learning disability is present. There may be an attribution of presenting features to the learning disability rather than the mental health disorder (Raghavan & Patel, 2005). A further consequence of this is that as people deteriorate, and sometimes the deterioration can be surprisingly fast, people are placed in younger disabled units or other somewhat inappropriate care provision, having been removed from their own home because people are no longer able to care for them. So, perhaps some of the quality requirements will enable services to be much more proactive in terms of helping people to maintain their place in their own home and to be supported in managing their condition as far as possible in their own home.

Quality requirement 2: early recognition, prompt diagnosis and treatment

Quality requirement 2 states:

> 'People suspected of having a neurological condition are to have prompt access to specialist neurological expertise for an accurate diagnosis treatment as close to home as possible. (DOH, 2005: pp. 4–5)

One issue that is particularly relevant here is the issue of epilepsy. The rationale states that misdiagnosis, or the challenge of trying to diagnose accurately certain neurological conditions, is difficult in the absence of clear and simple diagnostic features. The document further states that in conditions such as epilepsy there is a misdiagnosis in around one in four cases. The rationale states that an improved diagnosis can be the result of collaborative working between teams who then link with the neurologist. Staff who support people with learning disabilities are particularly experienced in collaboration with other professionals and can make an important contribution, not only to the diagnosis, but also to the understanding of the person. This is an essential part of a collaborative relationship that involves working with both the client and health and social care professionals responsible for the management of the condition.

Improved training in recognizing important symptoms is a crucial element for all staff likely to have contact with a person with a long term condition and this is particularly relevant for people with epilepsy and their carers. There is a real opportunity for LD nurses to stake a claim in providing this training and in becoming a source of expertise in terms of epilepsy knowledge and raising awareness. Increasingly, social care housing is managed without qualified staff on site 24 hours a day; unqualified staff may be supporting people who have epilepsy and may be uncertain about the importance of giving medication at the correct time. The importance of accurate recording of any seizure activity that is observed, and indeed understanding that what they are observing can be seizure activity, cannot be over-emphasized. With this in mind, improved training is highly important and arguably the LD nurse is well placed to provide this training.

Another issue with regard to epilepsy is the notion of people with a longstanding diagnosis that does not necessarily have a formalized record of how the diagnosis was achieved. Such an example would be case notes where people were diagnosed with 'epilepsy' several decades previously and are maintained on a dosage of medication that means they have not had seizures for many years, in some cases, and yet the same level of medication is continued (Shoumitro, 2000). Clearly it would be appropriate to try and address the issues of having clients referred for further assessment to establish whether the epilepsy medication itself is still required at the current level or if at all.

There is a significant issue concerning potential side effects of long term medication, particularly when people are being treated with polypharmacy (Robertson et al., 2000), i.e. more than one medication at a time. Possible complex interactions of such drugs and possible side effects need to be recorded. Again, this requires staff members who are adequately trained in terms of their awareness and are suitably clear about the need to report and record their observations. Within clinical practice, there are some clear examples, particularly in the case of people with learning disabilities, in terms of medication reviews. Some people do not have regular reviews and it states in the quality requirement that those taking three or more medicines should have a face-to-face review. A possibility here for LD nurses is that they can undertake a case load review to establish the people who are in receipt of a polypharmacy regime. They can then arrange the face-to-face reviews and support the person at the review with the specialist in order to ensure that the review takes place effectively. Alternatively, LD nurses with a prescribing qualification could carry out these reviews and determine the need for referral for a specialist opinion.

Another issue that is discussed in terms of early recognition is where conditions are present of a genetic origin. The NSF for Long Term Conditions (DOH, 2005) states that whenever a genetic condition is diagnosed or when a genetic opinion can form a diagnosis, the person needs to be referred to a geneticist. The person and their family can then be offered counselling and information about the implications so that they can make informed decisions about testing, treatment and other life choices; for example, potential effects on their future children.

Case study 1

A man of Pakistani origin with a moderate to severe learning disability and a genetically linked condition entered into an arranged marriage. He was married to a person from his own extended family. Over the course of time a child was produced who had inherited the same genetic condition as the father. The family was reluctant to receive any form of genetic counseling, stating that their religion forbade it, and decided continue to try for children because that was what was expected. The following year another child was born who also had the same genetic condition. Learning disability services attempted to offer advice and support but this was not accepted.

In terms of evidence-based markers for quality requirement 2 (DOH, 2005), the following issues should be considered:

- Improved access to specialist neurological expertise.
- Diagnostic services effectively designed and with sufficient capacity to enable a diagnosis.
- Improved access to appropriate treatments.
- Specialist nurses and practitioners with specific knowledge being available to support people with long term conditions in the community.
- Improved access to treatment reviews which ensure that people taking medicines on a long term basis have access to regular medication reviews.

Quality requirement 4: early and specialist rehabilitation.

The quality requirement is stated as:

'People with long term neurological conditions who would benefit from rehabilitation are to receive timely ongoing high quality rehab services in hospital or other specialist service settings to meet their continuing and changing needs. When ready they are to receive they help they need to return home for ongoing community rehab and support.' (DOH, 2005: pp. 4–5)

Again, a significant evidence-based marker for quality requirement 4 is that a seamless transition of care be provided through integrated working with other care professionals. In-reach and out-reach arrangements between different parts of the services should be provided and also specialist rehabilitation services to meet the needs of people with very severe and complex disabilities.

Quality requirement 5: community rehabilitation support

This requirement states that people with long term neurological conditions living at home are to have ongoing access to a comprehensive range of rehabilitation advice and support to meet their continuing and changing needs (DOH, 2005). Learning disability services are concerned with attempting to provide support for people to increase their independence and to help them to live as they would wish.

One of the evidence-based markers for quality requirement 5 is that providers of community rehabilitation and support services support people and their family members and carers to live with the long term condition and to develop knowledge and skills to manage the condition. These notions of self-efficacy and self-management are essential issues for people with long term neurological conditions. Professional and lay carers who are supporting them must also have the knowledge and skills to help them to manage their condition. This evidence-based marker refers to helping people to achieve a sense of well-being, which is a difficult concept to frame in a meaningful way, particularly in relation to people who have difficulties with communication. A sense of well-being is derived from achievement of satisfaction in a number of domains in life. The experience of good health is one such domain, which can often be compromised in the case of people with a learning disability and one that health and social care professionals may be instrumental in positively addressing.

Quality requirement 6: vocational rehabilitation

This requirement states the need for:

> 'people with long term neurological conditions to have access to appropriate vocational assessment, rehabilitation and ongoing support to enable them to find, regain or remain in work and access other occupational and educational opportunities.' (DOH, 2005: pp. 4–5)

There is a very clear opportunity here for people with learning disabilities because it is known from *Adults with Learning Disabilities in England 2003/2004* (Emerson et al., 2004) that the percentage of people in paid meaningful employment is very low and that services have traditionally struggled to find access to employment for people. A further issue is access to continuing education. The opportunities to access education are quite limited, particularly post-18 years.

The evidence-based markers of particular relevance are No. 1, 'Co-ordinated multi-agency vocational rehabilitation is provided which takes account of agreed national guidance and best practice', and No. 4, which refers to 'Specialist vocational rehabilitation services routinely evaluating and monitoring long-term vocational outcomes, including the reasons for failure to remain in employment' (DOH, 2005).

A particular issue for people with learning disabilities is that failure to remain in employment or for an employment situation to be attainable is because of perceived difficulties with their concomitant conditions. For example, their ability to understand rules, guidance or instruction within the context of risk management. Or, in the case of epilepsy, people who are at risk of having a seizure may be perceived as presenting a health and safety risk. If these reasons were to be transparent and documented in a comprehensive way, then this would be useful information to enable support workers to make a strong case for people remaining in employment.

Quality requirement 7: providing equipment and accommodation

This requirement states that:

> 'People with long-term neurological conditions are to receive timely, appropriate assistive technology/equipment and adaptations to accommodation to support them to live independently; help them with their care; maintain their health and improve their quality of life.' (DOH, 2005: pp. 4–5)

Once again services often struggle to provide assistive technology and equipment. There are usually long waiting lists and often difficulties in terms of the assessment process. One of the statements made within the NSFs is that no new extra funding will be provided and that funding must be provided from within existing resources. The fact that there is now a quality requirement stating that assistive technology should be supplied will enable people to make a stronger case for a person having access to whatever it is that they need. Particular examples may be mechanical hoists, adapted bathrooms, adapted kitchens and rise and fall beds.

This is supported in many ways by evidence-based markers No. 3, which states 'Assistive technology/equipment needs are documented in a person's integrated care plan', and No. 4, 'There are specific arrangements for joint funding of specialist assistive technology provision. For example, communication aids, electric standing frames and special seating aids' (DOH, 2005). In addition, marker No. 5 states that 'Social services work closely with housing and accommodation sectors and supporting people services to provide timely, suitably adapted or purpose built accommodation' (DOH, 2005). This hopefully will reduce the numbers of people living in inappropriate accommodation and being cared for without the support of the relevant pieces of assistive technology.

Quality requirement 8: providing personal care and support

This requirement states that:

> 'Health and social care services work together to provide care and support to enable people with long-term neurological conditions to achieve maximum choice about living independently at home.' (DOH, 2005: pp. 4–5)

A key difficulty is that once people are deemed to be facing difficulties living at home, one of the professional responses is to reassess their situation and move the person to more appropriate accommodation rather than trying to adapt the original accommodation to suit the person's needs. Evidence markers highlight how those living in supported accommodation should be in suitable settings for people with neurological conditions. Furthermore, care should be provided by appropriately trained staff members. There is a clear training issue in terms of people having access, not just to ad hoc sessions of awareness training, but to an ongoing programme of comprehensive training that meets the needs of people who are working with clients with long term neurological conditions.

A difficulty frequently encountered within care services is the high level of staff turnover. Managers can be faced with a situation where training provided for a staff group at the inception of a new unit will, within a short space of time, be redundant as a percentage of the staff will have left. This leaves a situation where new staff have to be recruited and training has to be delivered again; this clearly has cost implications. This is difficult in terms of managing services because there are only limited budgets available for training. Training packages should therefore be developed to provide in-house training, rather than having what might be referred to as 'inoculation-type' models of training where people go for training for one or two days in a month away from the actual care setting. It is also sometimes questionable as to how effective this type of training is. If training became a fundamental requirement and senior staff within a service had it explicitly stated in their job description that they would facilitate training, then a LD nurse could, on a regular basis, provide that training and support. This approach would be advantageous in terms of the achievement of evidence-based marker No. 3 for quality requirement 9.

Quality requirement 9: palliative care

Palliative care is an issue that has challenged LD services. There is a growing awareness of the importance of providing appropriate and suitable palliative care. Indeed, a number of national initiatives have been very successful in the last few years. The quality requirement states:

> 'People in the later stages of long-term neurological conditions are to receive a comprehensive range of palliative care services when they need them to control symptoms; offer pain relief and meet their needs for personal, social, psychological and spiritual support, in line with the principles of palliative care.' (DOH, 2005: pp. 4–5)

This quality requirement makes the point that NICE guidance regarding cancer patients requiring palliative care sets out a benchmark for palliative care services (National Institute for Clinical Excellence, 2004). The observation is made that the principles may be applied to other long term conditions, particularly in terms of cognitive and communication problems, which may, as it states, limit the person's ability to describe their experience, express choices or take part fully in counselling or other support. Equally there may be issues around mental capacity and consent and the need for advanced directives.

Quality requirement 10: supporting family and carers

One of the significant issues for the families and carers of people with learning disabilities is the difficulty of letting go and allowing people to move on to become independent. Learning disability services around the UK frequently face the rather uncomfortable task of accommodating people who may be in their forties, fifties or even sixties who have lived all their life with their parents. When their parents have died, the adult with learning difficulties may rapidly require access to services. The person's family may find it very difficult to allow their relative to enter services and may experience a perceived responsibility and duty to keep that person at home, however challenging that prospect may be. A significant evidence-based marker is No. 2, which states that 'involving carers is part of the planning process. All carers are treated as partners in care and helped to acquire the appropriate skills to support them in their caring role' (DOH, 2005). Arguably this is an ideal opportunity for collaborative working between LD services and parents and carers of people with learning disabilities. The idea of an effective and productive partnership work approach to the person-centred plan is crucial if services are to make real progress in meeting the complex needs of people with a learning disability.

Quality requirement 11: caring for people with neurological conditions in hospital or other health and social care settings

This requirement states that:

> 'people with long-term neurological conditions are to have their specific neurological needs met whilst receiving care for other reasons in any health or social care setting.' (DOH, 2005)

This focuses on the notion that people with long term neurological conditions may have complex health needs and may have multiple presenting conditions. There are perhaps few people working within LD services who would argue that their service user's needs are adequately represented within the context of the NSFs. There are working groups within PCTs and Acute Trusts who are tasked with meeting the performance indicator targets for each quality requirement. It is, however, worth questioning the degree of involvement in these groups from LD service representatives.

The Department of Health policy research programme has provided a funding scheme to explore research in long term neurological conditions. There are a number of different projects incorporated into this, the purpose being to establish an understanding of what the quality of current health and social care is and what the experiences of service users are. The project will consider the implementation of the NSF for Long Term Conditions and consider its effectiveness. One of the ongoing projects is led by Professor Gillian Parker from York University, who has secured £334,837 in order to examine integrated services for people with long term conditions. Another significant area of research is being led by Professor Lynn Turner-Stokes, who has secured £287,827 to research support for carers, particularly those who have multiple caring roles.

Conclusions

This chapter has set a number of challenges for LD nurses and other health care professionals involved in the support of those with learning disabilities to embrace the opportunities that are on offer within the context of the NSFs. There are clearly stated targets to deliver against the various quality requirements and these are demonstrably health focused; as such they seem to fall comfortably within the remit of the LD nurse and supporting colleagues.

The need to address the health issues of people with a learning disability has been clearly stated for several years and our understanding of the nature of those health needs has increased as new research evidence has been published. By developing work within the parameters of the NSF quality requirements, significant advances can be made in meeting the health needs of people with a learning disability.

The use of the audit form in Table 1 will hopefully provide the stimulus, if required, for services to more fully engage in the essential work of addressing health priorities through the mechanism of the NSFs.

References

Baker, M. (2000) *Making Sense of the NHS White Papers*, 2nd edn. Abingdon, Radcliffe Medical Press.

Block, M. & Justham, D. (2004) A study into nurses' awareness of the National Service Frameworks. *British Journal of Nursing* 13 (4): 205–214.

British Medical Association/NHS Employers (2006) *Revisions to the GMS Contract: Delivering investment in general practice*. London, British Medical Association/NHS Employers.

Buck, D., Smith, M., Appleton, R., Baker, G.A. & Jacoby, A. (2006) The development and validation of the Epilepsy and Disability Quality of Life (ELDQOL) scale. *Epilepsy and Behavior* 10: 38–43.

Checkland, K. (2004) National Service Frameworks and UK general practitioners: street-level bureaucrats at work? *Sociology of Health and Illness* 26 (7): 951–975.

Commission for Healthcare Audit and Inspection (2007) *Investigation into the Service for People with Learning Disabilities Provided by Sutton and Merton Primary Care Trust January 2006*. London, Commission for Healthcare Audit and Inspection.

Commission for Social Care Inspection & Healthcare Commission (2006) *Joint Investigation into the Provision of Services for People with Learning Disabilities at Cornwall Partnership NHS Trust July 2006*. London, Commission for Healthcare Audit and Inspection.

Davis, P. (2005) Long-term approach to long-term conditions. *Journal of Orthopaedic Nursing* 9: 59–60.

Department of Health (1997) *The New NHS: Modern, dependable*. London, Department of Health.

Department of Health (2000) *NHS Cancer Plan: A plan for investment, a plan for reform*. London, Department of Health.

Department of Health (2001a) *Valuing People: A new strategy for learning disability for the 21st century*. London: Department of Health.

Department of Health (2001b) *Carers and Disabled Children Act 2000: Carers and people with parental responsibility for disabled children. Policy guidance*. London, Department of Health.

Department of Health (2001c) *The Expert Patient: A new approach to chronic disease management for the 21st century*. London, Department of Health.

Department of Health (2002) *National Service Framework for Older People*. London, Department of Health.

Department of Health (2003) *Fair Access to Care Services – Guidance on eligibility criteria for adult social care*. London, Department of Health.

Department of Health (2004a) *National Service Framework for Children, Young People and Maternity Services*. London, Department of Health.

Department of Health (2004b) *Standards for Better Health*. London, Department of Health.

Department of Health (2005) *The National Service Framework for Long Term Conditions*. London, Department of Health.

Department of Health (2007) *National Service Framework Good Practice Guide*. London, Department of Health.

Department of Health and Social Services (1971) *Better Services for Mentally Handicapped People*. CMND No. 4683. London, HMSO.

Disability Rights Commission (2006) *Equal Treatment: Closing the gap*. London, Disability Rights Commission.

Emerson, E., Mallam, S., Davies, I. & Spencer, K. (2004) *Adults with Learning Disabilities in England 2003/2004*. London, National Statistics and Health and Social Care Information Centre.

Expert Advisory Group on Cancer (1995) *A Policy Framework for Commissioning Cancer Services 1995. A Report by the Expert Advisory Group on Cancer to the Chief Medical Officers of England and Wales*, Department of Health/Welsh Office, London.

Fyson, R. & Simons, K. (2003) Strategies for change: making valuing people a reality. *British Journal of Learning Disabilities* **31**: 153–158.

Healthcare Commission (2006) *The Better Metrics Project*. London, Healthcare Commission.

Institute of Health Research (2003) *'Key Highlights' of Research Evidence on the Health of People with Learning Disabilities*. Lancaster, University of Lancaster. http://www.library.nhs.uk/learningdisabilities/ViewResource.aspx?resID=34896 [accessed 17 July 2007].

Lancet (2007) Learning disability: a neglected concern (editorial). *Lancet* **369** (9566): 966. http://www.thelancet.com [accessed 4 June 2007].

Linehan, C., Noonan Walsh, P., van Schrojenstein Lantman de Valk, H. & Kerr, M. (2004) *POMONA Health Indicators for People with Intellectual Disability in Member States – Final report*. http://europa.eu.int/comm/health/ph_projects/2002/monitoring_2002_05_en.htm [accessed 20 April 2007].

Mencap (2004) *Treat me Right!* London, Mencap.

Mencap (2007) *Death by Indifference*. London, Mencap.

National Institute for Clinical Excellence (2004) *Guidance on Cancer Services. Improving supportive and palliative care for adults with cancer: the manual*. London, National Institute for Clinical Excellence.

Oliver, A. (2005) The English National Health Service 1979–2005. *Health Economics Journal* **14**: S75–S99.

Pickard, J. & White, B. (2006) National Service Framework for Long-Term Conditions – quo vadis. *British Journal of Neurosurgery* **20** (1): 6–8.

Raghavan, R. & Patel, P. (2005) *Learning Disabilities and Mental Health*. Oxford, Blackwell Publishing.

Reiss, S., Levitan, G.W. & Szyszo, J. (1982) Emotional disturbance and mental retardation: diagnostic overshadowing. *American Journal of Mental Deficiency* **86**: 567–574.

Robertson, J., Emerson, E., Gregory, N., Hatton, C., Kessissoglue, S. & Hallam, A. (2000) Receipt of psychotropic medicine by people with intellectual disability in residential settings. *Journal of Intellectual Disability Research* **44** (6): 666–676.

Rodgers, J. & Namaganda, S. (2005) Making information easier for people with learning disabilities. *British Journal of Learning Disabilities* **33**: 52–58.

Shoumitro, D. (2000) Epidemiology and treatment of epilepsy in patients who are mentally retarded. *CNS Drugs* **13** (2): 117–128.

Thompson, S. & Crome, P. (2002) The United Kingdom National Service Framework for Older People – one year on. *Journal of the American Medical Directors Association* **3** (5): 337–339.

Wanless, D. (2002) *Securing Our Future Health: Taking a long-term view*. London, HMSO.

World Health Organization (2007) *Epilepsy*. Geneva, World Health Organization. http://www.who.int/mental_health/neurology/epilepsy [accessed 4 June 2007].

Chapter 6

Mental health promotion: the key to the effective management of long term conditions

Maureen Deacon

Key points

- Highlighting the lived experience of having a long term condition
- Outlining the tasks that patients (and by implication, their family and social network) need to engage in for the purposes of effective self-management and in-context recovery (that is, to experience and maintain their optimal health status)
- Examining the argument that good mental health is a necessary condition for being able to carry out identified tasks
- Identifying how practitioners can promote the mental health of persons with long term conditions

---

Long term conditions, often referred to as 'chronic illness' in the literature, have been investigated from a range of scholarly perspectives. Broadly and very simplistically, these can be divided into biomedical and psychosocial viewpoints. However, if health and social care practitioners are to meaningfully engage in providing person-centred services (Department of Health (DOH), 2005) their work needs to critically apply a rounded range of knowledge to the person in their care. In relation to the psychosocial domain, Charmaz (2000: p. 278) notes how studies of illness have, over the last four decades, become increasingly focused on 'the experiencing subject'. This trend can also be seen in the biomedical field, where there has been growing attention paid to the 'expert patient' (Taylor & Bury, 2007). This idea has been taken up with enthusiasm by politicians, to the extent that, unusually, specific funding was made available to Primary Care Trusts (PCTs) for the development of Expert Patient Programmes (Taylor & Bury, 2007). The person/patient[1] then has, in theory at least, come to occupy centre stage. An important consequence of this trend has been a growing body of knowledge concerning the work that needs to be done by patients experiencing long term illness. This work can be usefully conceived of as a set of tasks to be undertaken, known here as a 'person specification'. The main interest here is in the relationship between the patient's mental health and their ability to successfully undertake these tasks. This is developed further into the argument that good mental health is a critical factor in the effective management of a long term condition and the practitioner's role in promoting mental health in this context is explored. The main discussion then proceeds by outlining two 'takes' on this patient work, one arising from a social science background (Charmaz, 2000) and the other from a biomedical standpoint (Von Korff et al., 1997). From this, in keeping with the person-centred goal of care, a holistic set of tasks are identified to be analysed further in relation to mental health.

The importance of mental health within the overall health agenda has been increasingly recognized and there are numerous initiatives designed, broadly, to promote mental health. The idea that mental health *should* be promoted is a relatively contemporary idea and standard 1 of the National Service Framework (NSF) for Mental Health (DOH, 1999a) makes it clear that health and social services should be doing this work. The notion of what we might call 'ordinary' mental ill health is now a commonplace topic of conversation when wrapped up in the metaphor of 'stress' (Radley, 1994), and we have a growing 'emotion industry' (Crossley, 2000). However, those who suffer from severe and enduring mental illness remain a stigmatized group (Social Exclusion Unit, 2004). The stigma associated with mental illness is a complex topic in its own right but for current purposes it should be noted that this affects the work of practitioners too. The mental health aspects of ill health are often neglected by non-mental health practitioners (Turner & Kelly, 2000), despite their obvious, enduring commitment to their patients. Personal enquiries about this matter have often revealed a fear of 'getting in too deep'. This appears to be a fear of triggering strong emotions that the practitioner will not be able to cope with; so, in practice, mental health is often overlooked. This may be wrapped up in common social fears of people with mental health problems and the worry of 'irrational emotion' and social disorder (Crossley, 2000: p. 281). Moreover it appears to involve practitioners' fears of inadequacy and helplessness in the face of mental distress.

However, there is growing evidence concerning the relationships between mental and physical health (DOH, 2001; Mentality & National Institute for Mental Health, 2004) and practitioners need to be challenged to reflect upon their fears and develop their mental health promotion practices as an essential component of their routine work. Guthrie (1996) found that between 20% and 25% of people with long term conditions had mood disorders, and there is a strong evidence base in the cancer field of a relationship between cancer and consequent mental ill health (Pitceathly & Maguire, 2003; Botti et al., 2006). Furthermore, research investigating the effects of depression in people with physical ill health shows that this results

---

[1] I have struggled with choosing between the use of 'patient' and 'person' throughout this chapter. On reflection, this dilemma seems very fitting with the topics under discussion here, not least the question that should be at the heart of all health and social care practice: how do I care for this patient in the context of their personhood?

in poorer health outcomes and greater use of health care facilities (Baune et al., 2007). There are numerous reasons, then, for practitioners to pay careful attention to promoting the mental health of their patients.

Action Learning Point

- Discuss with a trusted colleague your concerns about promoting mental health in your client group.
- Reflect on whether these concerns are based on real life experience.

Before unpacking the patient's work tasks in detail, I will consider this job in a more general sense first.

The patient's overall job description

The difficult work of managing a long term condition falls primarily on the patient and their family. Their measures of the 'effectiveness' of that work are likely to be very different from that of the professional team engaged in this collaborative effort (Turner & Kelly, 2000). These measures, too, are likely to be intersubjective: how we tell the story of our health status is a social production. For example, a family member may offer an alternative perspective on a health matter such as 'Oh, I think you've had a much better week' and go on to lay out their evidence for this assertion, in turn revising the current understanding of all concerned. Person-centred effectiveness measures, therefore, are complex and tenuous. Therein lies the potential for successful collaboration and effective management, or for misunderstanding and dissatisfaction.

Whatever the specific long term condition and the specific work in hand, it takes place in a temporal context (Radley, 1994). To live with a long term condition is a job for life and all the work that the patient does is situated within this conceptual, interpretive framework. So, for example, sticking to the recommended diabetic diet today requires little effort but tomorrow, or perhaps next week, it could be excruciatingly difficult for a multitude of different reasons. The day-to-day challenges of this work will go on for this person's forever, interacting with both the minutia and major milestones of their lived experience. Ricoeur (1984) argues that the use of narrative enables people to organize (and reorganize) their temporal existence as a sense-making strategy – 'I was doing this, then this happened and then I realized that what had happened before was due to this, etc.' Those with the appropriate cognitive ability will do the ongoing work of narrating their own story about their own long term condition. This unfolding story is the context in which the collaborating team has to work if they are to be person-centred, but it may be highly incongruent with the story required by the practitioner's employing authority and professional codes. It takes a skilled practitioner to effectively translate across these social divides and make the professional story promote the patient's health.

I will now turn from this broad context to outlining the themes from which a patient's tasks can be distilled. Charmaz (2000: p. 278) provides a useful analysis of a wide range of social and psychological studies concerning the lived experience of chronic illness. Importantly, she notes how investigators, despite many different starting points, have found:

> 'remarkably similar themes: ambiguity and uncertainty, autonomy and control, stigma and shame, isolation and connection and loss and reconstruction of self.'

These personal experiences are located by Charmaz (2000) within a series of issues to be tackled (these issues are distinguished for analytical purposes; in real life they will intersect). The patient's experience of developing a long term condition is placed in a context of their *prior assumptions about health and illness*. For example, given our enormous Western preoccupations with health and lifestyle, their moral overtones and injunctions for living a good life (Leichter, 1997), some people may feel shame and guilt at the point of diagnosis: 'this is all my fault – if only I'd eaten less/exercised more/given up smoking/taken more care of my diet, etc.' Others, of course, may have more fatalistic perspectives but whatever the specifics of the individual case, these prior assumptions will be an important part of the person's story and their ability to do their job. Building on the seminal work of Bury (1982), Charmaz (2000) discusses how a long term condition causes *biographical disruption*. The person's assumptions about who they are and the kind of life that they will go on to lead are often shattered by ill health. Loss then is a major theme that reverberates through the person's whole life from, for example, losing financial certainty to their sexual confidence.

In a very practical sense, the patient has to manage their illness. Charmaz (2000) explains how this involves learning what illness means, normalizing illness and regimes and developing illness management strategies. All the activities associated with these tasks assemble over time and lived experience. A person with rheumatoid arthritis has to learn what, for them, is the best balance of activity and rest, where to buy shoes that can be put on and taken off unaided, and how to carry on 'as normal' as best they can. Managing the social stigma of ill health is a specific illness management strategy that Charmaz (2000) considers in some detail. The rheumatoid arthritis sufferer may stagger when he stands up in the restaurant because his joint stiffness has unbalanced him but observers may think that he is drunk. He has to make decisions as to how he should manage what Goffman (1963) calls a 'spoiled' identity: should he explain himself to strangers? Should he make a joke of it? Should he just ignore it and try and not care what other people think of him? Learning which strategies fit best in different circumstances is vital work when living in a world where health is considered the social norm (Radley, 1994).

Von Korff et al. (1997: p. 1097) consider what they refer to as 'self-care' from a biomedical, behaviourally focused perspective and discuss the importance of developing care systems capable of delivering what chronically ill people require. Their discussion works from the premise that effective services are based on a collaborative effort between the patient, their family and the health care system. Based on a careful reading of a wide range of evidence they assert (pp. 1098–1099) that a number of 'essential elements' have to be in place for successful collaboration: a collaborative definition of problems, a system of targeting, goal setting and planning, a continuum of self-management training and support services, and active, sustained follow-up.

Despite the emphasis on collaboration, their work does appear to assume that there is a certain path to be established and followed. Their writing of matters such as poor treatment compliance and unhealthy habits which are to be tackled through the collaboratively identified strategies, indicate just who they think has the right to define the correct course of action. From a patient's standpoint this sense of certainty may be an important stabilizer within their shattered world, but it may not always be delivered in practice because the treatment of many long-standing conditions is an uncertain matter. On the other hand, it may deviate strongly from the patient's own measures of effectiveness and a life well lived. Nevertheless, their 'essential elements' offer useful ideas for practitioners. Clearly, to agree what the difficulties are to be worked on makes good sense, as does the idea of agreeing on goals (those measures of effectiveness) and how to achieve them.

Von Korff et al. (1997) argue that services need to be in place to teach self-management skills and to support patients in learning these skills. They emphasize that these efforts should be individualized and sensitive to patients' varying states of readiness and motivation. Their case that patient contact should be sustained over the long term includes evidence about an improved quality of life for particular groups of patients and a reduction in the use of inpatient services. These essential elements of collaborative management sit well with current policy (DOH, 2005) and the development of case manager and community matron roles (Murphy, 2004; DOH, 2006).

From this brief analysis of the papers by Charmaz (2000) and Von Korff et al. (1997) I shall now move on to developing a set of patients' tasks.

The tasks of self-managing a long term condition: the person specification

Comparing the work discussed above shows that resolving the issues raised by Charmaz (2000) is integral to the more behaviourally focused essential elements recommended by Von Korff et al. (1997). For example, in order to have a 'cool' and rational conversation about agreeing on the specific problems to be worked on, the patient requires a high degree of emotional equilibrium: they need to be able to listen carefully, to think calmly and constructively, to narrate their story cogently in a similar vein, and to have confidence in their own point of view whilst interacting with someone who they may perceive as having more social status and power than them. To achieve this meaning construction, a high level of intersubjective and interactional functioning is required and this is a 'big ask' of someone experiencing the emotional turbulence of major loss (Neimeyer & Anderson, 2002). Furthermore, the ability to agree on a set of goals assumes a comfortable clarity about future wishes and intentions. Again, we can see how huge a challenge this would be to a person struggling with biographical disruption. They may be angry, distressed and confused over the future direction of their life. Von Korff et al. (1997) recommend that goal setting should be small scale and realistic, on the face of it an eminently sensible idea but potentially problematic for the patient. Who, we might ask, is interested in discussing the achievement of a short walk into the garden, when previously it was this same person who created and maintained its vibrant beauty? Is it reasonable to expect a person who used to climb mountains to calmly discuss learning how to operate a wheelchair? With these examples in mind I propose the following tasks and consider how the resource of good mental health is a necessary condition for their pursuance.

For the purposes of positive self-management and in-context recovery (a process often referred to as adjustment), the patient/person (and their family) are required to do the following:

1 Review and revise their prior assumptions about health and illness.
2 Successfully mourn the multiple losses that their long term condition has forced upon them and contemplate further future losses.
3 Actively engage in learning what being ill means for them in a practical sense.
4 Actively engage in learning about their condition and what experts recommend for its management.
5 Keep things as normal as possible.
6 Develop new routines to accommodate compliance with prescribed medical regimes and actively engage in day-to-day problem-solving.
7 Deal constructively with the reaction of others to their ill health.
8 Make new plans for their life in light of changed circumstances.
9 Confidently express their point of view and negotiate goals with health and social care practitioners, giving reports of their progress and, if necessary, account for their non-progress.

This is not intended to be an exhaustive list, nor are these tasks assumed to follow on neatly from each other or be addressed to the same degree in every case: person specifications always have caveats! They are intended to provide an analytical framework for the consideration of mental health matters and now I turn to the argument that good mental health is a necessary condition for being able to carry out this work.

Action Learning Point

• Apply this 'person specification' to a known person with a long term condition.
• Consider their adjustment process and progress using this framework.

The necessary condition of mental health for meeting the person specification

There is much less written about mental health than mental ill health. The mental health of individuals is often associated with the idea of resilience (this is sometimes referred to as psychological hardiness), that is, the ability to cope with both the ordinary and extraordinary demands of living. To cope is to gain as much mastery as is possible over one's circumstances and wrapped up in this activity is hope. In this context, I intend by this a sense that it is worth struggling with the difficulties that the long term condition imposes because life still holds the possibility of joy and satisfaction. From the original work of Lazarus and Folkman (1984), psychological theory proposes that coping methods can be divided into two main strategies: problem-focused coping and emotion-focused coping. The former involves direct engagement with a problem. For example, a person newly diagnosed with diabetes makes a lot of effort to learn about her condition and carefully develops a diet plan that she knows is likely to be manageable for her. It is argued that problem-focused coping is more often engaged in when the person believes that they will be able to gain mastery over the difficulty they are facing, whereas emotion-focused coping is used in situations where there is no obvious solution (Wilkinson & Campbell, 1997). So, in the case above, the person with diabetes cannot make this go away. She decides to seek the support of her friends in listening to her talk about her frustration and sadness about her diagnosis and all its meanings for her. This narrative process – 'this is what has happened to me and this has changed who I am' – has the potential to enable a new life story to emerge. Effective coping is associated with a sense of 'self-efficacy', literally a belief that we have the capability and capacity to manage what is facing us (Wilkinson & Campbell, 1997). Again it is clear that this belief is cross-cut by the lived experience of hope and that our pre-morbid sense of self-efficacy and overall mental health status is implicated in the person's capacity for adjustment.

Neimeyer and Anderson (2002: pp. 48–51) propose that the personal reconstruction of meaning is essential for positive adjustment to loss. They argue that this process involves 'sense making', 'benefit finding' and 'identity reconstruction' and we can see how a sense of self-efficacy would be the engine for these challenging processes.

Mental health is implicated in how people feel about themselves and others, in their thinking and in how they make sense of the world around them. Furthermore, mental health affects our ability to learn and to express ourselves effectively (DOH, 2001). Drawing a clear line between mental health and mental ill health can be problematic, particularly in the boundary between the distress that can accompany a nasty life event and a depressive condition, but these distinctions are made routinely and patients/persons can largely be trusted to know the difference.

Having established what mental health is, we can now return to the person specification and 'unpack' its relationship to mental health.

Individual tasks in the person specification

Review and revise prior assumptions about health and illness

Achieving this task requires a measure of 'psychological mindedness' – that is, the capacity and motivation to reflect on thinking and feeling and, in this case, to do this in relation to their previous assumptions about health and ill health. For example, a person may have assumed that they would live to 'a ripe old age' because this is their family's normal pattern. Persons who have previously fully adopted the recommendations for a healthy life may be very angry and disappointed with their new status. They may feel a strong sense of injustice – 'it's not fair' and 'why me?' Chronic illness brings huge uncertainty and these previous assumptions are inevitably shattered. The person needs to rethink the implications of this change for their future and this is likely to involve bearing deep emotional pain. Facing distress requires self-efficacy; in this case, a belief that emotional pain can be endured and survived. This belief, too, is critical for the next task.

Successfully mourn the multiple losses that the long term condition has forced upon the person and contemplate further future losses

The experience of biographical disruption (Bury, 1982) reverberates into every aspect of the person's life and small matters can undo fragile emotional equilibrium, leading to what can feel like frightening emotional chaos. The losses sustained have to be mourned and this may be an untidy, episodic process, particularly so with the emergent nature of the morbidity associated with a long term condition. The work of mourning is tough; it requires the person to give themselves permission and support to grieve. This entails a sense of self-respect and a belief that grieving is a normal and natural process, not a character defect, a sign of moral weakness or a sign of madness. Hope, no matter how tiny and difficult to grasp, is intrinsic to this.

Actively engage in learning what being ill means in a practical sense

To be actively engaged in any activity requires energy and motivation. The latter is particularly important when the former is low, and facing the practical difficulties of a long term condition demands determination and persistence. Again it is clear how these emotional drivers are wrapped up in self-efficacy. A belief in the ability to reach a goal is what spurs a person on, but in this case people have to accept their limitations too. The person has to find a balance between the hard struggle of reaching a far off but attainable goal and accepting that some things can no longer be done. The latter necessitates self-respect and a concomitant willingness to reconsider their personal symbols of a decent life.

Actively engage in learning about the condition and what experts recommend for its management

Just how much a person wants to know about their condition and treatment is highly variable. However, co-operating with treatment plans does entail learning and this is more likely to be achieved when a person can 'think straight'. Nichols (1993: pp. 69–74) observes that there are many potential barriers to this, relating to current states of mental health. These include dislocation and confusion, emotional arousal and psychological shock, and selective listening and forgetting. The experience of fatigue may make concentration difficult. This task then is unlikely to be achieved in 'one go' and knowing enough to co-operate with treatment may take effort over a period of time, which, in turn, requires motivation.

Keep things as normal as possible

The need to keep things as normal as possible is related to the desire to minimize the experience of biographical disruption. Marris (1974) claims that the preservation of whatever aspects of personhood that can be hung onto is at the heart of grieving. This work of conservation enables the process of integrating the long term condition into the person's biography, rather than being completely engulfed by it – becoming, for example, a person with diabetes rather than a diabetic. This requires a sense of identity and some measure of confidence in that identity – something that we might call self-esteem.

Develop new routines to accommodate compliance with prescribed medical regimes and actively engage in day-to-day problem-solving

Developing new routines requires attention to detail. It entails the ability to organize yourself; to think through the steps required in complex activities and to remember to do things. This necessitates clear thinking and strong motivation and, as proposed above, the latter involves hope. The person has to believe that making the effort to do these things is worth it. This is unlikely to be a straightforward cost–benefit analysis and requires problem-solving. For example, taking a diuretic is simultaneously disabling and symptom relieving. Minimizing the former and living with the consequences may be preferable to the social difficulty on a day out of requesting frequent and inconvenient toilet stops. Being a patient also requires the task of accommodating appointments with health and social care practitioners. Despite the intentions of providing person-centred services, the reality is that patients, on the whole, have to co-operate with more powerful timetables. This seems to be particularly problematic in relation to care within the person's home, probably because this is where we most expect to be able to follow our own preferences. For example, a person may prefer to go to bed in the small hours and rise late but may have to fit in with something quite different if they are to receive personal care. Accepting these important inconveniences with good grace requires equanimity[2] – a state more likely to be reached having adjusted effectively to current circumstances.

Deal constructively with the reaction of others to ill health

Dealing with the stigma, curiosity and loving care of others is yet another challenge to be faced. Again, self-esteem is required if the person is not to be psychologically crushed by the consequences of stigma and stranger curiosity/embarrassment. Being ill changes relationships and their dynamics. A well-established balance of reciprocity maybe destabilized, the person may witness their partner struggling and feel helpless in ameliorating this. These changes have to be worked through, requiring the emotional capacity and motivation to engage with the arising difficulties.

Make new plans for the person's life in light of changed circumstances

Building a new future is embedded in the person's need to reconstruct their identity in the light of their long term condition. They are a changed person, now living a different life. Again this process requires self-efficacy: a belief that the future still

---

[2] I am not suggesting that this is what patients should do in these circumstance but have observed that this is normally what does take place.

holds promise and is worth planning for. This reconstruction process takes place through the routines of daily living and social interaction, whereby a new life story emerges over time.

Confidently express points of view and negotiate goals with health and social care practitioners, giving reports of progress and, if necessary, account for non-progress

As discussed above, mental health is implicated in the ability to communicate effectively. If patients are to be 'experts' in their own condition and to collaborate with care providers, they require interactional confidence. Nichols (1993: p. 70) refers to the 'socioeducational gulf' as a barrier to this communication. Patients need to be able to translate medical and organizational speak as a precursor to effective communication. It takes assertiveness to ask questions and to play an equal role in negotiating treatment goals and plans. It takes emotional strength to have a different point of view when in a position of enormous social and physical vulnerability. And it takes resilience to cope with the judgemental disapproval of practitioners when, perhaps for very good reasons, the patient has not stuck to the plan and gone off script.

In analysing the relationship of mental health to the tasks of effectively self-managing a long term condition, I have demonstrated how mental health is of fundamental importance. Mental health promotion therefore is a key part of practitioners' work in this field – it is not an added extra to be conducted by mental health experts (who are unlikely to be available); it is about engaging with the *person* who has a long term condition. The following section turns to how practitioners can promote mental health in this context.

Promoting the mental health of people with long term conditions

Initially I intend to consider the care of people who already have mental ill health prior to the onset of a physical long term condition.

It is well established that people with severe and enduring mental health problems (such as schizophrenia) are more likely to have physical ill health than the rest of the population and three times more likely to die early as a consequence (Rahka & McKeown, 2006). Moreover, this group are less likely to exercise as compared to the general populace for a variety of reasons including social isolation and difficulties with volition. These matters are now firmly on the agenda of mental health services and it should be acknowledged that this is an area of care in urgent need of development (DOH, 1999a; National Institute for Clinical Excellence, 2002). For the purposes of this current discussion, the important issue is that non-mental health practitioners involved with people who have long term conditions are likely to encounter those with co-morbid mental illness. Given the discussion above, it is evident that this group will face particularly acute difficulties with the goal of effective self-management for their long term condition.

The special measures required in promoting the mental health of this population involve their initial identification and collaboration across the health and social care network. The goal of the latter should be a collaboratively and systematically designed treatment plan that is co-ordinated and regularly reviewed by a named professional. The identification of this patient group may not always be straight-forward. The simplest way to approach this issue is directly: at the point of assessing a person with a long term condition, they can be sensitively asked if they are being, or have been, treated for a mental illness. It is unhelpful to avoid this issue, particularly if this avoidance is wrapped up in the social embarrassment embedded in stigma. A straightforward enquiry, delivered in a non-judgemental tone normalizes the issue and conveys its routine, non-threatening nature. There are many colloquialisms used to describe mental illness and these can be used to good effect to open up a line of enquiry. For example, 'Have you ever had any trouble with your nerves?' or 'Are you having any treatment for your mental health at the moment?' If the answer is positive in relation to current treatment, the assessment should pursue the patient's permission to make contact with their mental health worker (this person may be known to the patient as their 'care co-ordinator') and to try and understand what their difficulties are.

People with severe and enduring mental health problems who are in contact with secondary mental health services will be in receipt of a 'care programme' (DOH, 1999b). This refers to a systematic, multidisciplinary process whereby the person's mental health is assessed, a care programme delivered and regularly reviewed. The care co-ordinator is responsible for the systematic organization of the person's care and this includes consideration of their physical health. Care co-ordinators are usually community mental health nurses or mental health social workers. If it is difficult to establish who this is from the patient and their family it should be evident from their primary care notes. Another avenue is to contact the local mental health service and ask to speak with the person who is operating the 'single point of entry system'.

Having made this contact, a professional conversation needs to consider how best to collaborate in the patient's interest – what is the care package most likely to optimize the person's whole health? This is not a time to shy away from asking difficult questions. For example, does this person have a history of deliberate self-harm, suicide attempts, self-neglect, social withdrawal or violence? What is this patient's 'relapse signature'? This phrase describes what is known about the patient's prodromal state (Knight, 2002). For example, becoming perplexed and anxious may be a sign of impending acute psychosis; becoming much more talk-ative may signal a hypomanic episode. These prodromal symptoms usually appear two to six weeks prior to relapse. Recognizing them provides a window of opportunity for effective crisis resolution and it follows that the practitioner should know what to do in a crisis. Other important avenues to pursue include medication management, including possible interaction effects and psychological/cognitive issues that need to be worked with. For instance, the patient may have a short attention span and difficulties in absorbing new information. This has enormous implications for learning about their long term condition and its effective manage-ment. Health education may need to be parcelled out in small chunks; things may need to be repeated several times. The crucial issue is not to make assumptions about your ability to convey health information in a way that is useful to the person and their family – an issue for all patients, not just those with mental health problems (Radley, 1994). Those who are depressed and anxious may perceive health information in a negative way and have a low sense of self-efficacy. For example, a smoker who develops congestive obstructive pulmonary disease may see this as just punishment for their 'bad behaviour' and this perception clearly has ramifications for treatment concordance. A common attitude to people with debilitating and distressing conditions is 'well, no wonder they are depressed'. This belief is only useful for health promotion as a precursor to empathy and a therapeutic relationship, that is, if it leads to careful consideration of how to improve the person's mental health. Used as a 'counsel of despair' it leads to low treatment expectations and apathy in the care system; these prejudices can literally kill people.

Case study 1

A general practice nurse, Bob, was asked to see a new 64-year-old patient called John with regard to his newly diagnosed diabetes. On meeting him for the first time the nurse noticed that John seemed rather odd. He looked slightly dishevelled and generally unwell. He smelled of alcohol (though did not appear intoxicated) and his tremulous fingers were nicotine stained. Some of his conversation seemed out of place and he appeared unable to concentrate on the matters at hand. Bob was not confident that John understood the changes he urgently needed to make to his diet. John was repeatedly concerned about having to take 'more tablets'. Bob asked John what tablets he took and he replied that he took something for his nerves. This opened up a new line of enquiry and Bob found out that John was under the care of the local mental health service and John was able to give Bob the name of his psychiatrist. Bob reviewed John's medical record and found a recent letter from a mental health social worker who had added 'care co-ordinator' to her title. Bob sought John's permission to contact the social worker to discuss his needs but John initially was not too keen on this. However, when Bob offered to try and make contact in his presence John agreed and even when this strategy did not work out initially it seemed to reassure John that Bob just wanted to help. Contact was followed by a meeting between John, Bob and the social worker, and the latter was able to tell Bob about John's mental illness and treatment. Their meeting led to an updated care programme that included John's diabetic treatment and a list of signs that should alert the mental team to deterioration in his condition. They all took away a copy of the care programme and they agreed to review John's progress at a specific point in the future.

Given that good mental health is an essential condition for the effective self-management of long term conditions, it is critical to treat those who have mental ill health and, if necessary, to act as their advocate for treatment, particularly where other professionals may get caught up with the counsel of despair. In these treatment contexts it is important to be pragmatic rather than dogmatic. For example, cognitive behavioural therapy may have been shown to be as effective as antidepressants (National Institute for Clinical Excellence, 2004) but if there is a long waiting list for it locally and if it cannot be delivered in a way that is sensitive to the patient's physical ill health then the antidepressant will be a better option.

Providing conditions that enable self-efficacy and social support are the bedrock of mental health promotion (see below). The former can be achieved by constructively challenging destructive cognitions and collaborating in setting small, achievable goals alongside coping strategies. Working together in an 'experimental mode' can be useful: 'I wonder if trying X might help you feel just a tiny bit better – maybe you could experiment with that on two days this week and you can tell me if it helped or not. I do know it is likely to be really difficult for you – can you think of anything that would help you do it?' and so forth. Any success, no matter how small, should be celebrated and the patient's family should be drawn into this strategy as supporters. A lack of success can be supportively investigated, opening up opportunities for new problem-solving strategies, rather than being approached as a sign of hopelessness and a wilful lack of co-operation.

Working with people who have co-morbid mental ill health and physical ill health can present very particular challenges to the provision of an effective care package. The practitioner's sense of self-efficacy is critical too and assertive collaboration and confidence-building steps will help grow it.

Those patients who have a past history of mental ill health but who are not in current treatment may be very vulnerable to a further episode given the adjustment demands discussed above. It makes sense to get some detailed information about their previous problems, what helped them get better before, and to enquire how they feel their mental health is currently. A useful frame of reference here is context, functional disruption and timing: 'What do they think caused it? Was there anything upsetting going on in their life at that time? Did it interfere with their normal activities? Exactly how did it do this? How long did it go on for? Would anything indicate to them that it might be happening again?' This issue should be sensitively kept on the agenda throughout their care, enabling a rapid response if their mental health should deteriorate. In addition to these special measures, patients with previously identified mental health problems should receive the same mental health promotion activities as everybody else.

Wilkinson and Campbell (1997) argue that the best evidence for the factors that promote psychological hardiness (mental health) concern social support and self-efficacy. There is a growing evidence base, too, about the mental health benefits of exercise (Faulkner & Taylor, 2005) but clearly this needs careful, in-context consideration regarding the patient's long term condition. These activities can be positively engaged in and routinely promoted by practitioners. Practitioners underestimate the potential power of social support and are observed to minimize their efforts in this field. A case manager recently said to me 'I just listened – that's all'. This was in the context of a much improved situation for the person involved, including a dramatic reduction in emergency hospital admissions. If we do not listen, we cannot problem-solve. Social support does not make the problem go away. It does make it more bearable and it gives people the interactional and intersubjective opportunity to make sense of what has happened to them, to find benefit in what has happened to them and to reconstruct their identity (thus promoting their self-efficacy). The vehicle for this social support process is the patient's story (Murray, 1999; Neimeyer & Anderson, 2002) about *their* long term condition in the context of *their* life. The patient's tasks identified above could be conversational starting points. For example, 'Is the treatment causing you any problems? What have you managed to do this week that you are pleased about? What do you miss the most these days?' Practitioners, often most comfortable with 'doing', underestimate the health benefit of the social support that they are in such a good position to provide and promote from the person's social network. It can be useful to conceptualize the expression of distress as an important mechanism for adjustment, as opposed to something that should be stopped by phrases such as 'you need to be positive'. To listen and to comfort someone is a great gift but this can be hard to provide in the hurly-burly of practice. A lack of time is often perceived as a common barrier to this kind of work (Nichols, 1993; Botti et al.,

2006) but if it is not regarded as an essential component of effective care, the time will never be found. Even more compellingly, patients with good mental health will be better at self-managing their own condition and this, in turn, will free up the time of health and social care workers. Put simply, it is a good investment.

Practitioners should encourage the personal social support available to the patient and educate them about its enormous value. Not everyone will want to talk at length, some may hardly want to talk at all but this does not equate to a lack of concern with, or benefit from, social support. Learning how to get behind a person's emotional screen in a way that is right for them, just like any other skill, takes practice. This does not mean pressurizing people into disclosing things that they do not want to. It does mean inviting them to discuss things they would like to. This requires practitioners to practically demonstrate that *they* have emotional resilience – that they will not try and stop a person crying, expressing fear and distress or being angry. That they can bear to listen and share the person's hurt. That they will not turn away, use patronizing platitudes or use tactics to shut down the person's distress. It is crucial to trust patients to know what it is alright for them to talk about. Practitioners' fears of 'getting in too deep' are about themselves, not about their patients. It is useful to embrace the patient's story as a therapeutic act in its own right, rather than getting into feeling that solutions have to be found immediately. This is where a sense of inadequacy and helplessness can be self-generated – a poor condition for the practitioner's perceptions of self-efficacy.

A useful strategy for helping ambivalent people change their health behaviour is a process called 'motivational interviewing'. Originally developed for helping people with alcohol problems, interest has grown in its use, including in the field of diabetes (Welch et al., 2006). Ambivalence should not be regarded as a personality flaw. The effective self-management of a long term condition requires changes that are really difficult to make and it is only the patient that can do it. Motivational interviewing is aimed at enabling patients to examine and resolve their ambivalence about changing their behaviour (Rollnick & Miller, 1995: p. 325). Welch et al. (2006) note that motivational interviewing techniques are based on three underpinning ideas: (i) working in partnership; (ii) respect of the patient's independence and capacity to find solutions to their difficulties; and (iii) using interactive methods to encourage change. Probably the most important lesson for a practitioner to learn is that giving people who are ambivalent about behaviour change direct advice *does not work* (Rollnick & Miller, 1995). It follows that direct advice reduces, rather than enhances, self-efficacy. On the other hand, providing the non-judgemental opportunity for a patient to discuss the pros and cons of changing something gives them the chance to clarify what they should do and work out how they might go about it. Motivational interviewing also involves attending carefully to the patient's story and supporting their autonomy. This can be challenging when we think we know what is best for someone!

Relating to patients in the various ways described above demands a collaborative and shared expertise style and this does not come easily to all practitioners. Some people are more comfortable with the familiarity and associated procedural and practical paraphernalia of being the professional expert and feel very exposed when trying out new interpersonal strategies. Social support is important for a practitioner's mental health too. Botti et al. (2006) investigated the barriers that experienced nurses perceived in providing psychosocial support for patients with cancer. Although set in a particular disease and acute care context, their findings appear congruent for such support in many long term conditions. The barriers found were of a professional and personal nature. The professional barriers included high workload and a consequent lack of time. The nurses studied felt more comfortable using physical nursing tasks rather than direct enquiry as an entry into the person's psychosocial world. 'Doing' appeared to enable the practitioner to communicate with the patient but if time was short this tactic could be avoided. We can read into this that physical care was prioritized over psychosocial care in the face of a busy workload. A further barrier was a lack of knowledge regarding the patient's medical condition. The nurses expressed the view that a lack of knowledge led to a lack of confidence in engaging with the patient. Again, this points to a need to be 'in charge' of the interpersonal encounter. This lack of knowledge was also associated with communications within the interprofessional team. The nurses needed to be on top of what was going on with the person's treatment and care in order to be at ease with more personal encounters.

The research participants opined that continuity of care was the basis of building a trusting relationship with the patient and they saw this as the medium through which psychosocial care was successfully delivered. Given this model, they perceived that full-time practitioners had more of an opportunity to develop a relationship than those working part time. However, those managing to build such a relationship with their patient perceived that this increased their sense of isolation from their colleagues. Straying into this more personal territory was regarded as emotionally demanding and exposing and participants were concerned with how to do psychosocial care in a way that did not harm them. Back in 1960, Isabel Menzies studied the emotional work of nurses in a hospital setting and concluded that the social system of the institution operated as a defence against the anxiety that arises in nurse–patient relationships. These psychological barriers then are keenly felt but must be worked through if the mental health of patients is to be nurtured and promoted. It may be that case workers, as opposed to hospital-based nurses, have more malleable barriers because they can exert more control over their working environment. However, such practitioners need effective social support systems such as clinical supervision if they are to be able to effectively engage in mental health promotion work.

In situations where the mental health promotion efforts discussed above do not appear to be working, it is important to carefully assess the person's mental health and take appropriate action. For example, treating depression is clearly of critical importance. Depression erodes hope (Rowe, 2003) and hope is a necessary condition for healthy adjustment. Similarly, anxiety disorders will severely disrupt effective self-management. It is the antithesis of self-efficacy and needs to be treated robustly.

Action Learning Point

- Review your skills in mental health promotion and develop a plan for their further development.
- Ask a trusted colleague to give you some feedback on your listening skills and consciously practise them.

This section of the chapter has discussed various methods for promoting the mental health of people with long term conditions, including those who have mental illness. These methods promote self-efficacy and social support and these are the foundations of psychological hardiness. Being mentally healthy is a necessary condition for being able to successfully meet the person specification for the work of effectively self-managing a long term condition. This is undoubtedly a tough job for the person with the long term condition but mental health promotion efforts will make it more manageable. It is argued, too, that there are barriers to practitioners providing mental health promotion activities and note that growing through these barriers is also a tough job that requires adjustment, which, in turn, requires self-efficacy and social support.

Conclusions

This chapter has presented the argument that mental health is critical to the effective management of long term conditions. Consequently, the work of mental health promotion is regarded as an essential component of professional health and social care. By examining the lived experience of people with chronic illness from a psychosocial and biomedical perspective, the patient's role was conceptualized as a form of work. From this stance, a person specification, a list of tasks, was developed and the relationship between the patient's mental health and their ability to carry out this job was explored. Finally, the implications of this debate for the routine practice of mental health promotion was developed into recommendations for practice. This job description is a tough one too. It means stepping out of the safe, expert professional role and becoming a collaborative partner in the relationship. This may be uncomfortable until well practised and adjusted to, and practitioners will benefit from effective clinical leadership and clinical supervision in their efforts to gain more confidence in this important area of practice.

References

Baune, B.T., Adrian, I. & Jacobi, F. (2007) Medical disorders affect health outcome and general functioning depending on co-morbid major depression in the general population. *Journal of Psychosomatic Research* **62**: 109–118.

Botti, M., Endacott, R., Watts, R., Cairns, J., Lewis, K. & Kenny, A. (2006) Barriers in providing social support for patients with cancer. *Cancer Nursing* **29** (4): 309–316.

Bury, M. (1982) Chronic illness as disruption. *Sociology of Health and Illness* **4**: 167–182.

Charmaz, K. (2000) Experiencing chronic illness. In: G.L. Albrecht, R. Fitzpatrick & S.C. Scrimshaw (eds) *The Handbook of Social Studies in Health and Medicine*. London, Sage Publications, pp. 277–292.

Crossley, N. (2000) Emotions, psychiatry and social order. A Habermasian approach. In: S.J. Williams, J. Gabe & M. Calnan (eds) *Health, Medicine and Society. Key theories, future agendas*. London, Routledge, pp. 278–296.

Department of Health (1999a) *The National Service Framework for Mental Health*. London, Department of Health.

Department of Health (1999b) *Effective Care Co-ordination in Mental Health Services*. London, Department of Health.

Department of Health (2001) *Making it Happen. A guide to mental health promotion.* London, Department of Health.

Department of Health (2005) *The National Service Framework for Long-term Conditions.* London, Department of Health.

Department of Health (2006) *Caring for People with Long-term Conditions: An education framework for community matrons and case managers.* London, Department of Health.

Faulkner, G.E.J. & Taylor, A.H. (2005) *Exercise, Health and Mental Health. Emerging relationships.* London, Routledge.

Goffman, E. (1963) *Stigma.* Eaglewood Cliffs, NJ, Prentice Hall.

Guthrie, E. (1996) Emotional disorder in chronic illness: psychotherapeutic interventions. *British Journal of Psychiatry* **168**: 265–273.

Knight, A. (2002) Relapse prevention intervention in psychosis. In: N. Harris, S. Williams & T. Bradshaw (eds) *Psychosocial Interventions for People with Schizophrenia.* Basingstoke, Palgrave, pp. 130–142.

Lazarus, R.S. & Folkman, S. (1984) *Stress, Appraisal and Coping.* New York, Springer.

Leichter, H.M. (1997) Lifestyle correctness and the new secular morality. In: A.M. Brandt & P. Rozin (eds) *Morality and Health.* London, Routledge.

Marris, P. (1974) *Loss and Change.* London, Routledge and Kegan Paul.

Mentality & National Institute for Mental Health (2004) *Healthy Body and Mind. Promoting healthy living for people who experience mental distress.* London, Mentality and the National Institute for Mental Health.

Menzies, I.E.P. (1960) A case-study in the functioning of social systems as a defence against anxiety. *Human Relations.* London, Tavistock Publications.

Murphy, E. (2004) Care management and community matrons for long-term conditions. *British Medical Journal* **329**: 1251–1252.

Murray, M. (1999) The storied nature of health and illness. In: M. Murray & K. Chamberlain (eds) *Qualitative Health Psychology. Theories and methods.* London, Sage Publications, pp. 47–63.

National Institute for Clinical Excellence (2002) *Schizophrenia: Core interventions in the treatment and management of schizophrenia in primary and secondary care.* Clinical Guideline No. 1. London, National Institute for Clinical Excellence.

National Institute for Clinical Excellence (2004) *Depression: Management of depression in primary and secondary care.* Clinical Guideline No. 23. London, National Institute for Clinical Excellence.

Neimeyer, R.A. & Anderson, A. (2002) Meaning reconstruction theory. In: N. Thompson (ed.) *Loss and Grief. A guide for human services practitioners.* Basingstoke, Palgrave, pp. 45–64.

Nichols, K.A. (1993) *Psychological Care in Physical Illness*, 2nd edn. London, Chapman and Hall.

Pitceathly, C. & Maguire, P. (2003) The psychological impact of cancer on patients' partners and other key relatives: a review. *European Journal of Cancer* **39**: 1517–1524.

Radley, A. (1994) *Making Sense of Illness. The social psychology of health and disease.* London, Sage Publications.

Rahka, R. & McKeown, M. (2006) Health checks for those with SMI. *Mental Health Nursing* **25** (4): 10–13.

Ricoeur, P. (1984) *Time and Narrative*, Vol. 1. Chicago, University of Chicago Press.

Rollnick, S. & Miller, W.R. (1995) What is motivational interviewing? *Behavioural and Cognitive Psychotherapy* **23**: 325–334.

Rowe, D. (2003) *Depression. The way out of your prison*, 3rd edn. Hove, Brunner Routledge.

Social Exclusion Unit (2004) *Mental Health and Social Exclusion.* London, Office of the Deputy Prime Minister.

Taylor, D. & Bury, M. (2007) Chronic illness, expert patients and care transition. *Sociology of Health and Illness* **29** (1): 27–45.

Turner, J. & Kelly, B. (2000) Emotional dimensions of chronic disease. *Western Journal of Medicine* **172**: 124–128.

Von Korff, M.V., Gruman, J., Schaefer, J., Curry, S.J. & Wagner, E.H. (1997) Collaborative management of chronic illness. *Annals of Internal Medicine* **127** (12): 1097–1102.

Welch, G., Rose, G. & Ernst, D. (2006) Motivational interviewing and diabetes: what is it, how is it used and does it work? *Diabetes Spectrum* **19** (3): 5–11.

Wilkinson, J.D. & Campbell, E.A. (1997) *Psychology in Counselling and Therapeutic Practice*. Chichester, John Wiley.

Chapter 7

Managing long term conditions from the child's perspective: aspects of vulnerability and inequalities for children with complex needs

Ruth Thomas

Key points

- Outlining medical and technological advances and increased support for pre-term babies
- Identifying the fact that children suffering trauma and life-limiting conditions are experiencing increased life expectancy with subsequent challenges for their families
- Increasing awareness and recognition of children and young people who regularly provide care for others (who may be siblings) and their specific needs
- Examining issues of vulnerability and inequality
- Looking at developments in legislation and guidance ensuring the needs of identified children, young people and families are met 'seamlessly'
- Exploring the areas of inclusion and support, which can at times prove challenging for the agencies involved

Definitions and terminology

'Long term conditions' is a term that encompasses a wide range of chronic conditions with different levels of associated need. At one end of the continuum there may be a child with well controlled asthma which impacts minimally on their daily life and at the other end of the continuum a child who needs ventilation at home to keep them alive. The term 'complex needs' is often used interchangeably with 'disabled' and 'long term needs' and I shall use the terms interchangeably where appropriate. The child with complex needs may indeed have a disability. The different forms of legislation and guidance relating to children with complex needs will focus on a definition of disability relevant to the time and in context appropriate to its publication. For example, the definition of disability within the Children Act 1989 is:

> 'a child is disabled if he is blind, deaf or dumb or suffers from mental disorder of any kind or is substantially and permanently handicapped by illness, injury or congenital deformity or such other disability as may be prescribed.'

The term 'disability' may be used within this chapter when referring to children with complex needs as this is sometimes used in the literature.

This chapter will focus primarily on two areas that relate to longer term needs. Rather than focus on specific conditions, it will focus on children with complex needs. This may be children with physical, mental or learning disabilities requiring a complex package of care. The first area of focus is children with complex needs who have needs requiring care above and beyond that required by all children. The second area of focus will be on parents and siblings as regular carers of children with complex needs.

The term child/children will be used when referring generally to this patient/client group within this chapter to aid flow and consistency. The term young person/people will be used when specifically referring to those over 12 years of age but under 18. Young carers will be used when referring to children or young people who regularly care for others. Parent will be used when referring to mothers, fathers, adult carers and others with responsibility for caring for the child with complex needs. This chapter will also consider some perspectives of vulnerability and inequalities for children with complex needs.

Children with complex needs

There are estimated to be 11.7 million children aged under 18 years living in England (National Statistics, 2003) and there are approximately 700 000 disabled children aged under 16 years in the UK (Department for Work and Pensions, 2004). Due to the increased survival rates of premature babies and more children surviving trauma and serious illnesses, there are changing patterns of children's and young people's health needs emerging within society. Additionally, with developments in medical treatments, children with life-limiting conditions are now living longer (Farasat & Hewitt-Taylor, 2007). The fact that these groups of children have a diverse range of needs can help or hinder diagnosis and can make identifying appropriate support difficult. Over recent years the demand for community care has increased, with more children with complex needs being cared for in their own homes (Kirk et al., 2005). There are a growing number of children requiring long term ventilation to keep them alive who are now being successfully cared for at home (Kirk et al., 2005; Noyes, 2007). Recent government guidance has advocated care closer to home and the increase in the number of community children's nurses have all contributed to the growing expectation that children with complex needs should be cared for in their own homes. The government's care closer to home strategy aims to support patients, including children, to be nursed at home. *Making it Better: For children and young people* (Department of Health (DOH), 2007) outlines the reconfiguration of services to help meet the needs of children and young people.

Children with complex needs do not want to be seen as different from their peers and often adopt strategies to fit in with their peer group. The reality for families is that they often spend most of their time struggling to fit into 'normal' society (Carnevale, 2007). In addition to having to cope with their child's particular needs, there is also the need to address society's perceptions and expectations. Indeed ventilator-dependent children and their parents report a lower quality of life than their peers. KINDL (see www.kindl.org) measures four domains of quality of a child's life – 'psychological well-being, social relationships, physical functioning and everyday life activities'. This was used in one study (Noyes, 2007) to measure parents' and children's perceptions of the child's quality of life. Results included a significantly lower level of self-esteem than their peer group.

Parents can feel that their children are not high priority for health services due to their prognosis of life-limiting illness or due to longer term needs that will increase without the condition improving. Many may have to make decisions about whether their child's life should continue (Carnevale, 2007).

Underpinning legislation and guidance for children

Over recent years legislation has recognized children as individuals within society rather than as mini adults who are the property of their parents. The main areas of current legislation that recognize the rights of children are outlined below.

United Nations Rights of the Child 1989

The United Nations (UN) Convention on the Rights of the Child 1989 introduced a global Children's Rights Charter, which was an agreed set of principles outlining the best interests of children in order for them to reach their full potential. It advocates that although human rights apply to children as well as adults, children are recognized as a vulnerable group in society with specific needs. It concentrated on four main areas: (i) prevention (in terms of health care, harm, abduction and discrimination); (ii) participation (in decisions affecting the child); (iii) protection (from harm, conflict and exploitation); and (iv) provision (of basic needs, education and security). Though not legislation, it informed the 1989 Children Act and is still used as a benchmark for good practice today. It has been ratified by many countries as a measure of the basic quality of life for all children, acknowledging the best interests of the child as the primary concern. The main articles of the charter relating to children with complex needs are identified under the four headings in Box 1.

> **Box 1: The main articles of the UN Rights of the Child 1989 charter affecting children with complex needs**
>
> | **Prevention** | **Particapation** |
> |---|---|
> | Article 5 Parental guidance
Article 6 Survival and development
Article 18 Parental responsibility: state assistance | Article 12 Respect for the views of the child
Article 13 Freedom of expression |
> | **Protection** | **Provision** |
> | Article 2 Non-discrimination
Article 3 Best interests of the child
Article 4 Protection of rights
Article 19 Protection from all forms of violence
Article 34 Protection from sexual exploitation | Article 16 Right to privacy
Article 23 Children with disabilities
Article 24 Health and health services
Article 27 Adequate standard of living
Article 28 Right to education
Article 29 Goals of education
Article 31 Leisure, play and culture |

Human Rights Act 1998

Children's rights are further recognized within the Human Rights Act 1998 as having the same rights as all persons. The Human rights Act 1998 was implemented in October 2000 and incorporated the European Convention on Human Rights. The fundamental rights apply to all children including those with complex needs (Box 2). Children have historically been subjected to abuse in terms of physical punishment, which was perceived as culturally acceptable normal behaviour (Barber, 2007). Over the last 100 years, however, acknowledgement of children's rights has progressively developed and children's rights are now seen as being on a par with adults' rights (Davis, 2000). Furthermore, vast improvements in the health of children, children's nursing becoming a speciality in its own right, and the advent of the NHS with responsibility for the health and well-being of children and families, have all contributed to the increasing recognition of the importance and value of children and therefore the associated recognition of their rights (Davis, 2000).

> **Box 2: Fundamental rights of the Human Rights Act 1998**
>
> - The right to life
> - Freedom from torture, inhumane and degrading treatment
> - The right to liberty and a fair trial
> - A right to privacy
> - Freedom of conscience
> - Freedom of expression
> - Freedom of assembly
> - The right to marriage and a family
> - Freedom from discrimination

Children Act 1989

Based upon the UN Rights of the Child 1989, the Children Act 1989 provided a legal framework for ensuring all children's needs are met within England. Other parts of the UK have their own versions of the Children Act. It introduced the concept of paramountcy, whereby the welfare of the child is paramount. This recognized that the child's needs be put before parents' wishes in cases of protecting children from harm. Indeed the rights of the parent were overridden if there was risk of significant harm to the child (now superseded in the Children Act 2004, see below). The Children Act 1989 saw the introduction of the term 'child in need', which is defined as a child who is unlikely to (or have opportunity to) achieve or maintain reasonable health or development without local authority provision; or the child's health or development is likely to be impaired or further impaired without provision; or the child has a disability. In this definition 'development' is defined as physical, intellectual, emotional, social or behavioural development. The term 'health' refers to physical or mental health. Children who meet the criteria for being a 'child in need' are entitled to an assessment of their needs.

Special Educational Needs and Disability Act 2001

The area of education was not included within the Disability Discrimination Act 1995. The Special Education Needs and Disability Act 1995 (SENDA) was introduced to address this and is fundamental to enabling inclusion for children with complex needs within the education system. Part 1 of SENDA amends part 4 of the Education Act 1996. This removes the clause that prevented disabled children attending mainstream schools if they wanted to. Schools could utilize the clause of 'incompatible with the efficient education of other children', which prevented many children with complex needs attending mainstream education. Within the new SENDA amendment reasonable steps must be taken to include disabled children within mainstream education. In addition to 'reasonable adjustments' in terms of physical access within the school, general suggestions were made in terms of inclusive strategies such as teaching and learning strategies. This can include delivery of educational content, use of language and use of information formats. Formulating creative ways of delivering and managing teaching and learning can be of benefit to all pupils.

Children Bill 2004

The Children Bill 2004 was the first action to reform the child protection agenda following recommendations from the Laming Report (Laming, 2003). Lord Laming led the public inquiry into the untimely death of Victoria Climbie at the hands of her great aunt and her partner. Focus moved towards a preventative approach in safeguarding children alongside improving services and outcomes for children and families. The Children Bill 2004 is the main driver in implementing the guidance in the 'Every child matters' agenda (Department for Education and Skills (DfES), 2003a). Amongst the 108 recommendations from the Laming Report was the need for a champion for children, stronger responsibility and leadership within social services, and better information sharing between key agencies involved in safeguarding children (Laming, 2003). The introduction of the Children's Commissioner welcomed a champion for children's needs who was charged with leading on the Children Bill, which was the first step in transforming child protection following Lord Laming's recommendations. In relation to accountability and leadership, all local authorities have to appoint a director of children's services and a lead member for children. The formation of children's trusts is to encourage better collaboration of the key agencies. These function at strategic levels and include education, social services and health. Indeed it was suggested that social services and education amalgamate to enable improved accountability and leadership. The formation of a database to track the 11 million children living in England has proved to be problematic as each geographical area and each individual agency will need to have compatible systems. The use of electronic case files was advocated to help in sharing information and identifying problems and thus offering early interventions. In cases of child protection concerns, parents' rights are now overridden if there is 'any cause for concern'. This supersedes the Children Act 1989 where parents' rights were overridden if there was 'risk of significant harm'.

Children Act 2004

Although the Children Act 1989 still stands, the 2004 development incorporates new knowledge and understanding in children's rights and needs since that time. How social services function remains the same but delivery of social services changed with the implementation of the Children Act 2004 (which received royal ascent in November 2004). The Children Act 2004 provided the legal under-pinnings for the 'Every child matters' agenda. Local authorities have a duty to promote interagency working to help improve outcomes for children. Key agencies have to actively promote safeguarding of children. Local Safeguarding Children's Boards replaced the Area Child Protection Committees, with the focus on develop-ing policies and procedures to safeguard children. To enable better sharing of information, databases should be set up that can help track children within the key agencies. Each local authority has a duty to produce a 'Children and young people's plan' in collaboration with other key agencies that outlines agreed provi-sion to meet local need.

'Every child matters' agenda

'Every child matters' (ECM) is the government's initiative aimed at transforming children's services for 0–19-year-olds. It followed the Joint Chief Inspector's Report on safeguarding children (DOH, 2002) and the report on the public inquiry con-ducted by Lord Laming (Laming, 2003) following the death of Victoria Climbie. The government responded with *Keeping Children Safe* (DfES, 2003b) and subse-quently introduced the Green Paper *Every Child Matters* (DfES, 2003a). Consulta-tions with children, parents and carers, and practitioners working with children followed. The ECM agenda recognized the importance of supporting families to care for their children, early intervention was deemed necessary in order to protect children, and the needs of practitioners working with children were addressed. There are five outcomes for children that form the framework for implementing the ECM agenda. During the consultation exercises children reported that they wanted to:

1 Stay safe.
2 Be healthy.
3 Enjoy and achieve.
4 Make a positive contribution.
5 Achieve economic well-being.

In 2004 *Every Child Matters: Change for children* (DfES, 2004a) was published, which provided the national framework based on the five outcomes for implementing the transformation of children's services. There are numerous supporting documents widely available from the Department for Education and Skills website that aim to assist agencies in delivering the ECM agenda (see http://www.dfes.gov.uk/).

Every Child Matters: Next steps (DfES, 2004b) introduced the Children Bill 2004, which provides the statutory requirement of agencies to work together to improve outcomes for children (see above). It further identified four main areas of focus for implementing the ECM agenda that are aimed at improving the well-being of all children and families:

1 Supporting parents and carers.
2 Early intervention and early protection.
3 Accountability and integration.
4 Workforce reform.

National Service Framework for Children, Young People and Maternity Services 2004

The National Service Framework (NSF) for Children, Young People and Maternity Services (DOH/DfES, 2004) is a ten-year plan to improve the health and well-being of all children. It is concerned with the design and delivery of services focused around the needs of children and families. Key areas of good practice are apparent throughout the document and include:

- Increased involvement of children and families in decision-making.
- Promotion of healthy lifestyles.
- Enabling early interventions.
- Needs-led services.
- Tackling health inequalities.
- Promoting the safeguarding of children.

The NSF consists of eleven standards with the first five making up part 1 of the NSF. These are relevant for all children:

1 Promoting health and well-being, identifying needs and intervening early.
2 Supporting parenting (acknowledges 'parents with specific needs' and includes parents of disabled children who should have early identification of their needs and support via effective multiagency approaches).
3 Child-, young person- and family-centred services.
4 Growing up into adulthood (relates to improved access to services, particularly for disabled young people and those in special circumstances, which includes young carers).

5 Safeguarding and promoting the welfare of children and young people. (This is identified as a priority area for all agencies. Procedures and policies should be developed in line with national guidelines and legislation. It stipulates that each local authority is to have a 'Children and young people's plan' as advocated in the Children Bill. This outlines how the main agencies will effectively function as partners and integrated teams in safeguarding children, including responses to children who are actually harmed. In order to identify vulnerable children, a local population profile will be carried out, which will help areas target resources appropriately. Support in the form of supervision should be available for staff working with safeguarding children.)

Part 2 of the NSF comprises standards 6–10 and refers to children in particular circumstances:

6 Children and young people who are ill (children with long term conditions are referred to: 'high quality care is provided . . . which enables them [children with complex needs] to participate as fully as possible in everyday activities').
7 Children and young people in hospital.
8 Disabled children and young people and those with complex health needs (it is acknowledged that inclusion in terms of access to services, including transition to adult services, should be promoted for children with complex needs. It outlines the requirement of including children and families in decision-making and recommends that services are designed to meet the needs of children and families and to encourage inclusion).
9 The mental health and psychological well-being of children and young people (the focus is on inclusion).
10 Medicines for children and young people.

Maternity services (standard 11) are addressed in part 3 but are not considered within this chapter.

The implementation of this guidance is a ten-year plan which, as well as identifying the needs of vulnerable groups of children and young people, will help to address inequalities, particularly in terms of access to services (Box 3).

Although there is legislation and guidance in place to address the specific needs and promote inclusion, there are still additional issues in caring for children with complex needs. The specific issues of vulnerability and inequalities will be addressed in a further section of this chapter. Supporting families in caring for their child with complex needs is an important factor in helping families cope with the demands and challenges that the needs of their children present.

Action Learning Point

- How are government policy and guidelines being implemented in your local practice area to improve services for children with complex needs and their families?
- Consider how the 'Every child matters' agenda (DfES, 2003a, 2004b) and the NSF for Children, Young People and Maternity Services (DOH/DfES, 2004) have been implemented at the local level.
- What might you as an individual do to improve your practice in meeting this agenda?

Box 3: Main aspects of standard 8 of the NSF for Children, Young People and Maternity Services (DOH/DfES, 2004)

Standard

'Children and young people who are disabled or who have complex needs receive co-ordinated, high quality child and family-centred services which are based on assessed needs, which promote social inclusion and, where possible, which enable them and their families to live ordinary lives.' (DOH/DfES, 2004: p. 5)

Vision

'Services to be arranged around needs of the child. Children and families involved in decision making. Appropriate support to participate in family/community activities. (DOH/DfES, 2004: p. 5)

Interventions

- *Promoting social inclusion*: impact of poverty, access to services.
- *Early years/strong foundations*: early identification, integrated diagnosis and assessments, early interventions, co-ordination of health care.
- *Supporting parents/strengthening families*: short term breaks, key workers, information for parents and children, listening and responding to children and their families.
- *Expert Patient Programme.*
- *Education.*
- *Palliative care.*
- *Death of a child.*
- *Safeguarding children.*
- *Transition to adulthood.*
- *Planning and commissioning services.*
- *Training and development.*

Vulnerability and inequalities in health exist for some groups of children, including those with complex needs. The introduction of the ECM agenda and the NSF aim to address these issues by reviewing the ways services are designed and delivered. Services should be child-centred and focused on the whole child and family rather than be illness specific (DfES, 2003a; DOH/DfES, 2004). This is particularly important for children with complex needs who can have many visits to medical appointments for their various conditions (DOH/DfES, 2003). Early intervention is advocated as a preventative measure in terms of ensuring that appropriate help is offered at the right times for children and their families (DOH/DfES, 2003). Successful implementation of the NSF depends on the main agencies working closely together to improve the outcomes for children and their families.

Aspects of vulnerability and inequalities for children with complex needs

Staying safe

Children with disabilities are recognized as being at an increased risk of harm compared to their non-disabled peers (Box 4; Howe, 2006). This includes children with complex needs who have one or more disabilities. Vulnerability and risk are important considerations in safeguarding children. By identifying children and

> **Box 4: Possible factors associated with children with disabilities being at an increased risk of harm (DfES, 2006; Howe, 2006)**
>
> - Children exhibiting demanding behaviours
> - Children needing increased care and supervision
> - Children needing frequent medical/health care procedures
> - Poor child–parent attachment
> - Parents with low stress tolerance
> - Less outside contact than peers
> - Impaired capacity
> - Communication difficulties
> - Resist disclosure as do not want to lose services
> - Vulnerable to bullying and intimidation

families at risk of vulnerability or inequalities, then appropriate packages of care can be put in place. Vulnerability can be defined from differing perspectives. These can relate to the child's capacity to protect him or herself, which puts the responsibility of safeguarding onto the child (Cicchetti & Rogosch, 1997). This can be dependent on other factors. For example, Cicchetti and Rogosh (1997) identified that some children who had suffered harm appeared to be functioning appropriately due to protective factors such as high self-esteem. Barker and Hodes (2004) introduced a number of factors that may contribute to making families vulnerable. Situations (such as divorce and bereavement) leading to poverty and isolation add to family stress levels and thus to an increased risk of harm to the child. This can particularly relate to children with complex needs as the family situation can lead to a parent having to give up work to adopt the caring role, thereby reducing the family income. Many services within the community aimed at families are not geared towards children with complex needs in terms of access and availability. The factors of poverty and isolation can lead to increased stress within the family. When families are stressed they are less likely to cope with their already complex situation and there may be reduced uptake of preventative services, leading to additional stress.

There may be factors associated with poor child–parent attachments, which make children more vulnerable. An attachment refers to an affectionate bond between a child and its main care giver. Bowlby's (1969) theory of attachment focused mainly on the mother and child but he subsequently accepted the important role of significant others in caring for children. Positive attachments ensure protection, food and social interaction for the child. Young children ensure this occurs by using three different methods: signalling (e.g. cooing), aversive behaviour (e.g. crying) and the direct approach (e.g. reaching out). Howe (2006) discussed three different types of attachment relating to disabled children and abuse. Firstly, there are *secure attachments* where parents engage with their children and attend to their needs. Secondly, there are *insecure attachments* which can constitute avoidance measures by the parent (unwilling) and ambivalence (unable). There are many reasons why secure attachments may not occur between a child and parent. Problems within a relationship may affect how a parent relates to their child. Parents with mental health problems may not be able to address their child's needs. Parents with ill or disabled children may not pick up on the signals from the child, or the parents do not receive positive feedback from the child, and the child may then be considered unresponsive (Howe, 2006). The third type of attachment emerges during stressful situations and Howe refers to this as *disorganized*. The care giver who has an avoidant or ambivalent attachment with the child may behave in a way that does not allow the child to adopt their usual strategies. For example, if the care giver is acting in an abusive way or is personally distressed, this causes increased stress to the child who is unable to adopt their usual response.

Parents who understand their child's needs are more likely to parent in an appropriate manner. Where families have realistic expectations of their child and access appropriate support this may help to reduce stress within the family and therefore reduce the likelihood of harm to the child. Aspects of vulnerability and inequalities will be addressed below in relation to the five outcomes of the ECM agenda.

Being safe includes safeguarding children and protecting them from harm. Children are generally recognized as a vulnerable group within society. In this chapter vulnerability will be referred to in terms of being safe from harm. It is acknowledged that disabled children are more likely to be abused than their non-disabled peers (National Society for the Prevention of Cruelty to Children (NSPCC), 2003). The impact of abuse and neglect can not only affect the health and well-being of the individual during childhood, but the effects can continue into adulthood once the abuse or neglect has ceased (DfES, 2006). The additional factors associated with children who have complex needs often makes them more vulnerable than their peer group (Marchant & Page, 1992; DOH/DfES, 2004). Some children and young people may not have the level of intellectual ability to make decisions to keep themselves safe. They may be beholden to the perpetrator's demands and/or threats due to their level of understanding, or communication problems may mean there are difficulties in articulating concerns (NSPCC, 2003). Social services, health and education work closely together to formulate local policies and procedures that take into account the needs of disabled children and their families (DfES, 2006). As a child with disabilities is identified as being a 'child in need' then social services have a duty to undertake an assessment of the child's needs and provide the appropriate services under the Children Act 1989.

Being healthy

As outlined above, children with complex needs are recognized as a disadvantaged group in society. For these vulnerable children it is not only the particular disabilities and complex needs that relate to inequalities in their health, but also possible associated poverty, negative attitudes from society and limited access to services. 'Health inequalities' relate to variations in socioeconomic status, ethnicity, gender and location and can be articulated in terms of mortality rates, life expectancy, disease patterns and profiles. The government aims to improve the health of the population by increasing life expectancy and the number of illness-free years of individuals (DOH, 1999a). *The NHS Plan: A plan for investment, a plan for reform* (DOH, 2000a) reinforced the government's aim to reduce inequalities by trying to reduce the gap in infant mortality and morbidity between socioeconomic groups. Furthermore, *Tackling Health Inequalities* (DOH, 2001a) was concerned with reducing the relatively higher mortality rates in the manual groups of workers in society.

Arrangements made for disabled children must be included in the annual governors' report to parents.

3 *Special Educational Needs (SEN) Framework*. Local education authorities and schools already have obligations under the SEN Framework and these 'dovetail' with the amended Disability Discrimination Act 1995. It is an important framework, which disabled children and their families rely on to have their needs met. Children requiring SEN provision have largely been those with a learning difficulty. It is, however, also pertinent to children without learning difficulties who require provision above and beyond their peers in order to access education. The SEN Framework makes the assumption that disabled children can be supported in mainstream education, which equates to the government's view of increasing inclusion.

A child has a learning difficulty if he or she:

a) has a significantly greater difficulty in learning than the majority of children of the same age; or
b) has a disability which prevents or hinders the child from making use of educational facilities of a kind generally provided for children of the same age in schools within the area of the local education authority; or
c) is under five and falls within the definition of (a) or (b) above or would do so if special educational provision was not made for the child.' (Special Educational Needs and Disability Act 2001)

Making a positive contribution

There are many ways children with complex needs can make a contribution to society. One of the ways is by encouraging and increasing their contribution to decision-making about their own care. Obviously, it is important to include children and families in decisions about their care by asking and listening to them. To ensure their voice is heard, children and young people should be encouraged to contribute to consultations such as the current Good Childhood Inquiry being undertaken by the Children's Society (2006). Traditionally, children with disabilities and complex needs have been excluded from research studies about their needs (Watson et al., 2006). More recently there has been the recognition that more creative ways of obtaining data are one of the factors that enable this vulnerable group of children to be involved. Watson et al. (2006) recognize that there has recently been an increase in the involvement of disabled children in research studies about service delivery. They acknowledge, however, that including children with complex needs required further consideration. The challenges this presents are many and varied but, as with disabled children, families value the time afforded to listen to them.

Achieving economic well-being

In response to the 1998 Acheson Report on health inequalities, the government concluded that the poorer the person, the more likely that they would become ill and die younger (Acheson, 1998; DOH, 1999a). The index of multiple deprivation

(Office of the Deputy Prime Minister, 2004) is a measure of deprivation that consists of seven domains (income, employment, health deprivation and disability, education, skills and training, barriers to housing and services, crime and living environment). Each local authority has a score for each domain (dependent on specific criteria) and is given an overall rank within the country. This is one way of local authorities identifying areas of concern that require improvement. Families who have children with complex needs are more likely to live on benefits, which actually promotes social exclusion, the very opposite of recent government guidance on addressing the needs of these families. It has been recognized that it costs three times more to bring up a child with a disability than for children without disabilities, but families with disabled children have only 78% of the resources of all families with children (Roberts, 2000). The impact of caring can also be demanding on parents' physical and mental health. For many it means changes to their lifestyle, which can include financial implications, particularly if one or both parents have to give up paid employment to engage in a full-time caring role.

Parents' perspectives

When caring for a child with complex needs, changes in personal relationships can occur. This is not confined to partners but includes other members of the family, particularly other children and extended family members. Caring takes time and the main carer often does not have quality time on their own. Some carers may be susceptible to physical injuries such as back problems (Henwood, 1998; Hirst, 1998). Stress-related illnesses have been found to be apparent, particularly for female carers, those caring for a spouse and mothers of disabled children (Hutton & Hirst, 2001). Caring on a regular basis can lead to social isolation due to reduced time available to socialize. The role of parenting changes for the parents of a child with complex needs as the primary focus is on caring for their child's physical needs (Kirk et al., 2005). As the boundaries between caring and parenting blur, the parents may require emotional support in adapting to their new role. Indeed some parents may be coerced into accepting this caring role (Kirk, 2001). Respite care can be a valuable resource that helps take the strain from caring for an ill or demanding child and some families of children with complex needs use respite as a coping strategy (MacDonald et al., 2007). The availability of this service does, however, vary across the country with many providers offering differing levels of support. The problems associated with this are matching supply with demand due to factors such as training for workers and the costs of these services. For some families the type of respite care available does not match their needs and so is not utilized. MacDonald and Callery (2004) state that parental and service expectations may be very different; this in turn will affect the uptake of respite care.

One of the main challenges for parents of children with complex needs is that of social expectations. Although there are legislative acts to prevent discrimination within society (see above), wider views present a challenge for many parents. Indeed, many parents believe that generally society does not view their child's life as valuable compared to their peers. In 1963, Goffman introduced his theory of stigma, which has been widely discussed ever since and is still recognized as relevant today. Stigma is explained in terms of the social aspect of what is deemed as 'normal'. Although the original studies were undertaken in the context of physical disabilities, mental illness and sensory impairments such as deafness and blindness, this work can be related to children with complex needs in current society. Stigma is defined as an 'attribute that is deeply discrediting' and these qualities can relate to an individual's attributes or membership of a group (Carnevale, 2007). Individuals who are stigmatized may be discreditable, whereby the true extent of their 'difference' has not been made fully aware to society. To be 'discredited' means that society has already passed a judgement and has excluded the individual from 'normal' society (Carnevale, 2007). 'Passing' is a term used by Goffman to indicate strategies used for an individual to 'pass' as normal. This may include not revealing information about the disability to others. For the parents of children with complex needs this may mean not informing the child themselves of their particular needs. Thus for parents the dilemma is often choosing the right time to tell their child of their prognosis or the extent of their longer term needs.

Case study 1 is written by a mother who has a child with complex needs. Though written from a relatively positive perspective it also refers to the implications of caring for such a child. These include managing the diagnosis and prognosis, changes to lifestyle and family relationships, family economics and access issues. For this particular family it appears that appropriate services are in place in terms of education, equipment and respite care. It further highlights, however, the depth of need of the child and family and the related time and energy required from the parents and carers in meeting these needs.

Case study 1: Living with a child with complex needs

We are a family of four, consisting of my husband [aged] 38, our daughter [aged] 13, our son [aged] 5 and me [aged] 38. Our son has the condition spinal muscular atrophy type 1, a genetic condition that causes physical disability.

At 11 months old, we were given the devastating news that he would be lucky if he lived until his second birthday. However, he decided to defy the odds and although he has had a few major illnesses, he is doing extremely well and is stronger and more able than predicted. Today, at nearly six years old he drives a powered wheelchair and attends mainstream school.

Along the way, there have been many professionals involved in his care, to supervise and/or advise on how to care for our son. As a pyramid the apex would have to be given over to his main consultant, a neurological specialist, after that is a paediatric consultant and then a myriad of physiotherapists, occupational therapists, community nurses, orthotic technicians, dieticians, surgeons, general practitioners, health visitors and a social worker.

In the main this has been a positive experience. Many of those involved have provided invaluable help and direction. With the support of these outside agencies and in consultation with our needs, we have been able to provide a plan of care that addresses his needs from medical treatment through to vital equipment necessary for quality and sustenance of life. He has gastrostomy feeds, overnight ventilation and a cough assist machine. Through discussion and compromise we have been able to agree to more appropriate care, such as home care when he needs intravenous medication rather than repetitive hospitalization. We have always been able to have full involvement in his care and been given the opportunity to question every potential decision.

As a family unit, the condition has had a significant impact on us all. Our lives are totally different from how they would have been. In the beginning we all united in our grief, not just us, but also our extended family. Waves of emotion and sadness were overwhelming. Having to explain to our eight-year-old daughter the implications of the diagnosis was another momentous task.

However, as the months and years went by and we witnessed how well he stayed and how strong he was getting we were able to relax a little, although never allowing ourselves to become complacent. The miracle of that brought the implications of living with a disabled child, which then took over our lives.

Time in our house is short and we only have dinner times and weekends to chat or catch up with each other. Apart from a Friday night when we have an overnight carer, either my husband or I have to take him to bed, where we then stay with him until our bedtime. He requires turning approximately four to ten times per night and his overnight ventilator attending to. He needs help with every personal care need and someone's full-time attention. As his disability is purely physical, he also needs the same stimuli as every other boy his age. My husband works full time, but I am unable to work as I need to be available to care for him, to take him to his many appointments and if he is off school ill. Economically, this has had an impact on us and means we have had to cut back. We cannot always join in on social events due to lack of funds, but also due to the restraints of society and its lack of provision for wheelchair users. Just visiting friends and or family can pose problems due to lack of access and provision for him.

Our whole world has been turned upside down, with careful thought and plans evaluated every step of the way. We have learned to live with our life and despite everything, life is good. Our son is happy and healthy and a joy to be around. We now drive round obstacles, step out of the box and open alternative doors.

Action Learning Point

- In your area of practice, identify how the needs of parents and siblings of children with complex needs are addressed.
- Consider Case study 1. If this family lived in your area what local services could be put in place to support their needs?

Siblings as carers

Over recent years there has been growing recognition that some children and young people provide care for others, usually family members, on a regular basis. There are estimated to be between 20 000 and 50 000 young carers in the UK (DOH, 1999b), although according to the Children's Society there are 175 000 young carers in the UK today (Barnardo's, 2007). Doran et al. (2007) contextualized caring when analysing recent census data. For the first time in the history of the census, questions were asked in relation to the caring role. For the 5–15 year age group 61 000 girls and 53 000 boys were informal carers. This total of 114 000 children and young people equates to 1.4% of all the children and young people in the UK. Of these young carers, 18 000 were caring for over 20 hours regularly each week. Almost 9000 were providing at least 50 hours of care weekly. Individuals were also asked to rate their own health status and 773 under-16s who regularly provided at least 20 hours of caring weekly rated their own health as 'not good'.

Defining what constitutes a young carer can be problematic. Many young carers may just think they are doing their duty, subtly assume the caring role and do not perceive themselves as carers. Various definitions utilized today have the focus of 'restrictions' placed upon a young person's life because of their caring role. This may be helpful in terms of understanding the implications for young people and identifying areas requiring support. Disabled rights advocate that if individuals' needs were fully met then young carers would not exist. Newman (2002), however, suggests that young carers should be defined by the extent of their contribution (and implications of it) rather than the hours of input or the diagnosis of the person they are caring for. Becker et al. (1998) suggest a model of care in helping to understand how the concept of young carers has evolved. There are four aspects to the model (medical, social, young carers, family care) that show how society's views and understanding of disabilities have developed over time. In the 1950s, the medical model focused on the impact of disability and illness on family members. The 1970s brought the advent of the disability rights movement, which included a focus on discrimination and exclusion. Young carers were beginning to be recognized by the researchers in the 1980s, with their important contribution to the family being acknowledged. Currently, the family care approach incorporates the needs of the whole family with a shift away from children's and disability rights. In addition to their contribution to the family, it is also recognized that caring can have implications for the young carer's life. Education and leisure time can be affected due to the time and effort spent caring (which may include undertaking domestic tasks). In addition to not completing homework and coursework, not being able to socialize with the peer group can soon lead to isolation and exclusion (Dearden & Becker, 2002). Feelings of guilt and resentment may occur due to the young carer not being able to address their own needs. The national strategy for carers (DOH, 1999b) acknowledged the need for supporting young carers and recognized that their education should not be compromised by their caring role. The government recognizes the need to look after the health and well-being of young carers to ensure that their role of caring does not negatively impact on their lives (DOH, 1996a, 2000b). The 'Quality protects' initiative identifies that young carers should have the same life chances as their peer group (DOH, 1998).

Due to the possibility that young carers spend some, if not all, of their spare time caring means they are less likely to form relationships outside of the family. If they do not make relationships away from the home environment this may contribute to problems later on in adjusting to an adult world. Indeed it has been recognized that a child's health and potential to earn money are both linked to health outcomes in adulthood (Graham, 2000). Thus attention to the educational needs of young carers is recognized as particularly important in enabling them to enjoy and achieve, make a positive contribution and achieve economic well-being as outlined in the ECM agenda (DOH, 1996b, 1999b; DOH/DfES, 2004).

The Carers (Equal Opportunities) Act 2004 states that adult and children's services within local authorities should have a joint protocol that identifies and assesses the needs of young carers and their families. Interestingly, a child is more likely to receive an assessment of their needs if they are caring for a parent who is drug or alcohol dependent (Dearden & Becker, 2004). This may be because services for adult drug and alcohol misuse are more well established that those for children with complex needs.

Meeting the needs of children with complex needs and their families

The Children's Workforce

Within the ECM agenda, the *Common Core of Skills and Knowledge for the Children's Workforce* (DfES, 2005) outlines six areas of expertise that should be achieved by practitioners working with children. These are:

1 Effective communication and engagement with children, young people, their families and carers.
2 Child and young person development.
3 Safeguarding and promoting the welfare of the child.
4 Supporting transitions.
5 Multiagency working.
6 Sharing information.

Each category outlines the appropriate knowledge and skills required to fulfill that requirement (Table 1).

In providing effective outcomes for children and families, service managers should utilize this guidance in any single or multiagency training sessions. It can also be utilized for needs analysis for identifying individual training needs. It also has a role to play in workforce planning. In the future the government will ensure

Table 1 Knowledge and skills required in the 'common core'.

Common core category	Knowledge required	Skills required
Effective communication and engagement with children, young people, their families and carers	How communication works Confidentiality and ethics Sources of support	Listening and building empathy Summarizing and explaining Consultation and negotiation
Child and young person development	Understand context Understand how babies, children and young people develop Be clear about own job role Know how to reflect and improve	Observation and judgement Empathy and understanding
Safeguarding and promoting the welfare of the child	Legal and procedural frameworks Wider context of services Self-knowledge	Relate, recognize and take considered action Communication, recording and reporting Personal skills
Supporting transitions	How children and young people respond to change When and how to intervene	Identify transitions Provide support
Multiagency working	Your role and remit Know how to make queries Procedures and working methods The law, policies and procedures	Communication and teamwork Assertiveness
Sharing information	Importance of information sharing Role and responsibilities Awareness of complexities Awareness of laws and legislation	Information handling Clear communication Engagement

all training for the children's workforce will include the 'common core' (DfES, 2006). The government guidance on working together to safeguard children has recently been updated to include lessons from the Laming Report (Laming, 2003), findings from *Every Child Matters* (DfES, 2003a), consultation and subsequent guidance, and the updated Children Act 2004. It outlines the outcomes in addressing the concerns in relation to accountability, leadership and responsibility. Children's Trusts should operate at a strategic level whereby health, education and social services can make decisions on areas pertinent to children with complex needs such as pooled budgets. This is helpful in situations where it is not clear whether a need is a social, educational or health responsibility (DfES, 2006).

Action Learning Point

- Consider the role of interprofessional working in addressing the needs of children with complex needs and their families.
- Which other disciplines/agencies do you work closely with? Who should you work more closely with? How are relationships maintained?
- What might you as an individual do to improve communication within the wider interprofessional team?

Conclusions

In recent years there has been a continual growth in the number of children with increasingly complex needs. Legislation provided the legal thrust to ensure inclusive strategies are adopted for children with complex needs and their families – which includes being cared for at home and access to mainstream education. The government agenda provides a framework (in terms of the ECM agenda and the NSF) to enable the key agencies involved in children's services to work together to improve outcomes. Children with complex needs are deemed to be a vulnerable group within society due to additional factors associated with their needs, and as such are at an increased risk of suffering harm. Parents of these children have to deal with barriers to access within society, in addition to carrying out the main bulk of physical and emotional care of their child. Siblings can all too easily become socialized into the caring role, which can have implications for their own health and social care. Practitioners need to be aware of and address all these factors when negotiating care packages for such families.

References

Acheson, D. (1998) *Report on the Independent Inquiry into Inequalities in Health*. London, HMSO.

Barber, C.F. (2007) Abuse by care professionals. Part 1: an introduction. *British Journal of Nursing* **16** (15): 938–940.

Barker, J. & Hodes, D. (2004) *The Child in Mind: A child protection handbook*. London, Routledge.

Barlow, J., Wright, C., Sheasby, J., Turner, A. & Hainsworth, J. (2002) Self management approaches for people with chronic conditions: a review. *Patient Education and Counselling* **48**: 177–187.

Barnardo's (2007) Barnardo's Conferences. http://www.barnardos.org.uk/what_we_do/ working_with_children_and_young_people/young_carers.htm?campRef=060770 [accessed 8 July 2007].

Becker, S., Aldridge, J. & Dearden, C. (1998) Young carers and their families. In: A.M. Halpenny & R. Gilligan (eds) *Caring Before their Time? Research and policy perspectives on young carers.* Dublin, Barnardo's National Children's Resource Centre and Children's Research Centre.

Bowlby, J. (1969) *Attachment and Loss. Vol. 1: Attachment.* London, Hogarth Press.

Carnevale, F.A. (2007) Revisiting Goffman's stigma: the social experience of families with children requiring mechanical ventilation at home. *Journal of Child Health Care* **11** (1): 7–18.

Children's Society (2006) The Good Childhood Inquiry. http://www.childrenssociety. org.uk/what+we+do/The+good+childhood+inquiry/home.htm [accessed 12 November 2007].

Cicchetti, D. & Rogosch, F.A. (1997) The role of self-organization in the promotion of resilience in maltreated children. *Development and Psychopathology* **9**: 797–815.

Dahlgren, G. & Whitehead, M. (1991) *Policies and Strategies to Promote Social Equity in Health.* Stockholm, Institute for Futures Studies.

Davis, R. (2000) Achievements in child health over the first half of the 20th century. *British Journal of Nursing* **9** (1): 28–32.

Dearden, C. & Becker, S. (2002) *Young Carers and Education.* London, Carers UK.

Dearden, C. & Becker, S. (2004) *Young Carers in the UK. The 2004 Report.* London, Carers National Association.

Department for Education and Skills (2003a) *Every Child Matters.* London, Department for Education and Skills.

Department for Education and Skills (2003b) *Keeping Children Safe. The government's response to the Victoria Climbie Inquiry Report and Joint Chief Inspector's Report Safeguarding Children.* London, HMSO.

Department for Education and Skills (2004a) *Every Child Matters: Change for children.* London, Department for Education and Skills.

Department for Education and Skills (2004b) *Every Child Matters: Next steps.* London, Department for Education and Skills.

Department for Education and Skills (2005) *Common Core of Skills and Knowledge for the Children's Workforce.* Nottingham, Department for Education and Skills.

Department for Education and Skills (2006) *Working Together to Safeguard Children: A guide to inter-agency working to safeguard and promote the welfare of children.* London, HMSO.

Department for Work and Pensions (2004) *Family Resources Survey 2002–3.* http://www. dwp.gov.uk/mediacentre/pressreleases/2006/feb/drc-015-090206.asp [accessed 8 July 2007].

Department of Health (1996a) *Young Carers and their Families. A survey carried out by the Social Survey Division of ONS on behalf of the Department of Health.* London, Department of Health.

Department of Health (1996b) *Young Carers – Making a start.* London, Department of Health.

Department of Health (1998) *Quality Protects Initiative.* London, Department of Health.

Department of Health (1999a) *Saving Lives: Our healthier nation.* London, Department of Health.

Department of Health (1999b) *Caring about Carers: A national strategy for carers.* London, Department of Health.

Department of Health (2000a) *The NHS Plan: A plan for investment, a plan for reform.* London, Department of Health.

Department of Health (2000b) *A Jigsaw of Services: Inspection of services to support disabled adults in their parenting role.* London, Department of Health.

Department of Health (2001a) *Tackling Health Inequalities.* London, Department of Health.

Department of Health (2001b) *The Expert Patient: A new approach to chronic disease management for the 21st century.* London, Department of Health.

Department of Health (2002) *Safeguarding Children. A Joint Chief Inspector's Report on arrangements to safeguard children.* London, Department of Health.

Department of Health (2007) *Making it Better: For children and young people.* London, Department of Health.

Department of Health/Department for Education and Skills (2003) *Together from the Start – Practical guidance for professionals working with disabled children (birth to third birthday) and their families.* Nottingham, Department for Education and Skills.

Department of Health/Department for Education and Skills (2004) *National Service Framework for Children, Young People and Maternity Services.* London, Department of Health.

Doran, T., Drever, F. & Whitehead, M. (2007) Health of young and elderly informal carers: analysis of UK census data. *British Medical Journal* **327**: 1388.

Expert Patient Programme (undated) Looking after Me. http://www.expertpatients.co.uk/public/default.aspx?load=ArticleViewer&ArticleId=443 [accessed 14 November 2007].

Farasat, H. & Hewitt-Taylor, J. (2007) Learning to support children with complex and continuing health needs and their families. *Journal for Specialists in Paediatric Nursing* **12** (2): 72–83.

Fisher, H.R. (2001) The needs of parents with chronically sick children: a literature review. *Journal of Advanced Nursing* **36** (4): 600–607.

Goffman, E. (1963) *Stigma. Notes on the management of spoiled identity.* Englewood Cliffs, NJ, Prentice-Hall.

Graham, H. (ed.) (2000) *Understanding Health Inequalities.* Buckingham, Open University Press.

Hawley, K. (2005a) *Report on the EPP Parent Pilot Course, January 2004–January 2005.* http://www.expertpatients.nhs.uk/public/cms/uploads/PARENTS%20REPORT%20%20FINAL.DOC [accessed 8 July 2007].

Hawley, K. (2005b) *Report on the Expert Patient Programme for Children, January 2004–January 2005.* http://www.expertpatients.co.uk/public/cms/uploads/REPORT%20CHILDREN%20EPP%20FINAL.doc [accessed 5 November 2007].

Health Committee (1997) *House of Commons Select Committee. Health services for children and young people in the community: home and school. Third report.* London, HMSO.

Henwood, M. (1998) *Ignored and Invisible? Carers' experience of the NHS.* London, Carers National Association.

Hirst, M. (1998) *The Health of Informal Carers: A longitudinal analysis.* York, Social Policy Research Unit, University of York.

Howe, D. (2006) Disabled children, maltreatment and attachment. *British Journal of Social Work* **360**: 743–760.

Hutton, S. & Hirst, M. (2001) *Caring Relationships over Time.* York, Social Policy Research Unit, University of York.

Kirk, S. (2001) Negotiating lay and professional roles in the care of children with complex health care needs. *Journal of Advanced Nursing* **34** (5): 593–602.

Kirk, S., Glendinning, C. & Callery, P. (2005) Parent or nurse? The experience of being a parent of a technology-dependent child. *Journal of Advanced Nursing* **51** (5): 456–464.

Laming, H. (2003) *The Victoria Climbie Inquiry.* London, Department of Health.

MacDonald, E., Fitzsimons, E. & Noonan Walsh, P. (2007) Use of respite care and coping strategies among Irish families of children with intellectual disabilities. *British Journal of Learning Disabilities* **35** (1): 62–68.

MacDonald, H. & Callery, P. (2004) Different meanings of respite: a study of parents, nurses and social workers caring for children with complex needs. *Child: Care, Health and Development* **30** (3): 279–288.

Marchant, R. & Page, M. (1992) Bridging the gap: investigating the abuse of children with multiple disabilities. *Child Health Review* **1** (3): 179–183.

National Society for the Prevention of Cruelty to Children (2003) *It Doesn't Happen to Disabled Children. Child protection and disabled children. Report of the National Working Group on Child Protection and Disability.* London, NSPCC.

National Statistics (2003) *Census 2001.* http://www.statistics.gov.uk/cci/nugget_print. asp?ID=348 [accessed 8 July 2007].

Newman, T. (2002) 'Young carers' and disabled parents: time for a change of direction? *Disability and Society* **17** (6): 613–625.

Noyes, J. (2007) Comparison of ventilator-dependent child reports of health related quality of life with parent reports and normative populations. *Journal of Advanced Nursing* **58** (1): 1–10.

Office of the Deputy Prime Minister (2004) *Index of Multiple Deprivation 2004.* http://www.communities.gov.uk/index.asp?id=1128447 [accessed 8 July 2007].

Roberts, H. (2000) *What Works in Reducing Inequalities in Child Health? Summary.* Ilford, Barnardo's Publications.

Watson, D., Abbott, D. & Townsley, R. (2006) Listen to me too! Lessons from involving children with complex healthcare needs in research about multi-agency services. *Child: Care, Health and Development* **33** (1): 90–95.

Chapter 8

Psychosocial consequences of living with a long term condition

Diane Loggenberg

Key points

- Discussing how long term health problems impact on a person's quality of life
- Looking at how Parkinson's disease can work as an exemplar of a long term condition
- Defining 'quality of life'
- Outlining the physical challenges that affect quality of life
- The environment and its impact on quality of life issues
- Psychological aspects of quality of life issues related to long term conditions
- Exploring social complications, long term conditions and quality of life

Over the years, the agenda for the majority of researchers working with people with chronic conditions has been firmly embedded in the medical model. In general, the psychosocial consequences of living with a long term condition (LTC) seem to be viewed as peripheral and little consideration is given as to how people actually experience their disorder. The following chapter will attempt to redress this imbalance by integrating some of the known psychosocial sequelae of chronic poor health into a quality of life (QoL) framework. Then, given that many of the studies that look at QoL and long term illness only consider the perspective of the medical experts from any given field, this chapter will look further and present contributions from those who currently live with a long term condition.

What quality of life is and is not

In recent years, the term 'quality of life' has become popularized to the point of cliché. It is now generally accepted that QoL is as important as survival, and that a long life is not necessarily a good life. The term QoL has multidisciplinary applications and is frequently quoted by advertizing executives, journalists, medical professionals, psychologists, sociologists, health economists and even on billboards. Jones (1999: p. 337) noted that defining and measuring QoL has been 'one of the most ambitious undertakings that psychologists have engaged in'. She likened it to 'stress', in that the term is poorly defined but widely used.

Academia has also embraced the concept of QoL. There are books dedicated to QoL measurement scales (Bowling, 1995), paperbacks that give very detailed and wide-ranging coverage of QoL measures (Bowling, 1999) and bespoke journals for chronicling QoL research. However, despite a general acceptance of a QoL model, there is still little consensus regarding *who* should provide the definition of what gives a life quality, and against what criteria QoL should be assessed. Prutkin and Feinstein (2002: p. 3) reported on research undertaken to examine the history of the term QoL and its general acceptance by medical professionals. They found all of the following components of QoL in the studies reviewed:

'general health status, functional capacity, emotional function, level of well-being, life satisfaction, happiness, intellectual level, pain, nausea and vomiting, level of symptoms, fatigue, sexual functioning, social activity, memory level, financial status, and job status'.

One researcher who has dedicated her career to examinations of life quality is Ann Bowling. Together with seven other colleagues, Bowling et al. (2003: p. 270) carried out interviews with 999 British people, in a concerted attempt to definitively unpack the correlates of life quality. They reported that 'the concept and measurement of quality of life are dependent largely on expert rather than lay views of the important constituents', and that QoL was an amorphous concept reflecting both:

'macro societal and socio-demographic influences and also micro concerns such as individuals' experiences, circumstances, health, social well-being, values, perceptions and psychology . . . a collection of interacting and subjective dimensions'. (Bowling et al., 2003: p. 271)

To summarize, it seems that QoL, (and its successor, 'well-being'), has evolved into a subjective term that can be interpreted in different ways by different people. One of the known biases in QoL literature is that too many QoL questionnaires, particularly if linked to chronic illness, are no more than 'quality of health' indices. They are more likely to show 'levels of disability' than genuine quality of life with its concomitant richness and variety (de Boer et al., 1996). With these caveats in mind, we can look at the physical domain of QoL for people who live with long term health problems, before exploring the environmental, psychological and social domains.

The physical domain

Although this chapter is primarily concerned with chronicling the psychological and social challenges of living with long term health problems, without a solid understanding of the physical aspects relating to an individual's QoL, there can be little extrapolation to other, possibly more nebulous domains. Of the many questionnaires researchers can use to assess QoL, the World Health Organization (WHO) measure is especially robust and valuable. When originally developed, the WHOQoL measure was field-tested in 30 centres worldwide, in a variety of cross-cultural and longitudinal studies. There were two questionnaires developed, one a shortened version for people whose health might make it difficult to complete the more than 100 questions on the original.

'It [is] anticipated that the WHOQOL assessments will be used in broad-ranging ways. . . . [They] will be of value where disease prognosis is likely to involve only partial recovery or remission, and in which treatment may be more palliative than curative.' (WHOQoL Group, 1998a, p. 51)

In this chapter the WHOQoL-Bref[1] questionnaire, comprising just 26 questions, is the measure referred to throughout; this has seven questions relating to the physical domain. Examples of the types of questions used (Table 1), should illuminate the mechanics of how the WHO links health to quality of life. As can be seen in the extract reproduced in Table 1, the items on the WHO questionnaire are contextualized into the lives of those who are asked to complete it. By scoring the responses across each domain, a tally is produced which should accurately indicate the QoL for that particular person, with respect to one facet of their life. The most important detail to keep in mind about the WHO instrument is that it has been developed as a *global*[2] questionnaire for QoL and, although it may be used for measuring generic QoL for people with LTCs, it may not be sensitive enough to identify QoL difficulties for any one particular health disorder.

Table 1 A sample of the WHOQoL-Bref (WHO, 1993)

The following questions ask about **how much** you have experienced certain things in the last four weeks.

	Not at all	A little	A moderate amount	Very much	An extreme amount
3. To what extent do you feel that physical pain prevents you from doing what you need to do?	5	4	3	2	1
4. How much do you need any medical treatment to function in your daily life?	5	4	3	2	1

---

[1] The 26-item short form of the WHOQoL, called the WHOQoL-Bref, is used in this chapter. Power (1998: p. 14) stated that the 'need for a short form arises from the fact that a 100-item form is too long for use in many . . . studies in which QoL may be only one . . . part of the overall research focus'. Additionally, the 'Bref' questionnaire was developed so that even those with severe health challenges would be able to complete it without too much fatigue (WHOQoL Group, 1998a: p. 51).

[2] 'Global' here is used in its geographic context. To illustrate, the questionnaire is available in English, Chinese, Czech, Farsi, Indonesian, Polish, Russian and Thai (World Health Organization, 1994).

Parkinson's disease as an exemplar of a long term condition

One of the most deleterious LTCs affecting people in the UK today is known to be Parkinson's disease (PD). Because, as we advance into the 21st century, people are living longer, and because PD has a mean age of onset of 60 years for both men and women, there are serious concerns about the QoL for more and more people with a diagnosis of PD. Although the known figure for those with PD is currently 126 000, experts in the field consider this to be an underestimate, partly attributable to the difficulty of diagnosing the neurodegenerative disease. Parkinson's will be used as an exemplar of a LTC for the rest of this chapter for the following reasons:

- People with early-onset PD (diagnosed under the age of 55) may live for more than 30 years with ever worsening health challenges.
- These health challenges are compounded by the natural ageing process.
- The psychosocial difficulties for people with PD are relatively well documented.
- There is no universally acknowledged lifespan for people with PD; like many LTCs, the future is largely unknown and unpredictable.

Although a person's journey with PD is known to be particularly idiosyncratic, like many LTCs, there are commonalities within the progression that can usefully illuminate other chronic health challenges.

Action Learning Point

- Do you understand the difference between the medical model of health and the psychosocial model?
- How do you see a person's life as having 'quality?'
- Would your own definition of QoL differ from how the World Health Organization defines it?
- In what way is Parkinson's disease a good model of a long term condition?

Parkinson's disease, quality of life and the physical domain

In 2002, 247 people living in the UK, with a diagnosis of PD, were given the WHOQoL-Bref and asked to complete it (Loggenberg, 2005). This was so that the physical impact of the disorder could be statistically linked to QoL, and then improvements made to daily living with PD. The results for the physical domain can be seen in Table 2.

The most noteworthy aspect of Table 2 is that question 21, relating to sexual difficulties, is included in the physical domain. As can be seen, WHO designated this as a 'social relationships' issue. Because this was a research population with Parkinson's, the judgement had to be made as to whether the *physical* aspects of the LTC were likely to influence responses to item 21, and it seemed certain that this was the case.[3] Once the mean scores for all the physical questions are

---

[3] To investigate precisely in which domain the 'sex' question fits, a factor analysis was carried out. This is a statistical procedure used to link similar research areas. Question 21 was definitively subsumed within the 'physical domain'.

Table 2 Ranked means for 'physical' questions on the WHOQoL-Bref (lower scores = greater problems; thus items shown at the top of the table are the most problematical, those at the bottom of the table, the least problematical).

Question number	Mean score	Question content	Domain designated by WHO
18	2.15*	How satisfied are you with your capacity for work?	Physical
16	2.44	How satisfied are you with your sleep?	Physical
21	2.61	How satisfied are you with your sex life?	Social relationships
17	2.72	How satisfied with are you with ability for daily living activities?	Physical
3	2.75†	How much does pain prevent what you need to do?	Physical
10	2.87‡	Do you have enough energy for daily life?	Physical
15	2.91	How well are you able to get around?	Physical
4	3.77†	How reliant are you on medical professional treatment?	Physical

Overall mean: 2.71
*Where 1 = very dissatisfied, and 5 = very satisfied.
†Where 1 = not at all, and 5 = an extreme amount.
‡Where 1 = not at all, and 5 = completely.

calculated, it then becomes the responsibility of researchers/practitioners to consider possible implications.

Psychosocial implications of difficulties in the physical domain

Sexual difficulties

Of the 26 items on the generic WHO instrument, people with PD rated dissatisfaction with their sex lives as the third worst aspect of their Parkinson's, with only work and sleep difficulties superseding sex, confirming that sexual dysfunction was deleteriously affecting the quality of living for many people. In recent years, information has been accumulating that the sexual self-image of people with chronic illness is affected by societal attitudes and that fears of losing independence, or of being viewed as 'sick', can erode sexual confidence. Researchers are just beginning to understand that the importance of validating a person's sexual identity cannot be overstated (Basson, 1998).

One researcher who did not sideline sex issues was Simon (2000: p. 10), who alleged that although '60% of people with chronic health conditions live with some sort of sexual dysfunction . . . as few as 5% complain to their doctors'. Brown et al. (1990: p. 480) tried to define the mechanisms that have led to sex difficulties being largely ignored by medical professionals. They explained that 'the general lack of professional interest in the subject of sexual function . . . may relate to two main assumptions, neither of which are [sic] warranted'. They explained the first assumption as a belief that, because long term health difficulties are defined by physiological dysfunction, they must inevitably lead to sexual dysfunction. The second assumption was that 'patients are . . . either middle-aged or elderly, [and] not interested in . . . sex'. Clearly, any professional asked to work with an individual with a LTC should guard against making *any* similar generalized assumptions.

Literature searches clearly show that explorations of sexual function and LTCs represent a metaphorical hinterland. Fitzsimmons and Bunting (2001: p. 6) have alleged that 'this paucity of literature is [due to] the belief that if the motor symptoms are treated, psychosocial aspects of (any given) disease will spontaneously improve'. From the disability field, we learn from Perring (2001: p. 1) that the consequences of ignoring sexual needs may be severe:

> 'dissatisfaction and disappointment (with sex) . . . can lead to depression, a sense of isolation and an avoidance of any physical contact . . . as sense of self is lost, and needs to be grieved'.

Jacobs et al. (2000: p. 552) found that 'sexual problems . . . may particularly arise in couples where the partner is male' and that 'the male bias in distribution of sexual difficulties is related to state of employment'. Given that relatively few men with long term health difficulties are fully employed, this finding is particularly poignant.

Wenning (2000: p. 6), again working in the disability field, pinpointed the main known sex difficulties as 'infrequency, impotence and premature ejaculation' for men, and 'non-communication, avoidance, infrequency and non-sensuality' for women. He contrasted these with the traditional thinking that either physical disability and/or medical side effects were the main components of sexual dysfunction. Another difficulty suggested by Fitzsimmons and Bunting (2001), both registered general nurses specializing in PD, related to loss of perceived attractiveness. They believed that any one of the known PD side effects (cited as diaphoresis (profuse and excessive sweating), excessive facial oiliness and drooling) might diminish the sense of being attractive, and interfere with initiation of sexual contact.

Overall, the literature linking LTCs with some sexual difficulty tends to confirm what anecdotal accounts have raised over the years. It is apparent that most people with a chronic health challenge can expect to encounter some impediment to full sexual fulfilment at some point in the process of living with their disorder. The psychological corollaries of such struggles are largely disregarded.

Sleep difficulties

The WHO questionnaire asks only one question about sleep difficulties and Table 2 shows that life quality for people with PD, as may be true for many others with a LTC, is seriously compromised by sleep deprivation. It is difficult to imagine how severe sleep disturbances might fit into any model of living other than one that excludes salaried work and difficult, too, to exaggerate the profound negative impact on general QoL. This is felt by those with LTCs when they need to make special arrangements when away from home (either taking holidays or in hotels for business purposes) to accommodate disturbed sleep patterns and to ensure they do not disturb anyone who may need to accompany them. This hints to those with chronic health difficulties that they are a 'peculiar' group, a group that needs specialist provision in society and all such provisions have the potential to harm self-image. What practitioners may find when working with those who have chronic health challenges is that peaceful, uninterrupted sleep evades almost all people with chronic conditions, and good quality sleep seems to acquire an almost mystical elusiveness. For some, 'sleep' may become synonymous with the mythical 'Holy Grail': constantly talked about, remembered from the past, a common narrative for those with health difficulties and seen as comprising a transformative quality, that when found in life, would cure all other health-related struggles. It should always be remembered that, historically, sleep deprivation has been used as a method of torture.

When those with chronic illness talk about 'sleeping difficulties' it is useful to consider possible overlaps between their level of tiredness and their social lives. Too often LTCs can lead to impoverished social lives and produce the phenomenon known as 'premature social ageing'. This term was originated by Singer (1974) when studying people in the USA with LTCs. She noted that her population had fewer close friends than their healthy peers, had fewer social contacts, fewer leisure activities, and were more confined to their homes. She found that, typically, people aged 50 with a LTC had similar social calendars to those aged 70 but in full health.

A final psychological consequence that may follow sleeping difficulty is associated with loss of 'social identity'. If people are unremittingly weary and, hence, do not socialize to the extent that they did when fully healthy, then they cease to be the people they saw themselves as before they developed their LTC. There follows a period of 'identity renegotiation' as the chronically sick person redefines themselves in terms of their new health status. For some this may lead to a period of depression as the original self struggles to relinquish the healthy model and assimilate the new 'health compromised' model. Interestingly, although models of disability invariably include 'social identity' domains, there are no existing QoL models that do so. It seems that the 'domino effect' caused by physical challenges impacting on psychosocial arenas is largely trivialized, especially in the case of sleep worries. Yet,

> 'sleep disturbance, insomnia and its implications such as excessive daytime sleepiness are a major cause of impaired QoL. We need to be aware of the impact of sleep disturbance on patients' lives, and we should treat them with therapies shown to improve this problem'. (Chaudhuri, 2000: p. 1).

Difficulties with hospital admissions

It is the nature of chronic health conditions that those who endure them will generally spend more time as hospital inpatients than will their healthy peers (Weingart et al., 2000). Unfortunately, there is a mass of evidence to suggest that many people with LTCs experience poor outcomes from hospital admissions. Researchers looking at the possibly counterintuitive negative outcomes have struggled to explain exactly how and why hospitalization can be so detrimental to a patient's QoL (Harrold et al., 1999).

It seems that the immediate blow to life quality may be psychological, in that inpatients may experience feelings of isolation and marginalization due to their removal from familiar surroundings and the disruption of their normal daily routines. The 'patient' has lost their individuality and may inevitably feel they have no value. They may already have experienced a loss of identity through mechanisms such as loss of employment, reduction in social activities and reduction in number of friendships (Singer, 1974). One man with a LTC complained that, since his diagnosis, he had lost status, mobility, freedom (as he was no longer able to drive) and feelings of self-worth (Loggenberg, 2005). He attributed these losses to a combination of his health status, the repeated hospitalizations *and* his treatment by medical professionals. His future is likely to be clouded by the losses themselves and in a regrettably circular manner, also by the negative attitudes engendered by such losses.

Because so much health care in the UK is totally enslaved by the dominant medical professional model of well-being, this has led, in the past, to an over-reliance on hospital care. Practitioners state that a more holistic approach to LTCs was advocated almost twenty years ago. Despite such early recommendations for good practice, though, Bowman (2000: p. 7) found that people with LTCs represented a huge burden to the NHS; he stated that they tend to fall into a metaphorical 'black hole where patients [are] forgotten'. Rather alarmingly, Oxtoby and Williams (1995: p. 166), recognizing that 'going into hospital creates anxiety for most people', documented cases where patients were both 'poorly treated and neglected whilst in hospital' (Oxtoby & Williams, 1995: p. 168). As Timmins (2000: p. 25) noted: 'hospitals are dangerous places. One in 10 hospital patients contracts an illness during their stay'. The evidence that QoL tends to be impoverished by inpatient treatment should be foremost in practitioners' minds when making decisions as to whether or not a person with a LTC can remain at home or needs to be hospitalized. Clearly there will be times when there is no alternative to hospitalization but, even then, the receiving hospital should be informed of *all* the health complications that the individual may have. In particular, ward managers should be told of any medical professional input that is necessary for daily functioning.

Summary

In the preceding paragraphs three physical problems, commonly experienced by people with LTCs, have been explored in relation to life quality. Evidence has been presented that inextricably links sex difficulties, sleep worries, and the problems associated with hospital admissions with QoL. Each of these three focus areas is unpacked so that the mechanisms whereby functional problems translate into both psychological and social difficulties is made explicit, and the trajectory whereby LTCs track to diminished QoL is outlined. The psychosocial sequelae may include all of the following:

- Loss of confidence: dependence.
- Stigma: loss of social identity.
- The need to renegotiate self-identity: marginalization.

- Social and emotional isolation: premature social ageing.
- Compromised occupational identity: decrease in leisure activities.
- Perceived loss of attractiveness: 'peculiarity' of the group.

Action Learning Point

- List how many dimensions of the self might be affected by poor sexual function.
- Why is 'loss of confidence' important to the well-being of someone with a LTC?
- For all of the psychological consequences listed above, think of one non-medical intervention you could offer as help.
- Why is 'stigma' of relevance for those who have an LTC?

The environmental domain

Throughout this section, the term 'environmental' is used in the context outlined by WHO (WHOQoL Group, 1998b). When relating it to QoL, WHO saw 'environmental' as comprising:

- Financial resources.
- Freedom, physical safety and security.
- Health and social care: accessibility and quality.
- Home environment.
- Opportunities for acquiring new information and skills.
- Participation in and opportunities for recreation/leisure.
- Physical environment (pollution/noise/traffic/climate).
- Transport.

The eight environmental questions asked in WHOQoL-Bref are shown in Table 3. The mean scores imply that the people with a LTC who took part in this study (again, the example used throughout the text is Parkinson's disease) were 'moderately' happy with their *opportunities* for leisure activities, felt reasonably safe on a daily basis, lived in a fairly healthy environment and could mostly get hold of information when they needed it. They were not especially worried about personal finances, transport, nor access to health services, and expressed real satisfaction about their overall living conditions (mean 4.28 where a score of 5 would have indicated *total* satisfaction). The one caveat that should be taken into account, though, was that the factor analysis of these environmental items did not fully support the original WHO model of QoL. Question 14 (leisure activities) fell more into the 'social' domain than into the environmental and, interestingly, question 8 (safety in daily life) seemed to be interpreted as more about 'mobility' than environment. However, despite these slight contradictions, overall the WHO conceptualization of 'environment' was found to be reasonably robust for people with a chronic health challenge.

When relating the WHO environmental questions to those living with chronic health problems, it is vital to keep in mind that each specific health problem may impact on the questions in a very different way. This is especially true of disorders such as multiple sclerosis or, using our exemplar again, Parkinson's, because they

Table 3 Responses from people with Parkinson's disease to questions on the WHOQoL-Bref relating to the 'environmental' domain.

Question number	Mean score	Question content	Domain designated by WHO
14	2.93*	Do you have opportunity for leisure activities?	Environment
8	3.01*	How safe do you feel in your daily life?	Environment
9	3.54*	How healthy is your physical environment?	Environment
13	3.64*	How available is the information you need daily?	Environment
12	3.80*	To what extent do you have money for your needs?	Environment
25	3.81†	How satisfied are you with your transport?	Environment
24	3.87†	How satisfactory is your access to health services?	Environment
23	4.28†	How satisfied are you with your living conditions?	Environment

Overall mean: 2.99
*Where 1 = not at all, 3 = moderately, and 5 = completely.
†Where 1 = very dissatisfied, 3 = neither satisfied nor dissatisfied, and 5 = very satisfied.

tend to have highly proactive support societies to back them. These societies frequently have mission statements stating one of their aims as improving the QoL for people with the disorder. Through such charities, telephone information lines, help lines and web links are usually set up to improve access to information for their members, and ultimately improve QoL.

Because the WHO questionnaire is a generic, not disease-specific, QoL instrument, there is one area omitted that is known to distress many people with LTCs. This is the challenge of 'coming out' about compromised health status. 'Coming out' will be briefly unpacked in the following paragraphs, together with question 8, 'How safe do you feel in your daily life?'

Psychosocial implications of environmental difficulties

'Coming out' with a long term condition

For some living with a chronic health condition in the UK, it has been part of their life since birth. Unfortunately, however, the majority of those with a LTC will have had to navigate the turbulent waters of psychological adjustment and learn to live with newly diagnosed conditions that compromise health status. Few LTCs are totally invisible although clearly, some, like PD and multiple sclerosis, are more discernible than others. Where the health condition cannot be cloaked, it must seem entirely natural to 'deploy specific techniques to attract or deflect other people's attention to or from aspects of their bodies' (Seymour, 1998: p. 34). This is because the individual in modern society can be considered a 'performing self who is constantly on display and who is judged by his presentation in the public arena' (Öberg & Tornstam, 1999: p. 630). Goffman (1990) said the ability 'to perform' is fundamental when shaping a version of self that is socially valued rather than stigmatized. Following from this then, it is to be expected that many people with a LTC conceal their health difficulties from employers, friends and even, in some cases, close family. Such behaviours echo the actions of Wendell (1996: p. 8), who lived with ME[4] for a number of years and described how 'those of us who can learn to be, or be seen, as normal do so, and those of us who cannot meet the standards of normality usually achieve the closest approximation we can manage'.

Accounts of concealing LTCs can be seen in the press and on the internet. In a press interview, Cohn explained why she concealed her physical limitations: 'I've met obstacles, people not accepting me, job discrimination. People are afraid of difference and their own vulnerability' (Cohn, 2001: p. 5). Her comments were ratified relatively recently when Jerry Lewis was recorded referring to all people with chronic illness as 'half people' (Starkloff, 1999) and David Jones, the outgoing chief executive of Next, only disclosed his neurodegenerative diagnosis after 20 years of 'covering up' (Rankine, 2001: p. 33).

Work carried out by a welfare and employment rights advisor has shown that people with LTCs frequently conceal their health status because of uncertainties regarding income, or for fear of occupational marginalization, and that those most at risk due to their occupations are, invariably, the self-employed. If more people were able to feel totally secure about their employment prospects, even with their health disclosed, perhaps those feeling the need to 'conceal' might be reduced.

The implications for QoL in relation to 'disclosure' are largely unknown. However, findings from the Parkinson's study might usefully be extrapolated and considered here. Anecdotally, those who were confident enough to tell others immediately about their PD reported a good quality of life in response to their direct attitude, whereas the 'concealers', living in fear of being 'discovered', frequently talked about anxiety and a diminished QoL, which they felt was directly attributable to their subterfuge. Once a 'cover up' stance has been taken, a major decision then has to be made as to when might be the 'best' time to 'tell all'.

A really serious, pragmatic consequence of refusing to 'come out' may involve legal issues such as refused claims on insurance policies due to non-disclosure of a LTC. 'Coming out' may be handled either with caution or with an aggressive kicking down of the closet door. Israel (2001: p. 1) devised protocols to aid with disclosure. She directed that 'disclosures occur without drama, overwrought emotions, self-deprecating statements [and] taking into consideration others needs', adding that 'living with a secret can be torturous' particularly when 'many individuals become excessively obsessed with guilt' (Israel, 2001: p. 4; Human Rights Campaign Foundation, 2001). To aid with admission of health state, Sauerman (1995) published the following protocols:

1 Accept that some people may take the news as a temporary loss similar to the death of a person they love, so may feel denial, anger or depression.

---

[4]ME stands for myalgic encephalomyelitis – 'a debilitating neurological condition characterised by extreme fatigue; ME may last for many months or even years' (Sharpe, 2001: p. 118).

2 An initial state of shock can be expected. Be completely honest and explain that concealment would only harm interpersonal relationships.
3 Seek counselling where appropriate.
4 Break through any forms of denial – gentle prompting might be required.
5 Allow for different responses; often one person takes the lead and moves towards resolution ahead of others. Recognize that where couples are involved dysfunctions may occur in their own relationship.
6 Assure all concerned that no one has *caused* the health problems. Parents in particular may take on a burden of guilt and will need repeated reassurance.

Having enacted these protocols for herself , Sauerman (1995: p. 15) said:

'I've looked upon it as an unplanned journey. It was thrust upon us; we'd hardly have signed up for it if given the option of choosing something else. Unplanned however, does not mean unwelcomed. Today we can say, 'We're glad we know . . . Unplanned but not unwelcome.'

Action Learning Point

- For research purposes, how might the term 'environment' be used?
- Why is it important to consider the impact of environmental issues on people with LTCs?
- When is the optimum time for people with LTCs to 'come out' to family? To friends? To business associates?
- Why/how is access to 'leisure activities' an environmental issue?

The psychological domain

So much of what has already been written in this chapter could sit comfortably within the psychological domain, but for the purposes of continuity the WHO definition will be examined first. WHO proposed six definitive psychological questions for their QoL measure, but an additional three questions were found to relate to the domain (Table 4). Those items designated 'extra-domain' by WHO intuitively look like they should be conceptualized as relating to the emotions, but it was gratifying to have this confirmed by factor analysis.

As can be seen from Table 4, most of the WHO psychological questions ask, either directly or indirectly, about 'mood'. The exception to this is seen in question 11, relating to body image, and this will be unpacked in a later section, as once again the WHO designations were not fully applicable to people with a LTC. Perhaps this is the time to emphasize that generic QoL measures are notoriously poor at identifying psychological difficulties, and that disease-specific questionnaires are even worse. When deciding on which QoL measure to use (if any) with a particular patient group, the most important questions to ask are:

- For whom was this questionnaire developed?
- Is it totally reliable and fully validated?
- How were the topics on the questionnaire generated?
- Were people with the disorder (e.g. PD, multiple sclerosis, ME, etc.) consulted?

Table 4 Ranked means in response to 'psychological' questions on the WHOQoL-Bref.

Mean score	Question number	Question content	Domain designated by WHO
2.64*	26	How often do you have blue moods, anxiety or despair?	Psychological
2.87†	19	How satisfied are you with yourself?	Psychological
2.91†	27	How fed up do you feel?	Extra-domain
3.03†	7	How well are you able to concentrate?	Psychological
3.17†	6	To what extent do you feel life to be meaningful?	Psychological
3.20†	5	How much do you enjoy life?	Psychological
3.28†	1	How would you rate your quality of life?	Extra-domain
3.44†	11	Are you able to accept your bodily appearance?	Psychological
3.45†	28	How satisfied are you with your level of happiness?	Extra-domain

Overall mean: 3.11
*Where 1 = never, and 5 = always.
†Where 1 = very dissatisfied, and 5 = very satisfied.

- Was it generated by medical professionals working in the field of the specific disorder?
- Could there be a 'hidden agenda' with this questionnaire?
- Who funded its development?
- Is it fully applicable to the UK?
- Will the target population be able to manage the questionnaire without becoming over-tired?
- Is it easy to administer (logistically)?

Only by thoroughly screening any given QoL questionnaire can it be used to its full capacity. Once a practitioner understands its strengths and weaknesses, it can be used to its full potential and maximize the benefits to both patient group and practitioner. To clarify, the PDQ39 (Peto et al., 1995) is a Parkinson's disease-specific QoL questionnaire, comprising 39 questions, in eight named domains, which purport to definitively measure QoL for anyone with PD. The items on the questionnaire were generated by interviewing people with PD and asking each about their own individual lives with the disorder. The interviews continued until data saturation point had been reached, which is when no new topics are being raised. It is validated for use throughout the world and has proved to be, since its development, a really valuable research tool. However, the PDQ39 omits to ask people with PD about their sex lives, despite a plethora of evidence to say that 'sexual difficulties' can impact on QoL in an overwhelmingly negative way (PD Society, PDS6a). As Lloyd (1999: p. 20) found, 'sexual problems and sexuality issues often assumed major importance' for people with PD. The question to be asked then is: How could a global Parkinson's-specific QoL tool, the financial development of which was supported by the PD Society (UK), fail to recognize that sexual problems would certainly impact on QoL for people with PD? The answer is relatively straightforward. The questions on the PDQ39 were generated by interviews, carried out *by academics*, so those being interviewed were not sufficiently relaxed as to be able to talk about an immensely personal and private area of their lives.

Because many QoL tools disappoint when attempting to identify psychological difficulties for those with LTCs, the practitioner is forced to look to other methods. The skilled professional should hopefully be able to pick up on mood changes or alterations in behaviour in patients with health problems, but where there is no regular face-to-face interaction, then the questionnaire methodology could be supplemented by a qualitative methodology, such as direct interviews with those who are chronically sick. By carrying out interviews with people with a LTC, a researcher can legitimize the feelings of patients, and may lead to their talking about their social and psychological difficulties. This is indeed what has happened previously, where those with a LTC (in this case, PD) spoke about issues such as guilt, fear and anger/resentment (Loggenberg, 2005). Because of the dominance of these psychological problems in previous work, the areas of guilt, fear and anger/resentment will be fully explored in the following paragraphs, with links to more general LTCs.

Psychosocial implications of psychological difficulties

Guilt

Amongst medical professionals, there exists a general consensus that *any* chronic illness can lead to feelings of guilt, and that this guilt may manifest itself in myriad different ways. Michelson and Wynn (2001: p. 1) explained how guilt can be seen in 'the husband who has difficulty discussing the disease', the mother who 'cries often' or in 'family dynamics in a constant state of flux', whilst Seaburn (2001) pointed out that 'strong emotions' were all perfectly 'normal reactions' and should be embraced as part of a process of coming to terms with any diagnosis of chronic debility. Earlier, Garnett (1993: p. 1) had suggested that the only way to stop 'extreme guilt [and] suicidal thoughts' from exacerbating existing LTCs was to 'express [the guilt and] start toward resolution of the problem, [so that] long suppressed emotions do not resurface again and again'. In the context of any LTC, guilt can drain the quality of life for anyone closely involved with the patient, as well as for the patient him/herself.

The person with the health difficulties may feel guilty because of problems like depleted energy, extreme fatigue and lack of ambition; such feelings are more likely to be found in younger people. The most common reason for older people with a LTC to express feelings of guilt is that of 'becoming a burden'.

The psychological issues for carers can be highly complex. For example, in marriages where the male has generally taken a dominant, decision-making role but is now battling with health problems, it may be especially testing to allow the partner to take control and make all the key financial, legal and life choices. If the person with the LTC is elderly, the role reversal becomes even more problematic as the couple are already needing to make changes at an age when change is most difficult.

A relatively novel finding from the Parkinson's research field, that is entirely transferable to any other LTC, is that guilt tends to be highly resilient and often continues for many years after the person with health problems has died, and thus has the potential to impact on QoL for many decades. There is a dearth of literature devoted to ameliorating problems of guilt associated with chronic illness; evidently, there is a void to be filled. When scrutinizing the psychological consequences of living with a LTC, it might be worth keeping in mind the advice of Fitzsimmons and Bunting (2001: p. 1), who claimed that 'the concept of quality of life then goes beyond the dimensions of health functioning to performance of social roles, mental acuity, emotional states, subjective well-being and interrelationship'.

Fear

According to Pulst (2003: p. 2), the fears that tended to diminish QoL are 'worrying about how (your condition) will affect your life, concern about how quickly the disease will progress and what kinds of limitations to expect'. It may be relatively easy for people with LTCs to become morbidly preoccupied with their vulnerabilities and with the unfathomable implications of dying. But the point must be made that fear and caution should be clearly distinguished from each other. For people with chronic health challenges, fear is generally restrictive, preoccupative and, if not repressed, may become all-consuming (Young, 1999). Conversely, recent research has been able to show that caution, when sensibly exercised by a person with health problems, may prevent serious injury from falls, tumbles on stairs or may simply smooth the path of everyday life (Priddle, 2001).

Perhaps all people with LTCs could learn to combat their individual, highly personalized fears by adopting a similar attitude to that chosen by a medical professional doctor who himself had been forced to retire early from his profession due to having a LTC. McGoon (1990), knowing that 'fear' could preoccupy the minds of the chronically sick, suggested that fear and a LTC are mutually incompatible:

> 'We patients . . . should feel liberated from an excessive fear of death. We have, it seems, much less reason to dread the ultimate release from life's burdens. Let us enjoy our remaining lifetime to the limit of our restricted abilities, rather than forfeiting our remaining blessings and adding to our misery with inflated fears.' (McGoon, 1990: p. 145).

Fear of chronic illness is not a rare phenomenon, however the precise mechanisms of fear remain relatively unknown. The evidence suggests that *all* people with a LTC live with fear to a greater or lesser degree. Some people have adaptive mechanisms that help accommodate fear, whilst others are frightened of each new day. Although a search of extant literature sources failed to identify *why* those with a LTC might be frightened, there were better results from interviews and published case histories that were reviewed, as these did shed some light on the matter (Dakof & Mendelsohn, 1986; Barbosa et al., 1997; Baatile et al., 2000; Meyers et al., 2000; Heilman, 2001; Sunvisson & Ekman, 2001). The causes suggested were fear of the future, of dying, of symptom worsening, of choking to death, of depression and of cognitive decline. Fear and uncertainty have only one known antidote – information. If all people who newly join the corpus of people with a LTC were fully informed of their condition, in lay terms, many fears might well be tempered. Until such an ideal is realized, many people will continue to live with a psychological and emotional deprivation that removes the 'quality' from their lives.

Anger/resentment

Some of the psychological implications of living with a LTC raised in this chapter might represent new areas for practitioners to reflect on, whereas most people who have associated with those with chronic health challenges will recognize that both anger and resentment may raise their heads at any time. Although this anger/resentment (the terms are used interchangeably) might be expressed in personal and occasionally idiosyncratic ways, there is a small body of evidence to suggest that *all* people newly diagnosed with a chronic illness will inevitably feel some degree of anger about the change in their health status. Andersen (2002: p. 44) ascribed the origin of his 'anger' as rooted in a grieving process. 'Grief' he believes, must inexorably follow learning of 'a chronic debilitating disease' and will be expressed because 'the sense of being healthy . . . is lost, along with a part of one's identity' and 'such losses are not easy to digest'. Initially, Andersen's 'anger' was directed at the health problem itself, then he was angry at how unfair the world was, and finally he was extremely (and slightly illogically) angry with the doctor who had confirmed he was ill. Like Lester (2004: p. 2) who reported a patient's anger as an 'emotional, almost irrational outburst against the bio-medical professional community' due to the patient's 'bitter reaction and frustration and misdirected anger', Andersen initially found his changed health status 'not easy to digest', but ultimately he discovered that he was able to reconcile himself to the 'new reality, [and] adjust . . . creatively', until in due course he was able to resume life with renewed enthusiasm (Andersen 2002: p. 123).

Unfortunately, not everyone with a LTC will be able to positively adjust to their new status and much anger may be directed at those closest to the patient, hence the success of popular songs such as 'You always hurt the one you love'.[5] Knowing that the anger/resentment may ultimately prove destructive to personal relationships is no deterrent for many with LTCs and the impact on overall QoL is frequently dual-pronged. First, when angry and bad tempered, the bile is directed at those closest to the patient, thus potentially reducing the quality of the core relationship in the patient's life. Second, these same feelings of anger, when coupled with the physical limitations of the chronic health condition, may reduce social QoL as unresolved personal conflicts may stop people from socializing together. Ultimately, friends, family and carers may choose to enjoy their social and physical pursuits (walking, sailing, etc.) with other, more able-bodied and possibly more even-tempered, companions.

---

[5] 'You always hurt the one you love, The one you shouldn't hurt at all, You always take the sweetest rose, And crush it till the petals fall, You always break the kindest heart, With a hasty word you can't recall – So if I broke your heart last night, it's because I love you most of all' (Roberts & Fisher, 1944).

As previously stated, anger and resentment may naturally accompany diagnosis of chronic illness (sometimes termed a biographic disruption) because 'one of the most common reactions is anger' (Panicker et al., 1999: p. 144). As long as 'people defy the myth of perfection . . . defy the disciplines of normality and . . . attack everyone's sense of well-being and invincibility' (Hunt 1966: p. 155), there will necessarily be resentment. Unfortunately, little has been published to minimize the effects of resentment or anger. This omission has contributed to a 'culture of silence' where anger is 'submerged' and there exist no 'resources, vigour and vocabulary to expose it' (Freire, 1993: p. 12).

Fitzgerald (1995) strongly argued that the 'culture of silence' permeates much social policy and ensures that no one speaks. Much of the anger people with a LTC feel could be neutralized if people were more understanding. West (1992: p. 30) found that 56% of people with a LTC felt that they were treated differently, pre- and post-diagnosis. She noted that most 'normal'[6] people were uncomfortable with disability (one woman with a LTC felt her friends had become 'patronising baby sitters') and that there was a positive correlation between psychological well-being and how well people understood chronic health states.

The implications seem clear; if the anger associated with disability is neither owned nor treated, many people with LTCs must remain psychologically malfunctional and have diminished QoL for the foreseeable future. Society must now address its own prejudices and reconceptualize chronic illness. Whilst the majority of people continue to perceive LTCs as vile and pitiful illnesses, and people with the health problems continue to be seen as 'sufferers', then anger and resentment must, inexorably, exist. In time, maybe those with a LTC may be perceived as empowered, functioning individuals with real QoL. And if such perceptions create over-optimistic pastiches of life with LTCs, then at least there will be something to balance against the current, overwhelmingly negative focus the media insists on.

In summary, it seems that although the physical complications of LTCs tend to represent the major area of concern for most chronically ill people, the psychological problems inexorably follow on from those physical impediments. Given that so many medical professionals throughout the world devote their skills to improving the situation for those with a LTC through drug and surgical intervention, perhaps the time has come for the psychological sequelae to be recognized, and for QoL to be enshrined as the measure by which to manage the chronically sick and their complex health (physical and emotional) needs.

Action Learning Point

- Why is it vital for practitioners to consider the psychological health of their patients?
- Why should people *never* be called 'diabetic', 'parkinsonian', etc?
- Why might chronically sick people feel anger or resentment?
- What is wrong with the term 'sufferer'?

---

[6] Normal: 'conforming to that which is characteristic and representative of a group; not deviating markedly from the average or typical' (Reber, 1995: p. 498).

The social domain

Social relationships

The WHOQoL questionnaire used in the Parkinson's research, used as an exemplar in this chapter, asked about both 'social support' and 'personal relationships' for people with Parkinson's. Somewhat incongruously, WHO perceived the question 'How satisfied are you with your sex life?' as one relating to 'social relationships'. The statistical results of the study did not support this description, so a factor analysis was used to clarify how this question was interpreted. It seemed the item on 'sex life' was primarily tied to the 'physical', but also in part to the 'psychological'. One of the most interesting findings in this domain was that five of the 'environmental' issues were clarified by factor analysis as being more 'social', possibly due to their being seen as relating to 'social support'.

Importantly, whichever way they were interpreted, the mean scores for the 'social' questions on the WHO questionnaire showed that social problems were less problematic than physical. The single exception to this inclination was 'leisure activities', which bucked the general trend and highlighted a problem that a small body of literature has previously identified. Given that social researchers already know that people who have a LTC are those most at risk of reduced social contact (Singer, 1974), this result should be seen as quite alarming.

One final area of concern that emerged in the Parkinson's research (but during interview, not in response to a QoL questionnaire) and which could definitely be construed as 'social', referred to the quality of interpersonal relationships people had with their medical professional support teams. Because people with PD, and indeed any LTC, tend to have long term relationships with medical professionals,

Table 5 Responses to the WHOQoL-Bref relating to the social domain as supported by factor analysis.

Question number	Question content	Domain designated by WHO	Domain as result of factor analysis
14	Do you have opportunity for leisure activities?	Environment	Social domain (loss)
13	How available is the information you need daily?	Environment	Social domain (support)
20	How satisfied are you with your personal relationships?	Social relationship	Social domain
25	How satisfied are you with your transport?	Environment	Social domain (support)
24	How satisfactory is your access to health services?	Environment	Social domain (support)
22	How satisfactory is your support from your friends?	Social relationship	Social domain
23	How satisfied are you with your living conditions?	Environment	Social domain (support)

and because those with chronic health problems may have idiosyncratic, constantly changing needs, it seems entirely defensible to describe such long term care as a social issue.

Interpersonal relationships with medical professional teams

When talking to patients with a LTC there seems to be a raw underbelly of resentment that apparently rages against the medical profession. Interviews with patients and a plethora of case histories have illuminated a number of common complaints about medical professionals, including: unnecessary delays in diagnosis, patronizing attitudes, lack of time spent with specialists, over-reliance on medical professionals, and lack of continuity in consulting medical professionals. A common theme to emerge from all patients is that receiving a diagnosis of a LTC is a defining moment in their life.

Written case histories have confirmed that the majority of people with a LTC are, to a greater or lesser degree, unhappy with their relationships with their medical professional teams. Quindlen (2000: p. 1) asked only that professionals learn to see their patients 'as human beings – not as a pile of demographic statistics' or, in other words, 'without prejudice and without preconception'.

Noble (2000: p. 50) saw LTCs as a continual challenge to the medical profession because of the need for 'multidisciplinary initiatives to improve and sustain the quality of life'. She insisted that:

'practitioners need to be active problem diagnosticians and artful problem solvers. They must be ready to listen hard to the experiences of families.'

Because professionals are constantly being advised 'to improve the provision of medical professional support . . . [and to] prove the worth of services in today's cash-limited healthcare systems' (Clarke et al., 1995: p. 288), Clarke et al. suggested that medical professionals should be seen to work together to achieve common goals.

Although many professionals agree that best practice for treating LTCs should always include a referral to a multidisciplinary team, few of those with chronic health difficulties actually benefit from such a referral. However, 'a multidisciplinary team . . . and GP should discuss and agree . . . working practices which should be endorsed by all, including patients' (Bhatia et al., 1998: p. 478). Godwin-Austen and Hildick-Smith (1982: p. 14) felt that 'specialist review at intervals . . . would give the patient the best of both worlds', and Oertel and Ellgring (1995: p. 78) recommended that 'neurologists, psychiatrists, psychologists and other professionals' should all be involved. Unfortunately, the evidence suggests that access to a multidisciplinary team for those with LTCs is the exception rather than the rule. Because of this 'absence', there is a corresponding decrease in QoL for people who are not referred.

One aspect of the relationship between patient and medical professional that tends to be overlooked is the fact that most health professionals (doctors, nurses, physiotherapists, speech and language therapists, etc.) are trained to consider their profession as a curative profession; this may lead them to see palliative care as a compromise. They have full knowledge of the very worst complications that might develop for patients with LTCs (including depression, regular hospital admissions, disrupted employment patterns and even, in neurological disorders, cognitive decline), so perhaps it is to be expected that they are not always encouraging when interacting with patients who have chronic health needs. An alternative way to look at the difficult relationships might be to view the dilemma as attributable to a lack of support for medical professionals themselves. Repeatedly, research has shown that medical professionals have dangerously elevated stress levels (Rose & Rosow, 1993; Rout & Rout 1993; Rout et al., 1996; Avallone et al., 1997), yet despite the evidence little has been done to relieve such pressure.

Perhaps the most disturbing evidence relating to 'relationships with medical professional teams' and QoL is that few people with LTCs see their medical professional team as a harmonious whole; ultimately this undermines confidence in the system. The result is that those with the health difficulties lament the quality of their contact with medical professionals whilst, simultaneously, researchers in the field of chronic ill health berate their fellow professionals for not adopting a multidisciplinary approach to care. There seems to be just the one mutual goal. Perhaps if a circular solution were pursued whereby medical professionals were better supported professionally, and people with long term health needs were listened to assiduously, then a way forward might be found. But until the voices of the patients are valued and acted upon, the gulf between 'them' and 'us' must remain.

Social life and chronic health challenges

Oxtoby (1982: p. 38) analysed the social activities of 261 people with a LTC in Britain. She regretted that 15% 'actually wrote "nothing" or "no activities" when asked about leisure pursuits', and she concluded that 'days filled with boredom are a very potent source of unhappiness' for patients with LTCs. Whilst acknowledging that 'it is very difficult in any survey to obtain valid measures of social isolation', her study did show that 'more company' was the thing most frequently identified as being needed 'most of all' by people with a LTC (Oxtoby, 1982: p. 43). She identified the negatives of social living with a LTC as: days filled with boredom, difficulty with leisure activities, embarrassment about eating or drinking in public, children taken into care, and a saddening 58% of patients deferring holidays due to their condition. Reading, watching television and napping were the main activities of those who took part in the Oxtoby study. The destructive impact of such problems on QoL should not be overlooked.

A decade later, West (1992: p. 31) also found from a study of 49 people with a LTC that, 'specific difficulties inhibited socialising and . . . that a saddening 65% felt their social life had been curtailed by their disorder'. Additionally, West established that many chronically ill people saw others as being 'uncomfortable in their presence, until inevitably, the worse they become, the smaller becomes their social life' and this despite the fact that 'contact with others seemed to have a beneficial effect . . . and enhanced psychosocial well-being'.

A robust finding from the research of Oertel and Ellgring (1995: p. 78) was that 83% of people with a LTC felt *stressed* about their social life, so the research team recommended that intervention strategies be taught to enable 'the patient to solve these psychosocial problems'. Rather depressingly, no intervention strategies were ever developed though, so that Sunvisson and Ekman (2001: p. 44) had to report: 'an overriding sense of "being enslaved by illness" characterizes the daily lives of patients [who have] . . . little control over family, social situations or their future'.

Thankfully, the patient reality of a social life with a LTC is not *all* negative. There may be excellent environmental support, first-rate personal relationships and strong family scaffolding to shore up the lives of patients. However, what does seem clear from the assembled evidence is that, despite all this apparent goodwill, patients still tend to experience 'premature social ageing' (Singer, 1974: p. 143).[7] Although, originally, it was Singer who characterized and gave name to the impoverished social lives of people with LTCs, she has not been a lone voice in the wilderness. Dakof and Mendelsohn (1986: p. 375) noted that 'a compelling set of concerns . . . has received scant attention, namely, how individuals experience the impairments and limitations imposed by their neuropathology'. They explained that the 'paucity of psychosocial data' was a natural result of the dominance of the biomedical professional paradigm with its focus on 'reduction of capacity . . . and deteriorating function'. Lack of psychosocial research for LTCs has also been highlighted (Lee et al., 1994; Livneh & Antonak, 1994; Abudi et al., 1997; Diaz & Larrachea 1997; Brod et al., 1999; Noble, 2000; Schreurs et al., 2000; Sunvisson & Ekman, 2001). The calls for more social research have been plentiful but, to date, the responses have been limited. Andersen (1999: p. S26) has explained how,

> 'effective adaptation [to a LTC] demands that patients . . . elaborate coping strategies that empower them and promote a more salutary orientation to formidable psychosocial difficulties and thus, perhaps, blunt or prevent depressive responses.'

An active and satisfying social life must be encouraged so that patients may 'seize the initiative in terms of promoting an acceptable life-style . . . breaking through, rather than breaking down'.

Social identity

Although 'social identity' was not a domain used on the WHO questionnaire, the results of the factor analyses carried out on the QoL measure produced a grouping that defied any other description (Table 6). Any matters that caused a person to question their existing self-schema were classified as belonging to 'social identity'. The responses to the WHO questionnaire seemed to highlight that for many people with a LTC there were a number of losses to their lives following diagnosis, and that these appreciably detracted from good QoL. Had it not been for the detailed factor analyses performed on the quantitative database in the Parkinson's study, the domain of 'social identity' for those with LTCs might have remained in

---

[7] According to Singer, 'premature social ageing' describes the reduction in social activity and close friendships experienced by most people with PD (Singer, 1974: p. 143).

Table 6 Responses to questions on the WHOQoL-Bref questionnaire that comprised a new 'social identity' domain as supported by factor analysis.

Question number	Mean score*	Question content	Domains	Factor loadings
15	2.91	Are you able to get around?	Social identity/physical	0.31, 0.74
14	2.93	Opportunity for leisure activities?	Social identity/physical	0.53, 0.43
16	2.96	Satisfaction with your sleep?	Social identity	0.53
8	3.01	Safety in your daily life?	Social identity/physical	0.50, 0.46
7	3.03	How well can you concentrate?	Social identity	0.61
6	3.17	How much is life meaningful?	Social identity/psychological	0.42, 0.50

Overall mean: 3.00
*Where 1 = not at all, 3 = a moderate amount, and 5 = extremely.

obscurity. It was only when the additional unidentified domain was thought of in terms of 'losses' that it became clear that the items from the questionnaire were connected to the social identity of someone with a LTC. The evidence showed that physical losses can and do have an enormous detrimental effect on sense of self. Patients seemed to 'lose' the person they used to think they were, and were forced to negotiate a new identity for themselves – one which incorporated the 'sick self'.

The 'losses' reported via the WHO questionnaire focused on getting around, getting out (leisure activities), sleeping and physical safety; and then focused on the more abstract losses such as 'concentration' and a 'meaningful life'. The true nature of the losses was not entirely clear until all the results were analysed. It then became apparent that almost all people with a LTC pass through a period of identity crisis, with the timing and severity of the crises varying from person to person. Construction and negotiation of social identity for people with chronic illness is not new; identity and identity confusion have been addressed by social scientists since the earliest times (James, 1890; Allport, 1955; Harré, 1976; Tajfel, 1981; Breakwell, 1983, 1992). However, few health researchers have considered social identity to be important, presumably, again, because of the supremacy of the biomedical professional model, and none has incorporated it into a QoL model.

Social identity and body image

The WHO questionnaire asks just one question about levels of satisfaction in the area of body image, and Table 7 shows how people with Parkinson's responded to it. Although the mean score on question 11 indicated that the people in this study were moderately able to accept their bodily appearance, this might not be

Table 7 Responses to question 11 on the WHO questionnaire. The WHO assigned this to the psychological domain.

Question number	Mean score*	Question content	Domains	Factor loadings
11	3.44	Can you accept your bodily appearance?	Identity (loss)/physical	0.26, 0.50

*Where 1 = not at all, 3 = a moderate amount, and 5 = completely.

an accurate indication of their body image as such. The results of the factor analysis suggested that this question was interpreted as a 'mobility' issue (eigen value 0.50) from within the physical domain, rather than a psychological or social identity issue. Fortunately, there were ample interview data to supplement the WHO findings and these data were used to augment the slightly ambiguous questionnaire results. When massed together, the findings from the PD study showed that the changes to the body resulting from the LTC caused many people to despair, and wrecked life quality for many of those who took part in the research. Because this was such a damaging problem for so many people, and possibly difficult for those of us with healthy, fully-functioning bodies to comprehend, a number of quotes from the original PD study have been selected to illustrate, in the following case studies, how people with a LTC felt about their bodies.

Case study 1

Don (pseudonym) had led an especially active life prior to having PD and was a keen mountaineer, hiker and rock climber. He was one of the men who was most vociferous about his physical appearance. He commented:

'Parkinson's gives you a right "Charlie" on your back. If I see myself in a shop window, when I'm out, I look like an old man. I've got a right "Charlie" . . . It drives you down. If I wasn't ill, I wouldn't even think about age. Parkinson's shrinks you . . . It drives you and it shrivels you . . . It shrinks your body, and I didn't realize that until one morning. I woke up and I was really off . . . and I felt *that* small [index finger and thumb stuck together]. I felt like a hedgehog curled up . . . that's Parkinson's . . . it really shrinks you.'

(Don, transcript lines 339–346)

What was especially surprising about Don's statement was that this was a completely unsolicited comment. No questions had been put to him about his physical appearance, most especially since, when the interview started, he was utterly frozen (by his disorder) into immobility. A further surprise was to follow, when the subject of physical appearance and body image was raised again at a group interview. Once again, it was a man who seemed most distressed about perceived changes to his looks (Case study 2).

Case study 2

Jack (pseudonym) virtually exploded with indignation when talking about how he felt. He was dressed extremely well and looked both youthful and healthy, but still felt that:

'Before I was diagnosed . . . well I've got other problems. But nobody knew about them . . . if I didn't tell them. I feel that, overnight, I've gone from a young, fit, able man into . . . an old man. I walk like an old man. I think I look like an old man in the mirror . . . I actually despise looking in a mirror now . . . It really does get to me, that. It does, yes. . . . very much so . . . It's how it feels.'

(Jack, transcript lines 185–192)

One of the most articulate female interviewees was Martha. As a retired (due to ill health) professional woman, she seemed to have considerable insight into how she might appear to others (Case study 3).

Case study 3

'It is very difficult to feel, or even make yourself look attractive, in the later stages of the disease. Feeling old and decrepit . . . hardly able to put one foot in front of the other . . . dribbling and drooling, shaking from head to foot – all this is enough to turn anyone off . . . and it must be distressing for a loving partner . . . to live with this type of deterioration. How does one ever truly accept it . . . how to accept the new 'status quo' gracefully? The breakdown of a close and loving relationship through illness is worse . . . possibly . . . than an actual bereavement . . . a living hell in fact!

(Martha, transcript lines 84–89)

From the extracts quoted, it is clear that body image issues are not confined to the fashion industry, nor do they show a gender bias, but both men *and* women with LTCs have been vitriolic about the changes their bodies undergo whilst making the journey occasioned by a LTC. Given that in the PD work, more men than women mourned the loss of previously robust body image, it might be argued that women are more resilient in their responses to body image disruption, possibly because from puberty onwards hormonal fluctuations can lead to constant flux.

Working with another LTC, Williams and Barlow (1998) investigated body image in relation to arthritis and found that self-concept, and belief about oneself, were central tenets of mental health and that society idealized the attractive, fully-functioning, controlled body. Given that most people with a LTC could be considered to be the antithesis of such body ideals, the inclusion of a body image (physical appearance) category within a QoL model must be justified. The ever-increasing significance given to physical appearance and bodily presentation in recent years (Featherstone, 1991; Turner, 1994) has resulted in a reification of the 'healthy, attractive body' (Salter 1997: p. 1) and, ultimately, to the ascendancy of the 'myth of bodily perfection, in which we can and should strive to achieve perfect bodies' (Stone 1995: p. 413).

Reporting at the same time as Salter, Barron (1997: p. 230) also underlined the importance of 'still feeling attractive'. He pointed out that the prevailing norms of physical beauty 'play an important part in how people view themselves, as physical appearances are an important part of the identity'. Furthermore, that 'having a physical impairment may mean having to come to terms with a body that departs from cultural norms of attractiveness' (Barron, 1997: p. 229). There can be little doubt that the mass of evidence linking body image and social identity has far-reaching ramifications for those who feel less attractive due to a LTC. In terms of QoL, the physical self is affected in predictable, reasonably well documented ways, but the impact to the psyche is more challenging to measure. It may be seen in reports of diminished confidence or in the changes to frequency, or type, of leisure activities. Clearly, both social lives and social relationships may be influenced by feeling unattractive, so health professionals who work with people with a LTC need to bear in mind that poor body image can have far-reaching consequences. Where problems of this nature do arise, then the work of Kelly and Field (1996), who outlined a 'negotiation model' to aid those with chronic illness, might prove useful. According to Williams (1996: p. 32), this model allows individuals 'to take positive (practical and symbolic) actions . . . to realign the relationship between body, self and society'.

Social identity and loss of confidence

Few people would doubt that confidence levels can be compromised by living with LTCs, but the QoL literature ignores 'confidence' altogether. This is rather disappointing as a number of research projects investigating the correlates of confidence and performance have shown that 'any negative event will affect the self-confidence in individuals and will make it difficult for them to perform' (Cox, 1998: p. 48). Even for people with perfect health and fitness levels, confidence tends to be highly abstract and subjective. Confidence has the synonyms of belief, certainty, assurance, poise and buoyancy, but it would be somewhat counterintuitive if people with LTCs were to choose to use such positive descriptors to depict themselves. Reassuringly, though, there is some evidence that confidence lost through health challenges may be regained after identity renegotiation has been successfully traversed.

After studying and pondering statements from people with LTCs about confidence, it seems to be the case that although losing one's confidence might superficially be seen as a 'psychological' construct, there is evidence, too, that confidence is linked to 'social identity' for some of the chronically sick. Where confidence levels are linked to job performance, and the job performance itself involves interpersonal interaction, then there appears to be a clear, discernible correlation between the two. The implications, especially for younger people with a LTC, suggest that employment status and job satisfaction might be diminished and, therefore, QoL could be lowered appreciably by this seemingly minor problem.

The other main implication for QoL and confidence is that when confidence is battered by feelings of unattractiveness, then core interpersonal relationships might be damaged. This is where the work of health professionals might prove crucial. If patients are seen to be losing confidence, then they should be referred to an appropriate specialist (psychologist, psychotherapist, cognitive behavioural therapist, occupational therapist or perhaps a counsellor) who may help them develop a number of attitudinal coping strategies.

Social identity and employment

Being employed, whether full time, part time or voluntarily, is known to affect perceptions of happiness. Kahneman et al. (1999) showed that employment status positively impacted on self-esteem, attitude, mood and general satisfaction with life. They suggested that lack of satisfactory employment inevitably leads to boredom, poor mental health, higher suicide rates, increased depression and even alcoholism. Because, during the course of the journey with a LTC, *all* those who are ill will have personal physical battles to fight, it seems unfair to burden them with employment problems too. The WHO questionnaire includes just one question about 'capacity for work' and the responses from people with Parkinson's can be seen in Table 8.

Although those who took part in the PD QoL study saw this question as primarily a mobility query (therefore from within the physical domain), they did show by their responses that they also saw it as having a psychological element. Perhaps this was not the most interesting dynamic here though; with a mean score of just 2.15, 'capacity for work' was reported to be *the* most serious issue to compromise QoL for people with a LTC. Unfortunately, there is no possible way of deconstructing the precise mechanism that caused 'capacity for work' to decrease life quality for those who took part in the study, but we should recognize that WHO chose their wording for this item very carefully indeed. This was not simply about employment, but could also be interpreted as 'work' in relation to daily chores such as gardening, housekeeping, walking to collect the newspaper, etc. By thus broadening the interpretation of question 18 on their QoL questionnaire, the compilers have designed an instrument that is sufficiently sensitive to be able to pick up subtle constructs of 'work'. Arguably this makes the questionnaire particularly valuable for people with LTCs who might not be formally employed in work but who, nevertheless, have work to do each and every day of their lives.

Evidence in the disability literature suggests that many people with LTCs who remain in formal employment do so by virtue of concealing their health status from their employers. This is a potentially perilous practice, as people may discover when they attempt to call in any occupational insurance policies – these are invalidated by non-disclosure of serious health conditions. Those who choose to retire early due to their health may consciously reject part-time or fractional employment opportunities 'for fear of losing social security and public health-care benefits' (Rabasca, 1999: p. 3). Some of the chronically sick might benefit from flexible working patterns, although, again, they run the risk of occupational marginalization. In the USA, McDonough and Amick (2001: p. 135) picked up that men were

Table 8 Responses to question 18 on the WHOQoL-Bref questionnaire. The WHO assigned this to the psychological domain.

Question number	Mean score*	Question content	Domains	Factor loadings
18	2.15	Satisfaction with capacity for work?	Physical/psychological	0.75, 0.19

*Where 1 = very dissatisfied, and 2 = dissatisfied.

'vulnerable to the labour market effects of poor health' and, interestingly, that 'black men were less likely to leave the labour force than white men'. Arrow, also investigating 'at risk' groups. found that 'people with previous patterns of unemployment were high risk for redundancy' (Arrow, 1996: p. 1651). Employment patterns reflect differential access to disability pensions/work-related benefits, therefore detailed analyses of trajectories for health and employment are clearly called for. 'Work comes in many forms: part-time, temporary, home-working, voluntary work, working for oneself, working for others, providing services, running bureaucracies, or entertaining' according to Porteous (1997: p. 3). Porteous noted that whilst, for some people, work was an activity to be avoided, others admitted that work was their main source of pleasure and satisfaction.

Wendell (1989) claimed that work and identity were inextricably linked in terms of productivity and achievement, yet there is a general understanding that all those with a LTC will, at some time, have to adapt 'productivity' levels to fit the demands of their disorder (Wermuth & Cox, 1996). Loss of status, which for some is synonymous with loss of employment, can frequently lead to deficiency of self-image and ultimately complete loss of self-worth. In addition to financial benefits, work can also provide important psychological rewards by helping to build self-esteem and general feelings of well-being (Kagan et al., 1997). Poarch (1998: p. 130) found 'a community of work' when researching, and suggested that if this 'community of work' is disrupted by diagnosis of chronic disease, the problem of threatened identity arises.

In 1994/5, a US census of unemployed people with disability found that 70% were jobless, despite three-quarters of these people saying they would prefer to work. Üstun and Sartorius (1996: p. 11) noted that 'attitudes towards those who are not employed outside the home remain atavistic . . . creating misery in those who do not hold a formally established job'. Sartorius alleged that a number of valuable social attributes were now lost, specifically 'the rearing of children, creative art and many other activities . . . [which] are accorded incomparably less attention, respect and rewards than success in one's work'. He recognized that paid work has been enshrined as the crowning achievement in the Western world. In Britain, Kagan et al. (1997: p. 2) discovered that 'work and home life may be in conflict, but in our culture both are essential for a full life'.

In general, the body of psychosocial research that addresses the needs of people with LTCs ignores the universal need for people to maintain their self-esteem and self-identity by contributing to the workforce and thus have robbed people of an important aspect of QoL. According to people with PD in the UK, 'satisfaction with work' is *the* most important component of QoL and therefore should never be flouted by those who purport to care for individuals with a LTC.

The reasons why people with LTCs are dissatisfied will generally be varied – physical limitations may lead to frustration with energy levels, there may also be a lack of information on reducing working hours or taking early retirement. Those who are unhappy due to decreased energy levels might realistically benefit from counselling therapies. If they are given help that enables them to align their work expectations with the reality of their health state, then levels of disappointment and frustration might be lowered and their overall QoL improved. Where there is a constant 'falling short' of planned 'work' (in its broadest sense), there will tend to be much frustration; if this is allowed to continue and fester, it must eventually decimate QoL for all those who are chronically sick.

For the second problem identified, where little information is offered to people with respect to alternatives to the full-time work model, the inference seems clear. Should these practices be continued, then many people who could contribute to the workforce in a meaningful way will be retired too early and against their wishes. Those being coerced into premature retirement due to a LTC are highly likely to represent the most experienced sector of any workforce, given that they will probably be older, and may well be reaching their peak productivity age. Clearly this trend ought to be arrested as soon as possible and those with LTCs should be enabled to work, full or part time, until they feel unsuited to do so. If necessary, employers who limit the productive lives of their employees by using discriminatory practices against those with health limitations should be prosecuted to the full extent of European law.

Those people with a LTC who do manage to remain in employment will, of necessity, have made significant sacrifices in order to align impaired health with employment practices. The evidence suggests a greater reluctance to retain men with LTCs than women, even where the men have specialist skills. Although a person's expertise may be channelled into charity work (possibly working for a society linked to their own health challenge), there must still be resentment that skills developed in a lifetime of employment are dismissed so easily. This suggests, again, that more time, money and legal expertise need to be dedicated to supporting people with LTCs who wish to continue with formal employment contracts.

In the past, many people with LTCs have reported feeling highly vulnerable when discussing their own future with their employer; they spoke of resentment towards managers who asked them to make career choices when they were still cognitively compromised due to recent diagnosis. Roessler et al. (1998: p. 189) investigated such effects together with how the chronically sick managed work decisions. They found that the two most important factors for maximizing career opportunities were: (i) ability to explain any special adaptations necessitated by their disorder (self-efficacy); and (ii) belief that they would retain employment as a result of their own efforts (outcome expectations). Other recommendations for successful adaptation were: (i) having resilient role models who had already coped with 'career problems created by chronic illnesses' (Roessler et al., 1998: p. 261); (ii) reduction of workplace barriers; (iii) objective assessment of barriers to productivity; (iv) career interventions to reduce or remove barriers (Roessler & Rumrill, 1999: p. 26); and (v) 'active labour market policies and employment protection [to] increase the opportunities for people . . . to remain in work' (Burstrom et al., 2000: p. 435).

There have been some interesting reports from neighbouring European countries where correlations of chronic illness and employment have been investigated. LaRocca et al. (1996: p. 37) found that people with chronic illness were unlikely to 'take advantage of job-retention services until an employment crisis develops'. LaRocca et al. recommended that all consultations should be organized sooner rather than later in the disease process.

Finally, if it is accepted that Table 8 above metaphorically 'shouted' the importance of work for people with a LTC, and that QoL was blighted by dissatisfaction in this area, then the full context of the work–family interface must be considered and changes brought about. As early as 1993, Cooper and Lewis were advocating that a more flexible approach to work patterns would improve overall QoL for all people, not just for those with impairments. They suggested the widespread implementation of flexitime, glidingtime, variable days and maxiflex[8] (Cooper & Lewis 1993: p. 121). A similar way forward was offered by Golini (2001: p. 35) who maintained that 'the labour market has to be changed . . . encouraging horizontal mobility', suggesting as a possible solution that employers learn 'to adapt the organisation of work . . . to the changing capacities of workers' (Golini, 2001: p. 38).

The White Paper *European Social Policy* (European Union, 1994: p. 5) called for a 'reconciliation of professional and family life' and pointed out that 'changing demographic trends mean that the responsibility for elderly dependants is moving up the social agenda'. This paper acknowledged that 'both men and women are likely to have caring responsibilities throughout all or much of their working lives' (Cooper & Lewis, 1993: p. 31). If these issues are considered in the context of LTCs, then the ramifications of ignoring the needs of patients become apparent. If regulations that protect the employment of those with chronic illness were fully enforced and a commitment were made to alternative models of employment, rather than the dominant 'male model',[9] then the chronically sick might feel empowered when making work choices, rather than dis-abled (Lewis, 1997). Although people do occasionally become litigious over employment rights, they are only able to act when they are familiar with the vagaries of the law; those who do not speak out about their work needs are unfortunately overlooked. Until those with chronic illness are legitimized with what Neal et al. (1993) branded a 'sense of entitlement'[10] then workplace discrimination against those with LTCs will linger.

Inferences must be drawn from such robust findings; future research must elucidate *why* the work area is so problematical and how the future for the chronically ill can be improved. Potential employers must be made to face up to the reality of living with chronic illness; with most health problems, the 'capacities' of workers do, in fact, vary, but they are certainly not lost altogether. Where those with a LTC wish to retain high levels of activity, whether work-related, home-related or leisure, they should be encouraged and enabled so to do.

Action Learning Point

- What, precisely, is 'social identity' and in what ways does it contribute to the well-being of those with LTCs?
- How can practitioners help people, whose bodies have changed – or are changing – due to a health condition, feel positive about themselves?
- Why is it important to consider 'opportunities for work' when talking to those with a LTC?
- What are the dangers of concealing a LTC at places of employment?

---

[8] Glidingtime: start and finish times may vary each day. Variable days: the number of hours worked each day may vary provided that all employees are present for a minimum core period. Maxiflex: daily hours are varied to suit the employee with no 'core period' requirement.

[9] The 'male model' of work prescribes full-time, continuous work from the end of education until retirement without any concessions to the demands of family (Cook, 1992).

[10] 'Sense of entitlement': whereby people are entitled to voice their needs and ask for modified working practices.

Conclusions

Because, over many decades, so much research into LTCs has been dominated by the biomedical professional model, there is a paucity of information with regard to either the psychological or the social corollaries of chronic poor health. This chapter redresses the balance by linking LTCs to the World Health Organization model for QoL, called the WHOQoL-Bref. This latter, which is a globally resilient instrument, comprises 26 questions segregated into four domains: physical, environmental, psychological and social. Throughout the chapter, Parkinson's disease is used as an exemplar of a LTC, although it is acknowledged that neurological disorders do not typify the multiplicity of LTCs that health professionals encounter in their work, rather that the psychosocial sequelae associated with PD are relatively well documented.

Three problematic areas linked to the physical domain were identified and discussions on sexual difficulties, sleep difficulties and hospital admissions followed. Within the environmental domain, just one topic is deconstructed and this is the difficulty of 'coming out' with a LTC. The first debate raised in the psychological domain is about the guilt that is frequently coupled with living with a LTC. The second topic covered is fear, and finally anger/resentment were handled as a single theme. As in all the previous sections, these are linked to the WHOQoL model and all include recommendations for health professionals as to how to manage such complications.

The final section relates to two areas that are subsumed within the social domain. Both social relationships and social identity are examined and further split so that, overall, five topics linked to LTCs are evaluated in respect of QoL. These are: (i) interpersonal relationships with medical professional teams; (ii) a social life with a LTC; (iii) body image; (iv) loss of confidence; and finally (v) employment and LTCs. The chapter is presented in a manner that should challenge existing beliefs about caring for people with LTCs and in a way that puts the *people* before the *condition*.

References

Abudi, S., Bar-Tal, Y., Ziv, L. & Fish, M. (1997) Parkinson's disease – patients' perceptions. *Journal of Advanced Nursing* **25**: 54–59.

Allport, G.W. (1955) *Becoming: Basic considerations for a psychology of personality*. New Haven, CT, Yale University Press.

Andersen, S. (1999) Patient perspective and self-help. *Neurology* **52** (7): S26–S28.

Andersen, S. (2002) *Chronic Disease and Grief*. London, Unwin Hyman.

Arrow, G.T. (1996) Socioeconomic Factors and Mortality. www.wnmeds.ac.nz/academic/dph/Publicationsreports/Blakely [accessed 5 September 2002].

Avallone, F., Arnold, J. & Dewettee, K. (eds) (1997) *Job Stress in the Primary Care Team in England*. Quaderni di Psicologia del Lovoro No. 5. Milan, Edizion, Angelo Guerini e Associati Spa, pp. 393–399.

Baatile, J., Langbein, W.E., Weaver, F., Maloney, C. & Jost, M.B. (2000) Effect of exercise on perceived quality of life. *Journal of Rehabilitation, Research and Development* **37** (5): 529–534. http://www.vard.org/jour/00/37/5/baati375.htm [accessed 17 August 2004].

Barbosa, E.R., Limongi, J.C.P. & Cummings, J.L. (1997) Neuropsychiatry of the basal ganglia. *Cognitive and Behavioural Neurology* **20** (4): 769–790.

Barron, K. (1997) The bumpy road to womanhood. *Disability and Society* **12** (2): 223–239.

Basson, R. (1998) Sexual health of women with disabilities. *Canadian Medical Professional Association Journal* **159**: 359–362.

Bhatia, K., Brooks, D.J., Burn, D.J. et al. (1998) Guidelines for the management of disease. *Hospital Medicine* **59** (6): 469–480.

de Boer, A.G.E., Wijker, W., Speelman, J.D. & de Haes, J.C.J. (1996) Quality of life in patients with Parkinson's disease: development of a questionnaire. *Journal of Neurology, Neurosurgery and Psychiatry* **61**: 70–74.

Bowling, A. (1995) The Assessment of a Quality of Life Instrument. www.cjnr.nursing.mcgill.ca/archive/ 30/30_4_williams.html [accessed 3 September 2002].

Bowling, A. (1999) *Assessing Quality of Life*. Oxford, Oxford University Press. www3.open.ac.uk/learners-guide/careers/toolkit/careers_statement [accessed 3 September 2002].

Bowling, A., Gabriel, Z., Dykes, J., Marriott-Dowding, L., Fleissig, A., Banister, D., Evans, O. & Sutton, S. (2003) Let's ask them: a national survey of definitions of quality of life and its enhancement among people aged 65 and over. *International Journal of Ageing and Human Development* **56** (4): 269–306.

Bowman, C. (2000) Economic and quality of life impact study. Presented at the European Disease Association Conference, 9–12 November 2000, Vienna, Austria. http://www.shef.ac.uk/misc/groups/epda/viennar.htm1 [accessed 8 July 2001].

Breakwell, G.M. (ed.) (1983) *Threatened Identities*. Chichester, John Wiley.

Breakwell, G.M. (ed.) (1992) *Social Psychology of Identity and the Self Concept*. London, Surrey University Press.

Brod, M., Mendelsohn, G.A. & Roberts, B. (1999) Patients' experiences of disease abstracts. *Social Gerontology* **53B** (4): 213–222.

Brown, R.G., Jahanshahi, M., Quinn, N. & Marsden, C.D. (1990) Sexual function in patients with Parkinson's disease and their partners. *Journal of Neurology, Neurosurgery and Psychiatry* **53**: 480–486.

Burstrom, B., Whitehead, M., Lindholm, C. & Diderichsen, F. (2000) Inequalities in the social consequence of illness: how well do people with long-term illness fare in the British and Swedish labour markets? *International Journal of Health Services* **30** (3): 435–451.

Chaudhuri, R.K. (2000) Sleep disturbances overlooked in Parkinson's patients. Presented at the International Congress of the European Federation of Neurological Societies, 14–18 October 2000, Copenhagen, Denmark. http://www/.talkaboutsleep.com.news/Parkinson's.htm [accessed 8 July 2001].

Clarke, C.E., Zobkiw, R.M. & Gullaksen, E. (1995) Quality of life and care. *British Journal of Clinical Practice* **49** (6): 288–293.

Cohn, J. (2001) Inclusion: The US Art Magazine. http://www.vsarts.org/gallery/exhibits/athletes/inclusion.html7–11 [accessed 17 September 2001].

Cook, A.H. (1992) *Cooperative Managerial Style*. New York, Cornell University Press. courses.csusm.edu/hist331mj/womenandtheworkplace/ [accessed 5 September 2002].

Cooper, C.L. & Lewis, S. (1993) *The Workplace Revolution: Managing today's dual-career families*. London, Kogan Page.

Cox, R. (1998) *Sports Psychology: Concepts and applications*. Missouri, McGraw-Hill.

Dakof, G.A. & Mendelsohn, G.A. (1986) The psychological aspects of a chronic illness. *Psychological Bulletin* **99** (3): 375–387.

Diaz, F. & Larrachea, E. (1997) Psychosocial research in Parkinson's disease. *Journal of the Neurological Sciences* **150** (Suppl. 1): S182.

European Union (1994) European Social Policy. www.ecu-activities.be/1995_1/quest.htm [accessed 5 September 2002].

Featherstone, M. (1991) The body in consumer culture. In: M. Featherstone, M. Hepworth & B. Turner (eds) *The Body: Social Process and Cultural Theory*. London, Sage Publications, pp. 170–196.

Fitzgerald, J. (1995) When 'quality of life' becomes quality or life, it's time to challenge the concept. *Health Issues* **42**: 19–22.

Fitzsimmons, B. & Bunting, L.K. (2001) *Quality of Life Issues with Parkinson's Disease.* http://pspinformation.com/disease/quality.shtml:1–12 [accessed 18 July 2001].

Freire, P. (1993) *Pedagogy of the Oppressed.* London, Penguin.

Garnett, D. (1993) Coping with chronic illness. *Lifeline* **XI** (1): 1.

Godwin-Austen, R.B. & Hildick-Smith, M. (1982) *Parkinson's Disease: A general practitioner's guide* (revised edition 1991). London, Parkinson's Disease Society of Great Britain.

Goffman, E. (1990) *Stigma: Notes on the management of spoiled identity.* London, Penguin.

Golini, A. (2001) Employment, Labour and Social Affairs. www.oecd.org/pdf/ M00017000/ M00017726.pdf [accessed 5 September 2002].

Harré, R. (ed.) (1976) *Personality.* Oxford, Blackwell Publishers.

Harrold, L.R., Field, T.S. & Gurwitz, J.H. (1999) Knowledge, patterns of care, and outcomes of care for generalists and specialists. *Journal of General Internal Medicine* **14**: 499–511.

Heilman, H. (2001) *Learning How to Give Bad News.* http://www2.tulane.edu/ EditorialNewsDetails.cfm?EditorialID=477 [accessed17/10/04].

Human Rights Campaign Foundation (2001) *Resource Guide to Coming Out.* Washington, Human Rights Campaign Foundation.

Hunt, P. (ed.) (1966) *Stigma: The experience of disability.* London, Geoffrey Chapman.

Israel, G.E. (2001) Why Bother Coming Out? http://www.firelily.com/gender/gianna/why. come.out.html [accessed 8 January 2001].

Jacobs, H., Vieregge, A. & Vieregge, P. (2000) Sexuality in young patients with disease: a population based comparison with healthy controls. *Journal of Neurology, Neurosurgery and Psychiatry* **69** (4): 550–552.

James, W. (1890) *Principles of Psychology.* New York, Holt.

Jones, J.J. (1999) Quality of life measurements. *The Psychologist* **12** (7): 337–338.

Kagan, C., Lewis, S. & Heaton, P. (1997) *The Context of Working and Caring for Disabled Children.* IOD Occasional Papers. Manchester, Interpersonal and Organisational Development Research Group (IOD).

Kahneman, D., Diener, E. & Schwarz, N. (1999) *Well-Being: The foundations of hedonic psychology.* New York, Russell Sage Foundation.

Kelly, M.P. & Field, D. (1996) Medical professional sociology, chronic illness and the body. *Sociology of Health and Illness* **18** (2): 241–257.

LaRocca, N.G., Kalb, R.C. & Gregg, K. (1996) A program to facilitate retention of employment amongst persons with multiple sclerosis. *Work, A Journal of Prevention, Assessment and Rehabilitation* **7** (1): 37–46.

Lee, K.S., Merriman, A., Owen, A., Chew, B. & Tan, T.C. (1994) The medical, social and functional profile of Parkinson's disease patients. *Singapore Medical Professional Journal* **35**: 265–268.

Lester, J. (2004) Why the Anger? http://neuro-www.mgh.harvard.edu/forum05/07/04 [accessed 22 February 2005].

Lewis, S. (1997) Family-friendly policies: a root to changing organisational change or playing around at the margins? *Gender, Work and Organisation* **4**: 13–23.

Livneh, H. & Antonak, R.F. (1994) Review of research on psychosocial adaptation to neuromuscular disorders: cerebral palsy, muscular dystrophy and Parkinson's disease. Psychosocial Perspectives on Disability, special issue. *Journal of Social Behaviour and Personality* **9** (5): 201–230.

Lloyd, M. (1999) The new community care for people with Parkinson's Disease and their carers. In: R. Percival and P. Hobson (eds) (1999) Parkinson's Disease: Studies in Psychological and social care.

Loggenberg, D. (2005) *Negotiating the Great Divide: Theorising a new quality of life framework for people with Parkinson's disease.* Library Archive Q6579372. Manchester, Manchester Metropolitan University.

McDonough, P. & Amick, B.C., III (2001) The social context of health selection: a longitudinal study of health and employment. *Social Science and Medicine* **53**: 135–145.

McGoon, D.C. (1990) *The Parkinson's Handbook*. New York, Norton.

Meyers, A.R., Gage, H. & Hendricks, A. (2000) Health-related quality of life in neurology. *Archives of Neurology* **57**: 1224–1227.

Michelson, R. & Wynn, S. (2001) The emotional implications of chronic illness. *MHE Coalition Newsletter* **5**, 1–32.

Neal, M., Chapman, N., Ingersoll-Dayton, B. & Emlen, A. (1993) *Balancing Work and Caregiving for Children, Adults, and Elders*. Newbury Park, CA, Sage. www.upa.pdx.edu/IOA/pubs2.html [accessed 5 September 2002].

Noble, C. (2000) Parkinson's disease: the challenge. *Nursing Standard* **15** (12): 43–51.

Öberg, P. & Tornstam, L. (1999) Body images among men and women of different ages. *Ageing and Society* **19**: 629–644.

Oertel, W.H. & Ellgring, H. (1995) Medical professional education and psychosocial aspects. *Patient Education and Counselling* **26**: 71–79.

Oxtoby, M. (1982) *Parkinson's Disease Patients and their Social Needs*. London, Parkinson's Disease Society.

Oxtoby, M. & Williams, A. (1995) *At your Fingertips*. London, Class.

Panicker, D.M., Deshpande, N., Pinto, C. & Vas, C.J. (1999) Coping with dementia. *Bombay Hospital Journal* **4101**: 143–148.

Percival, R. & Hobson, P. (eds) (1999) *Studies in Psychological and Social Care*. Leicester, British Psychological Society.

Perring, M. (2001) Parkinson's Disease and Sexuality. http://www.partnertherapy.com/PartnerTherapy/144 [accessed 18 July 2004].

Peto, V., Jenkinson, C., Fitzpatrick, R. & Greenhall, R. (1995) The development and evaluation of a short measure of functioning and well-being for individuals with Parkinson's disease. *Quality of Life Research* **4**: 241–248.

Poarch, M.T. (1998) Ties that bind: US suburban residents on the social and civic dimensions of work. *Community, Work and Family* **1** (2): 25–148.

Porteous, M. (1997) *Occupational Psychology*. London, Prentice Hall.

Power, M. (1998) WHO's who in quality of life: a World Health Organization perspective. *Health Psychology Update* **32**: 13–16.

Priddle, M. (2001) Chronic Disorders: Classic Care Pharmacy (Pharmawise). http:/www.classiccare.on.ca/newsletter1.html [accessed 12 December 2001].

Prutkin, J.M. & Feinstein, J.R. (2002) Quality-of-life measurements: origin and pathogenesis. *Yale Journal of Biology and Medicine* **75** (2):79–93.

Pulst, S.M. (2003) Coping with the Emotional Aspects of Disease. www.cedars-sinai.edu/3035.html [accessed 6 July 2004].

Quindlen, A. (2000) Untitled. http://www.revjm.com [accessed 17 September 2001].

Rabasca, L. (1999) Knocking down societal barriers for people with disabilities. *Monitor Online* **30** (10): 1–4.

Rankine, K. (2001) After 20 years, it is time to break the silence. *Daily Telegraph* 26 May, p. 33.

Reber, A.S. (1995) *Dictionary of Psychology*, 2nd edn. London, Penguin.

Roberts, A. & Fisher, D. (1944) 'You Always Hurt the One You Love'. http:www.rienzihills.com [accessed 29 November 2004].

Roessler, R.E. & Rumrill, P.D. (1999) New directions in vocational rehabilitation: a 'career development' perspective. *Journal of Rehabilitation* **65** (II): 26(i).

Roessler, R.E., Reed, K.L. & Brown, D. (1998) *Transition of Adolescents with Chronic Illness*. dept.kent.edu/rehab/cmcv.htm [accessed 5 September 2002].

Rose, R.D. & Rosow, N.I. (1993) Physicians who kill themselves. *Archives of General Psychiatry* **29**: 800–805.

Rout, U. & Rout, J.K. (1993) *Stress and General Practitioners*. London, Kluwer.

Rout, U., Cooper, C.L. & Rout, J.K. (1996) Job stress among British general practitioners: predictors of job satisfaction and mental ill-health. *Stress Medicine* **12**: 155–166.

Salter, M. (1997) Introduction. In: M. Salter (ed.) *Altered Body Image: The nurse's role*, 2nd edn. London, Balliere Tindall, pp. 1–29.

Sauerman, T. (1995) *Outproud – Be yourself*. Philadelphia, Philadelphia Friends of Lesbians and Gays.

Schreurs, K.M.G., de Ridder, D.T.D. & Bensing, J.M. (2000) A one year study of coping, social support and quality of life. *Psychology and Health* 15, 109–121.

Seaburn, D. (2001) How Can Chronic Illness Affect the Family? http://www.aamft.org/families/ConsumerUpdates/ChronicIllness.asp [accessed 11 December 2005].

Seymour, W. (1998) *Remaking the Body: Rehabilitation and change*. London, Routledge.

Sharpe, M.C., Archard, L.C., Banatvala, J.E., Borysiewicz, L.K., Clare A.W., David, A., Edwards, R.H. Hawton, K.E., Lambert, H.P., Lane, R.J. et al. (1991) A report: chronic fatigue syndrome: guidelines for research. *Journal of the Royal Society of Medicine*, 84 (2): 118–121.

Simon, J. (2000) Overcoming sexual dysfunction: Parkinson's disease. *Living Well* 2 (1): 10.

Singer, E. (1974) Premature social ageing: the social-psychological consequences of a chronic illness. *Social Science and Medicine* 8: 143–151.

Starkloff, M. (1999) Max Speaks Out. http://www.allsupinc.com [accessed 17 September 2005].

Stone, S.D. (1995) The myth of bodily perfection. *Disability and Society* 10 (4): 413–424.

Sunvisson, H. & Ekman, S.L. (2001) Environmental influences on the experiences of people with chronic disorders. *Nursing Inquiry* 8: 41–50.

Tajfel, H. (1981) *Human Groups and Social Categories*. Cambridge, Cambridge University Press.

Timmins, N. (2000) Shake-up of care for elderly can ease NHS ills. *Financial Times* 5 June, p. 25.

Turner, B. (1994) Preface. In: P. Falk (au.) *The Consuming Body*. London, Sage Publications.

Üstunn, T.B. & Sartorius, W. (eds) (1996) *Mental Illness in General Health Care: An International Study*. Wiley-Blackwell, Oxford.

Weingart, S.N., Wilson, R.M., Gibberd, R.W. & Harrison, B. (2000) Epidemiology and medical professional error. *British Medical Professional Journal* 320: 774–777.

Wendell, S. (1989) Toward a feminist theory of disability. *Hypatia: Journal of Feminist Philosophy* 4: 104–124.

Wendell, S. (1996) *The Rejected Body: Feminist philosophical reflections on disability*. London, Routledge.

Wenning, S. (2000) Overcoming Sexual Dysfunction. www.bringhealth.com/impotence_cause_cure.html [accessed 4 September 2004].

West, K. (1992) *Assessing the Needs of Parkinson's Disease Sufferers and their Carers*. http://james.parkinsons.org.uk/StudentProjects/DinksProjectBook.pdf [accessed 5 September 2002].

WHOQoL Group (1998a) *User Manual*. Geneva, World Health Organization.

WHOQoL Group (1998b) Development of the World Health Organization WHOQOL-BREF quality of life assessment. *Psychological Medicine* 28: 551–558.

Williams, B. (1996) The vicissitudes of embodiment across the chronic illness trajectory. *Body and Society* 2 (2): 23–47.

Williams, B. & Barlow, J.H. (1998) Falling out with my shadow: lay perceptions of the body in the context of arthritis. In: S. Nettleton & J. Watson (eds) *The Body in Everyday Life*. London, Routledge, pp. 124–141.

World Health Organization (1993) *World Health Organization Quality and Life Study Protocol*. Geneva World Health Organization (MNH7PSF/93.9).

World Health Organization (1994) *New Horizons in Health*. Manila, WHO Office for the Western Pacific.

Wermuth, N. & Cox, D.R. (1996) *Multivariate Dependencies – Models, Analysis and Interpretation*. London. Chapman and Hall.

Young, R. (1999) Update on chronic illness. *American Academy of Family Physicians* 15 April: 2155–2169. http://www.aafp.org/afp/990415ap/2155.html [accessed 12 January 2007].

Chapter 9

Redocumenting home and managing long term conditions: the social organization of place and space

Eileen Fairhurst

Key points

- Identifying the social organization of place and space and relevance to home
- Examining how policy documents relevant to long term conditions treat the idea of home
- Looking at the social construction of home as an environment of risk in professional practices – of designers of sheltered housing and/or health and social care workers
- Implications of the professional perspectives on home for the meaning of home for individuals with a long term condition

The policy of community care has implicitly identified the home as an 'appropriate' place of care. Higgins (1989) criticized community care policy for its neglect of the meaning of home. She called for the abandonment of the term 'community care' from social policy and for its substitution with the distinction between home and institution. Yet, it is only more recently that the category of 'home' has explicitly entered policy discourse. Few would dissent from policy aims to put the patient at the centre of care so that independence is gained. The overall intention is that the home becomes the primary place of care. In so doing, the home is contrasted with the hospital as a place of care. This is evident in the policy mantra of 'care closer to home' (Department of Health (DOH), 2006). The home as a 'place' becomes a derivative of place of care. In parallel with these changes has come an emphasis on reducing health inequalities. Quality of care has been one of the matters focused upon under that wider topic. National Service Frameworks (NSFs) were established to address variations in quality of care received by individuals in different parts of the country. The purpose of establishing standards of care was to lay out what people could expect no matter where they lived in England. Inevitably, perhaps, where public policy is characterized by achieving centrally driven targets, emphasis is placed on identifying systems and processes for achieving those standards of care. These system and process mechanisms facilitate monitoring and audit, which are used to indicate progress towards the achievement of standards.

From the perspective of those individuals with long term conditions, their management becomes part and parcel of everyday life and is situated in their own homes. How and in what ways individuals manage their long term condition in the context of their own homes has received little attention (Oldman & Beresford, 2000; Percival, 2002; Imrie, 2004). Given these points, it can be suggested that the policy of home as the preferred and primary place of care treats the home as a 'black box' (Fairhurst, 1997a). The lived experience of 'being' in one's own home has been hardly studied. This chapter explores the implications of those managing long term conditions at home, for the meaning of home and everyday life, especially where impairment affects mobility.

There are three major themes in this chapter. Initially, I will outline literature on the social organization of place and space in relation to the category of home. Then, the social construction of home evident in selected policy documents and finally professional practice will be examined. The *National Service Framework for Older People* (DOH, 2001) and the *National Service Framework for Long Term Conditions* (DOH, 2005a) and the consultation document *Independence, Well-Being and Choice* (DOH, 2005b) are the chosen policy documents. In relation to professional practices some of my previous research (Fairhurst, 1993, 2000; Fairhurst & Vilkko, 2004) is used to identify the ways in which architects designing sheltered housing and health and social care professionals conceptualize the category of home. I will show how the outcome of a risk assessment in terms of safety may result in professional personnel recommending changes to the physical layout of a home and its fabric so that it is socially redocumented. Much of the material I will use in this chapter is drawn from studies relating to later life. Since these studies had a general concern with consequences of physical impairments for mobility, their salience to many long term conditions is apparent. Whilst the NSF for Long Term Conditions has an emphasis on neurological conditions, it is not restricted to them. Indeed, explicit reference is made to much of the NSF's guidance having applicability to all long term conditions (DOH, 2005a). Finally, the chapter concludes by considering the implications of all these professional perspectives for the meaning of home to individuals with long term conditions.

The social organization of place and space

The starting point for this section is the rather abstract claim that any form of home pertains to a physical space that may be bounded by either physical or symbolic markers (Fairhurst, 2000). There is a long tradition in the social sciences of connecting physical space, boundaries and social activity. There is the literature relating to the general field of urban life. Early studies of urban sociology were characterized by the ecological approach of the Chicago School of urbanism. This assumed that in cities individuals were sorted into specific spatial areas to which they were 'best suited' (Park, 1952). Such mechanisms, derived from the processes of competition, invasion and succession characteristic of biological ecology, enabled the mapping of cities into areas of distinct and contrasting social characteristics. A contemporary variation of this ecological approach can be seen in urban regeneration plans where spatial areas of cities are developed as 'creative' or 'knowledge' zones and so on. Bus drivers and traffic wardens, whose occupations are carried out in the street, assign particular meanings to spatial areas and individuals' activities found there (Richman, 1980). Even queuing, which might be thought of as entailing no physical boundaries, is not exempt from social organization. For instance, Lee and Watson (1992–3) showed how in France and England queues were organized according to clearly recognized rules used by those individuals in the queue. Concerns with the significance of space for general social matters are evident too in the work of Goffman. Goffman's (1966) observations of visitors approaching isolated crofters' cottages on the Shetland Isles led him to develop the distinction between 'front' and 'back' stage activity as concepts for understanding general social action.

More specifically for the concerns of this chapter, there is the literature focusing on the home as a spatial environment. Social anthropologists' interest in domestic architecture and homes reflects Durkheim and Mauss (1963) in their pursuit of the classification of social life. They distinguished between symbolic classifications of a moral or religious nature and technological classifications referring to practical schemes of distinction. They argued that these ideas were based on models of society held by different cultures. Social anthropologists have focused on the linkage between homes and houses and social structure. They have conceptualized domestic architecture and homes as representing models of society so that the number of separate rooms within a home reflects the complexity of a society. For instance, Donley-Reid's (1990) critique of technological determinism, as a key for interpreting domestic organization rather than stressing symbolic and social values, suggests that the floor plan of the Atoni house conveyed social structure from one generation to another. We will return to this matter of technological determinism later when examining the social construction of home in policy documents. Tambiah (1969) studied a northeast Thailand village in which age, gender and social intimacy and social distance were reflected in social relations sanctioned around the household's east–west line of orientation.

Douglas's (1972) reference to the physical layout of houses and social relations along north–south or east–west axes as indicators of genealogical and age distinctions is not a phenomenon found only in non-Western cultures, for it has been noted in the British Isles. Arensberg and Kimball (1965, 1968) identified the phenomenon of the 'west room' in rural areas of western Ireland. This was that part of the farmhouse where the 'old couple' moved upon the marriage of their eldest son. The west room was where sleeping and living took place. The old couple's move to the west room not only involved both a change and reduction in living space but also marked the father's retirement from running the farm and the son's social maturity in assuming control of it. Whilst anthropological study of domestic space in Western cultural contexts has maintained its focus on symbolic significance of spatial arrangements and decoration (Cieraad, 1999), it has also adopted a more metaphorical turn. Douglas (1991: p. 290) contends that home is a kind of space where 'the ideas that persons are carrying inside their heads about the lives in space and time are realised'.

Other analysts, seeking to elaborate the social significance of home, have started with the notion of physical space. They have theorized how particular kinds of social relationships are associated with particular types of physical space. A distinction is made between public and private space in which different kinds of relationships are apparent. For instance, Saunders and Williams (1988) viewed home as constituting and reproducing elements of the public and private spheres of social life. The concepts of privacy, privatism and privatization are three distinctive but related aspects of the home as a private sphere. For them, home, since it is at the centre of a whole complex set of relationships and is the crucial medium through which society is structured, denotes a range of diverse meanings. Saunders and Williams identified three different ways in which the meaning of home may vary. Firstly, between household members, so that it is here that age and gender relations are articulated. Secondly, between different types of households according to social class, household composition, ethnicity and housing tenure; and thirdly, according to different regions and/or societies.

Allan and Crow's (1989) edited collection on the meaning of home also centred on the distinction between public and private, but especially on the connection between home and family in contemporary society. For them and their contributors, home was portrayed as a physical location, constructed around the 'family' and where the modern domestic ideal of home and family are synonymous. In this collection, the home was akin to a black box, the unpacking of which was pursued primarily, though not exclusively, via an examination of gender relations.

One of the most comprehensive examinations of home is offered by Mallet (2004). She notes that interest in the meaning of home has come from disciplines such as sociology, social anthropology, psychology, architecture and philosophy. She formulated her focus on understanding home in the following terms:

> 'Is home (a) place(s), (a) space(s), feeling(s), practices, and/or an active state of being in the world? Home is variously described as conflated with or related to house, family, haven, self, gender, and journeying. Many authors also consider notions of being-at-home, creating or making home and the ideal home.' (Mallet, 2004: p. 65)

Mallett's purpose in her critical review of a wide range of different disciplinary literature, some of which has been referred to previously, was to map out a programme of interdisciplinary studies of home intended to answer the questions of how home is, should or could be understood. Such wide-ranging concerns, though, are beyond the scope of this chapter.

In contrast to the academic writings referred to so far, our everyday usage of home is that it is *both* a physical location and a location in space. Depicting the home as a physical location involves its conceptualization as a structure bounded by a perimeter such as a wall or garden or, for homeless people sleeping on the street, possibly a tarpaulin or cardboard. The fabric of the home, its walls and boundaries, serve as a marker between home and non-home. Examining the home as a location in space rests upon ideas about a building in the context of the built or natural environment. The home, as a physical location, is a place that carries meaning dependent on events which occur within its walls/symbolic boundaries but, as a location in space, it is part of something else and is defined in terms of its relationship to its surroundings.

Conventionally home is a space in which material objects such as furniture, pictures, books and domestic equipment are placed and social activity takes place.

Social construction of home and policy documents

Now that we have seen some of the differing approaches to social space and the social organization of the home and domestic space we can turn to consider the ways home is conceptualized in policy documents. I want to suggest that the *National Service Framework for Older People*' (DOH, 2001), *National Service Framework for Long Term Conditions* (DOH, 2005a) and *Independence, Well-Being and Choice* (DOH, 2005b) are recent English policy documents that construct the home as a place of risks. The NSF for Older People, in common with others, was intended to:

'set national standards and define service models for a defined service or care group; put in place strategies to support implementation; and establish performance measures against which progress within an agreed time scale will be measured.' (DOH, 2001: p. 9)

Emphasis is placed upon quality of service provision. Three of the eight standards have particular relevance to our concerns.

- *Standard 2* focuses on patient-centred care such that:

'NHS and social care services treat older people as individuals and enable them to make choices about their own care. This is achieved through the single assessment process, integrated commissioning arrangements and integrated provision of services, including community equipment and continence services.' (DOH, 2001: p. 12)

- *Standard 3*, intermediate care, outlines the intended outcomes of the previous standard:

'Older people will have access to a new range of intermediate care services at home or in designated care settings, to promote their independence by providing enhanced services from the NHS and councils to prevent unnecessary hospital admission and effective rehabilitation services to enable early discharge from hospital and to prevent premature or unnecessary admission to long-term residential care.' (DOH, 2001: p. 12)

- *Standard 6* refers to the prevention of falls:

'The NHS, working in partnership with councils, takes action to prevent falls and reduce resultant fractures or other injuries in their populations of older people. Older people who have fallen receive effective treatment and rehabilitation and, with their carers, receive advice on prevention, through a specialised falls service.' (DOH, 2001: p. 13)

Similarly, not all of the quality requirements (QRs) of the NSF for Long Term Conditions are relevant to our interests here. For our purposes we shall restrict our interest to QR5, QR7 and QR8. These are as follows:

- *Quality requirement 5*, community rehabilitation and support:

  'People with long-term neurological conditions living at home are to have ongoing access to a comprehensive range of rehabilitation, advice and support to meet their continuing and changing needs, increase their independence and autonomy and help them to live as they wish.' (DOH, 2005a: p. 4)

- *Quality requirement 7*, providing equipment and accommodation:

  'People with long-term neurological conditions are to receive timely, appropriate assistive technology/equipment and adaptations to accommodation to support them to live independently, help them with their care, maintain their health and improve their quality of life.' (DOH, 2005a: p. 4)

- *Quality requirement 8*, providing personal care and support:

  'Health and social care services work together to provide care and support to enable people with long-term neurological conditions to achieve maximum choice about living independently at home.' (DOH, 2005a: p. 5)

The are a number of similarities between these two NSFs in that both refer to rehabilitation as a mechanism to enable individuals to live at home (standard 2 of the NSF for Older People and QR5 of the NSF for Long Term Conditions); both identify adaptations to accommodation and equipment as promoting independence (standard 6 and QR7, respectively); and both emphasize the exercise of choice about care (standard 2 and QR8, respectively). There is, though, one notable difference between these two NSFs. Unlike the NSF for Older People, the NSF for Long Term Conditions offers a definition of home:

'"Home" in this context means the place where the individual *chooses* [emphasis in the original] to live, which may be their own accommodation or a residential or care home.' (DOH, 2005a: p. 5).

This is another way in which home is viewed unproblematically in these policy documents. Adopting this meaning of home assumes equivalence between these different types of home. Evidence from studies of registered care homes for the elderly suggests otherwise. For instance, Willcocks et al. (1987) show that the provision of a 'homely' setting in residential homes is difficult to achieve as institutional rather than domestic patterns of care persist, nor is this likely to be reversed, even in smaller (less than four places) residential homes. Peace and Holland (2001) found that, despite proprietors expressing feelings of affection for their residents, the home is also their business. They continued:

'The "homeliness" of small homes centres on their scale, informality and physical appearance, but, as a result of public accountability it is constantly under pressure to move towards formality and "organised" living. Activities and the division of domestic labour within small homes are more like the pattern in larger residential care settings than in "normal" domestic homes'. (Peace & Holland, 2001: p. 407)

Whereas the notion of risk and its assessment are implicit in the NSFs, the consultation document, *Independence, Well-being and Choice* (DOH, 2005b), had an explicit focus on the management of risk. Two major themes are apparent in the document. Firstly, the management of risk so that a balance should be achieved between 'supporting people to manage risk in their lives and the need for protection at appropriate times' (DOH, 2005b: p. 21). Secondly, consumer sovereignty, by:

'putting people at the centre of assessment, increasing direct payments and the introduction of individual budgets. Direct payments are a system whereby individuals receive money and they decide for themselves what services or help they need. The purpose of individual budgets is to promote independent living. This is not just about being able to stay in your own home but is also about providing people with choice, empowerment and freedom.' (DOH, 2005b: p. 34)

I want to argue here that these policy documents treat the home as a taken-for-granted category. Home is considered in relation to hospital as an alternative place of care. Despite an emphasis on 'person-centred care' and 'fitting services around people's needs', there is little recognition in the NSFs that 'home' is more than a black box. On the contrary, from a sociological perspective home does not have an existence of its own to which 'things can be done' but is subjectively experienced. Whilst there are over 300 references in the *National Service Framework for Older People* (DOH, 2001) and over 200 in the *National Service Framework for Long Term Conditions* (DOH, 2005a), not one has an explicit focus on the social significance of home.

A house in the sense of 'bricks and mortar' can have 'things done to it'. A house can be added to by building an extension. Similarly, functional features of it can be adapted. The replacement of a bath by a walk-in shower or the installation of a hoist still enables an individual's body to be washed but the means through which this is achieved differs. In everyday life we are unlikely to refer to adding to or adapting our homes. It is only through examining the lived experience of individuals with long term conditions that the meanings of care at home can be delineated.

Sociologists talk about these kinds of matters in terms of 'agency'. By this is meant that individuals are capable of thinking and acting so that they interpret social situations rather than reacting to external stimuli. Some instances of this line of thought are found in Kelly and Charlton's (1995: p. 83) critique of the social model of health in health promotion and Allen's (2000) cautioning about viewing individuals as 'physiological dopes' in the study of illness and housing. Let us explore the ways in which this matter of an individual's 'agency' is addressed in these policy documents.

The *National Service Framework for Older People* (DOH, 2001: p. 41) claims that: 'Many older people want alternative care to hospital admission'. This is based upon a recent review of the evidence of patient preferences for location of care (Luff et al., 2000). An examination of this review raises, however, more questions than are answered. Luff et al. (2000: p. 103) note on the one hand, 'a preference for alternatives to long-term hospital and institutional care was found amongst elderly people' and, on the other, 'in several service areas, notably, terminal care, hospital at home, and long term care of the elderly, there appear to be discrepancies or potential conflicts between carer and patient preferences'. The conflation between the home as an entity contrasting with hospital and as a category situated in social relations is apparent here.

The focus on falls in standard 6 of the NSF for Older People depicts the home as a hazardous environment containing potential risks such as 'poor lighting, particularly on stairs, loose carpets or rugs and inaccessible lights or windows' (DOH, 2001: pp. 78–79). With appropriate interventions such as the provision of equipment, adaptations or repairs, the risk of falls can be reduced and, thereby, home can be made safer. The NSF (DOH, 2001: p. 36) enumerates and specifies these matters so that, for instance, there will be 'an extra 35 000 items of hoist and lift equipment in older people's homes' and '250 000 more older people with walking aids'. There is, then, an assumed determinism between such pieces of technology and safety. The presence of the former leads to the latter.

Beck's (1992) analysis of risk adds to the understanding of risk as a social construct. He argues that risk is about the probabilities of physical harm occurring as a result of technological or other processes. Technical experts – health and social care workers in the case of the NSF – are given licence to outline the boundaries of risk. Similarly, as Scott and Williams (1992) have pointed out, the belief in the control of both nature and people for the greater good results in experts of the state keeping 'danger at bay'. Striving to contain these dangers means, in the case of policy documents, addressing the predictability of accidents in order to make them 'avoidable'. Hence, danger is controlled. Overall, the policy documents' reliance upon a predominantly medical model of care and underpinnings of technological determinism present a decontextualized view of individuals and health and social care at home. The approaches of policy-makers to risk are rather abstract.

Social construction of home and professional practices

Designers of sheltered housing

Although ideas of risk and its assessment in the context of home have come to the fore in recent policy documents, they have also been implicit in the practice of architects designing sheltered housing (Fairhurst, 2000) These professionals orientate to older people primarily in terms of the ageing body; its physical decline renders them vulnerable and the architect's task is to 'protect' them from harm stemming from the inherent dangers of the built environment. I showed how designers applied the category of 'vulnerability' in relation to older people. In the 1960s vulnerability was assumed to be an aspect of the ageing body. Old age was seen as an adversity to be overcome as physical decline predisposed older people to become vulnerable to accidents within the home: the home was a source of danger. Incorporating the principles of 'comfort, convenience and safety' into housing design was seen as a way of reducing, if not controlling, such danger. That focus on the ageing body and its implied physical degeneration, with its attendant restriction of social life, underpinned the ways in which designers approached their task. They assumed a reduced living space would be needed by older people so that architects emphasized its ergonomic usage in order to make life 'as easy as possible' *within* the home. By the 1990s the view of vulnerability as consequent upon activity *outside* the home shifted designers to a concern not so much with protecting old people from themselves but from others, particularly vandals. Since designers did not have access to knowledge of unique features of potential residents, design could only be informed by abstract knowledge of 'what older people are like'. A consequence of this was that ideas about space and its utilization remained at a rather general level. I went on to demonstrate how older people's meanings of domestic space usage rested upon ideas such as being able to entertain family and other visitors and to have adequate space to display treasured objects (Percival, 2002).

Home visits and rehabilitation of older people

We have already noted that home is a physical and social space in which social interaction takes place. Let us examine some of the issues raised by this in the case of an older person discharged from hospital to home. I will sketch out a possible discharge scenario and show how a complex array of social relationships may arise which have implications for subsequent 'life at home'.

Sociologically, rehabilitation is an activity that is done by different sorts of individuals with different perspectives, in different ways and in different places. These multiple interpretations have their genesis not only in occupational training but also in terms of features of organizational routines. Later, these varying occupational interpretations of rehabilitation are related to the ways occupational therapists and social workers redocument a suitable home environment. Rehabilitation claims to be concerned with attaining maximum independence for older people. It might be assumed that retaining some semblance of 'the familiar' to the individual is important in encouraging independence in daily living. Examining 'the familiar' and how an individual copes with this ostensibly underpins the purpose of a home assessment visit.

The final stage of a rehabilitation programme is discharge from hospital. Assessments of an individual as 'more' or 'less' independent are crucial in decision-making about discharge. That independence may mean different things in different contexts is implied by the use of a home visit as part of assessing independence. A home visit may be either to the patient's own home, that is, the one from which the patient was admitted to hospital or to a prospective home, for example a relative's or residential home. Although an individual may be mobile and have successfully completed an 'activities of daily living' assessment in hospital, the purpose of a home visit is to demonstrate the individual's ability to live in their own environment. The significance of this for future living is not lost on older people who may refer to a home visit as a 'test' which can be passed or failed. A rehabilitation programme in the hospital is in some senses a practice for the 'real thing'. Underlying such a course of action is the belief that features of an environment may enable an older person to remain independent. As a consequence, therefore, some environments are more suitable than others.

The first point to note, following Schutz (1964), is that any individual who comes home from a period away returns home as a 'stranger'. Thus, the home to which one returns is not the same as that which one left and its significance, its meaning, has also changed. Such changes are likely to be amplified in further ways for it is probable that an individual will return with altered physical functioning and, as outlined above, there may be changes in the physical layout of the home.

This process may be seen as the redocumentation of a normal environment (Fairhurst, 1993). It is a consequence of the way in which occupational therapists view their task as, firstly, assessing risk and, secondly, reducing risks presented to older people by objects found in the home. The purpose of such a process is to make the home a suitable physical environment. The identification of a suitable environment rests not only on recognizing a normal environment, but also on redocumentation of a normal environment.

Whilst still in hospital, an older person will be assessed for their ability to carry out a range of activities of daily living, for instance dressing, mobility, cooking, etc. Typically before discharge, a home visit will be arranged, the purpose of which is to ensure than an older person can function in their own environment, their own home; in other words, that independence has been achieved. Upon arrival, he or she may be asked to make a cup of tea or undertake a similar everyday task. Such activities are used to check out an individual's physical capability to light matches or to turn taps on his/her own sink, or to ascertain that a person is not disoriented in such a way as to be unaware of the kitchen layout. Attention is paid to the age of the house, whether it be a flat, bungalow or multi-storey accommodation, its layout and structure. Thus, for instance, the existence of a step down into the kitchen or the absence of a banister on the stairs, the depth of a stair tread and access to the bathroom and toilet are all noted. On the basis of such a visit, alterations to the house may be made and adaptations provided for the person.

In everyday life we do not routinely need to justify why we want to live in our homes but for older people being discharged from hospital that everyday, taken-for-granted legitimacy becomes problematical. They need to demonstrate to occupational groups that they can be independent in their own homes. It is in this way that 'strangers' acquire legitimate interest in what goes on in the home. Furthermore, such strangers can transform the category of home into a place of risk and danger. We shall return to the implications of such matters in a later section of the chapter.

Schutz's reference to the stranger is doubly pertinent. Firstly, any absence from home, however short, puts one into the position of stranger, for the homecomer is not the same person who left. As a consequence, 'the old accustomed surroundings have received an added meaning derived from and based upon our experiences during our absence' (Schutz, 1964: p. 110). We shall see how this operates in the case of older people being discharged from hospital. Secondly, doing a home visit involves the entry of strangers into an older person's home. Social workers and remedial therapists, by virtue of their occupational membership, have their status as strangers legitimized so that their presence in somebody's home becomes acceptable. Such is the extent of this legitimization that the 'strangers' may not only assess the appropriateness of the arrangement of objects within the home as a physical space but also go on to rearrange that spatial location – thereby making home itself strange to the returning homecomer and also enhancing his/her strangeness to the once familiar environment.

For occupational therapists, an older person's home is cast as an environment of physical objects. They interpret the suitability of the physical environment with reference to safety, specifically the ways in which physical objects present a hazard or potential hazard. A contrast is then made between the home as a safe or a hazardous environment. Danger is seen as an inherent feature of a home. A cooker or gas fire is more than a functional object to cook food or provide heat. They are a source of possible danger for an individual who has arthritis or has some kind of physical impairment after a cerebral vascular accident. The on–off controls may be difficult to manipulate so that there may be a time lag between turning the gas supply on and its ignition. A fireside rug originally may have been put on to the floor to 'add some colour' to a room, but to an occupational therapist it becomes something over which an older person may trip. Similarly, stairs are not solely a functional device for linking two levels of a structure, but rather potential obstacles. A banister-free and/or ill-lit staircase with steep stair treads becomes a danger that may prevent an individual from going upstairs to sleep or to wash and toilet. It is in these kinds of ways that household objects, long familiar to the occupant, take on specific kinds of significance for those charged with assessing an older person's independence. In relation to the above examples, maintaining an older person's independence would depend upon altering any, all or a combination of them. Consequently, a new cooker or fire would need to be installed, or it might be recommended that, with modifications such as putting a bathroom or toilet downstairs, an individual could live on the ground floor of their home and, in effect, reduce the boundaries of its occupation. The extent of safety offered by the physical layout of the home reflects not just a normal environment but rather a redocumented safe environment. Thus, for a home to become a safe environment is contingent upon its transformation from a hazardous environment.

Recognizing home as a suitable environment: a case study

Recognizing home as a suitable environment rests on the 'right' combination of physical and social features. An appropriate physical or social environment, on its own, is seldom sufficient for identification as a normal environment. For this to happen the two distinctive categories – safe and supportive environment – are joined together to allow the redocumentation of a normal environment. The case conference report of a home assessment visit in Case study 1 shows how the absence of this linkage of categories precludes the process of reinterpretation of normality and hence makes 'independence' problematic.

Case study 1

The occupational therapist's report was prefaced by the comment that she had a 'sad tale to tell'. She went on to note that the woman's flat was 'ideal'. She could dress herself and had been 'very good during flat training' but she had a spatial difficulty: she had walked past her stove. The occupational therapist thought the woman would not be safe at home. She needed a lot of support: people to 'keep an eye on her'. The woman had no contact with her neighbours and her daughter appeared unwilling to help her mother.

The social worker's report elaborated upon the social contacts available to the woman. The social worker considered the woman's daughter to be aggressive. The latter did not think her mother should have been taken on a home visit. Although initially the daughter had helped her mother, she now felt she could not continue with this. The social worker suggested that there was not a very good relationship between the mother and daughter for they no longer spoke to each other. In addition, the woman had not lived in the area for very long so could not be expected to have built up relationships with neighbours. In the event, the woman was placed on a waiting list for a place in a local authority home.

The actual outcome is less important than what we can glean about how the bonding of the two categories, safe and supportive, is necessary for the redocumentation of a normal environment. The occupational therapy and social work emphases on safety and social support are salient here. The occupational therapist made much of the suitability of the woman's physical environment and of her ability to care for herself. Whilst such matters are necessary parts of the assessment of 'being independent', their presence was inadequate once the woman was observed in her own home. Her unawareness of a potentially dangerous object, in this case a cooker, raised the issue of safety. This matter of safety assumed added significance because the woman was seen as someone who lacked the support of family and neighbours: without such support she did not have a normal social environment. The absence of this feature of normality underpinned the social worker's description of the home visit. She accounted for the lack of social support in term's of the daughter's aggressive personality (had had 'enough' of caring) and the woman's status as a relative newcomer to the area. The conditions required to provide a normal social environment could not be met from a social work perspective.

From this report of a home visit we can see how, from the standpoint of a rehabilitation team, this process of redocumentation is situated in a concrete social context. In the context of the hospital, the woman had reached the stage of her rehabilitation career where her independence needed to be assessed in her own environment. She was considered 'ready for a try out'. As has been outlined, though, once in her own home her actions were interpreted as 'unsafe'. The earlier appearances of her as independent were reinterpreted. In addition, the unavailability of willing carers prevented the categorization of the social environment as supportive. The combination of these two matters meant the woman's home could not be identified as a safe and supportive environment and, consequently, its redocumentation as normal.

Garfinkel (1967) refers to the way in which the documentary method, as a set of interpretative procedures, allows for the retrospective–prospective sense of occurrence. Not only does it involve looking back to reinterpret actions but also setting up future patterns of behaviour. The purpose of a home visit is precisely of such concern for it is an attempt to predict how an individual will manage once discharged from hospital. From the occupational perspectives of occupational therapy and social work, the categories of safe and supportive are crucial in assessing independence in the future in a particular context, i.e. an individual's home. Unless the general categories of physical and social environments can be transformed into the more specific ones of safe and supportive, the prediction of an individual's future as one of independence cannot be made.

Implications of professional practices for the meaning of home for individuals with a long term condition

So far we have seen that the consideration of home as a place of care in policy documents is underpinned by notions of technological determinism and that professional practitioners cast home as a physical location in which matters of risk are paramount. Now we can return to those ideas about the social organization of space and place with which this chapter started and consider their implications for individuals with a long term condition living at home. We know that home has great social significance for people in later life (Askham et al., 1999). Moreover, there is a literature that pinpoints the importance of objects as a source of memories for the preservation of an older person's identity (Csikszentmihalyi & Rochberg-Halton, 1981; Hazan, 1989; Percival, 2002; but see Fairhurst 1997b, 2005 for an alternative perspective on memories). Given this kind of evidence, it might be assumed that actions requiring the removal of objects in order to make a home safe may have consequences for an older person's sense of well-being in that such a course of action may be a source of distress to them. The extent to which an older person might be willing to 'trade off' keeping treasured objects for a 'safe' environment is an empirical matter.

If home is considered in terms of a location in space then individuals may not necessarily wish to stay there 'at all costs'. For instance, if the significance of home is assessed in the context of the type of neighbourhood in which it is located, then by virtue of noisiness of the neighbourhood or lack of cleanliness, it may be considered to be 'unsafe' and people may wish to move away from their current home (Fairhurst, 2000).

Arguably, the portrayal of home in the policy documents and professional practices outlined in this chapter is one that objectifies space so that it is construed as an external structure 'containing and constraining action'. This is at the expense of recognizing that 'material arrangements of space and place and embodied competencies for their use are organised in, through, and for, the accomplishment of action' (Crabtree, 2000). This perspective on the social organization of space has profound implications for care at home that is contingent on the use of equipment or other material aids and adaptations.

Aids and equipment literally 'take up' space and adaptations 'redraw' space. Just as Albert (1990) has identified the strategy used by home care givers of 'drawing lines' between care-giving tasks and non-care giving aspects of the household to prevent its radical reorganization, a similar process may occur in the case of equipment and adaptations. For instance, how is space which is 'taken up' by equipment defined and what are the consequences of less space for the meaning of home? Moreover, the possession of aids by individuals does not guarantee their use. Although I have not systematically gathered evidence on this, health care professionals have indicated to me that walking aids may be 'pushed in a corner' and rarely used. Similarly, does the 'redrawing' of space, following alterations, mean that particular caring activities are tied to specific spatial areas?

Aids and equipment may not only take up space but also, of themselves, be socially organized. Kontos' (1998) research in a supported housing agency cautions against reliance upon aids as some kind of technological 'fix' guaranteeing 'independence'. She notes a concern for older people's management of a deteriorating body by being cautious and attempting to avoid falls by weighing up the costs and benefits of getting out of a chair and using a walker to go and get something. One way in which individuals with a physical impairment may organize their daily lives is by the use of 'energy saving strategies' (Imrie, 2004: p. 759).

McCreadie and Tinker's (2005) research on assistive technology (AT) and older people offers further pointers on these kind of matters. They note that while alterations to the home and the installation of aids may be preferable to moving, some in their study viewed assistive technology as an 'intrusion' that altered their meaning of home. Some older people commented adversely on raised lavatory seats and plastic hand-rails. In this sense, trade offs between 'staying put' at home and an individual's sense of their *own* home result.

In our everyday life particular kinds of activities are routinely linked to particular domestic spaces. In doing this we make moral assessments about the 'right and proper place' to do certain activities. For instance, we have ideas about sleeping upstairs rather than downstairs and sharing a bed with one's partner (Fairhurst, 2007). Washing and toileting are other daily activities that are conventionally restricted to specific locations within the home. The separation of such activities reflects our cultural classifications of dirt and danger. Following Douglas (1974), dirt is 'matter out of place'. Living at home with a long term condition may disrupt such taken-for-granted matters. Imrie (2004) has shown that the provision of aids and alterations to homes of people with a disability is no permanent guarantee of independence: bodily impairment is not static but inevitably changes with processes of deterioration so that its meaning is located in a domestic context. His research further demonstrates the inadequacy of technological determinism as a route to individual independence: such decontextualized 'solutions' inevitably ignore the social significance of domestic environments.

So far I have suggested a number of ways in which policies on care at home may have implications for changing the meanings of space and objects. Let us finish with one further matter: that the home becomes a place of work for health and social care workers. Studies of health care, given within the home, have shown that generally it is undertaken in a different way to that done in conventional medical settings. Sankar (1986) demonstrated that the interaction of medical students on home visits to the chronically ill reflected features of a guest–host relationship, so that the former had less control over communication.

Others have outlined the strategies used by health workers to do their work in homes. Bowers (1992) offers an ethnomethodological analysis of how community psychiatric nurses accomplish a home visit. He showed how typifications of 'being a friend' and 'being a nurse' inform 'being in the home' and are the ways in which the community psychiatric nurse exerts control over work. Coffman's (1997) exploration of paediatric nurses' experience of working in the homes of technology-dependent children emphasized the nurse's presence as a 'stranger in the family'. More recently, Ward-Griffin and McKeever (2000) have focused on how the relationships between community nurses caring for older people at home and family care givers develop and change. They outline how the shifting boundaries in nursing and care work result in changes in the nurse–family care giver relationship. These are evident in four separate but connected types, which are those of nurse–helper, worker–worker, manager–worker and nurse–patient.

Whilst all of these materials help us to understand the issues that are presented to health professionals who carry out their work in an individual's home, we have limited understanding of what it might mean from his/her perspective. Although there is evidence of consequences of caring in the home for care givers (Gubrium & Sankar, 1990) and of how older people may be involved in defining quality home care (Raynes et al., 2001), we know little about how social space within the home may be redefined by recipients of care. To be cared for by professional staff in a person's own home requires that the professionals enter that person's own physical and social space to do their work. A person's own home, then, becomes a place of work for others. Managing space as a boundary between work and family is a dilemma for home workers (Sullivan, 2000), but what might happen when the home of a person with a long term condition becomes the workplace of health and care workers? Some indications of what this means to disabled people have been given by Imrie (2004), who reports that carers may be seen as akin to strangers. How individuals, themselves, manage and give meaning to social space when health and care professionals enter it to do their work remains to be outlined.

I noted earlier that health and social care policies are underpinned ostensibly by ideas about choice and independence for individuals. Therein lies a paradox: between the needs of individuals as individuals and the goals of public policy. The latter emphasize quality assurance and standards but also a clear monitoring and performance management structure (Peace & Holland, 2001). This is a process which has been referred to as 'surveillance' (Dingwall & Robinson, 1990). The extent to which such 'surveillance' of activities within the private area of the home, in order to achieve public policy, is acceptable to individuals living at home with a long term condition is yet to be ascertained. The call in the *National Service Framework for Long Term Conditions* (DOH, 2005a) for the inclusion of qualitative studies to assess the impact of its guidelines on quality of life for individuals promises the possibility that such matters may be addressed.

Action Learning Point

- Imagine you have a long term condition that affects your mobility.
- List those areas of your home where you do particular activities, identify if that space is public or private and why you think it is public or private.
- Identify if there are any objects or possessions in your home which have a special significance to you and why.
- How would you feel, and why, if a health professional wanted, in the interests of your safety, to come into your private space, identified above, to do their job and/or suggested removing one of your treasured possessions, also identified above.

References

Albert, A. (1990) The dependent elderly, home health care and strategies of household adaptation. In: J. Gubrium & A. Sankar (eds) *The Home Health Care Experience: Ethnography and policy*. London, Sage Publications, pp. 19–36.

Allan, G. & Crow, G. (eds) (1989) *Home and Family*. London, Macmillan.

Allen, C. (2000) On the 'physiological dope' problematic in housing and illness research: towards a critical realism of home and health. *Housing, Theory and Society* **17**: 49–67.

Arensberg, C. & Kimball, S. (1965) *Culture and Community*. New York, Harcourt and Brace.

Arensberg, C. & Kimball, S. (1968) *Family and Community in Ireland*, 2nd edn. Cambridge, MA, Harvard University Press.

Askham, J., Nelson, H., Tinker, A. & Hancock, R. (1999) *To Have and to Hold: The bond between older people and the homes they own*. York, Joseph Rowntree Foundation.

Beck, U. (1992) *The Risk Society*. London, Sage Publications.

Bowers, L. (1992) Ethnomethodology II: a study of the psychiatric nurse in the patient's home. *International Journal of Nursing Studies* **29**: 69–79.

Cieraad, I. (ed.) (1999) *At Home: An anthropology of domestic space.* Syracuse, Syracuse University Press.

Coffman, S. (1997) Home care nurses as strangers in the family. *Western Journal of Nursing Research* **19** (1): 82–96.

Crabtree, A. (2000) Remarks on the Social Organisation of Space and Place. http://www. mundanebehavior.org/issues.vlnl/crabtree.htm [accessed 30 May 2007].

Csikszentmihalyi, M. & Rochberg-Halton, E. (1981) *The Meaning of Things.* New York, Cambridge University Press.

Department of Health (2001) *National Service Framework for Older People.* London, Department of Health.

Department of Health (2005a) *National Service Framework for Long Term Conditions.* London, Department of Health.

Department of Health (2005b) *Independence, Well-Being and Choice.* London, Department of Health.

Department of Health (2006) *Our Health, Our Care, Our Say.* London, Department of Health.

Dingwall, R. & Robinson, K. (1990) Policing the family? Health visiting and the public surveillance of private behaviour. In: J. Gubrium & A. Sankar (eds) *The Home Care Experience: Ethnography and policy.* London, Sage Publications, pp. 253–274.

Donley-Reid, L. (1990) A structuring structure: the Swahili home. In: S. Kent (ed.) *Domestic Architecture and the Use of Space.* Cambridge, Cambridge University Press, pp. 114–126.

Douglas, M. (1972) Symbolic orders in the use of domestic space. In: P. Ucko, R. Tringham & G. Dimbleby (eds) *Man, Settlement and Urbanism.* London, Duckworth, pp. 513–521.

Douglas, M. (1974) *Purity and Danger.* Harmondsworth, Penguin.

Douglas, M. (1991) The idea of a home: a kind of space. *Social Research* **58** (1): 287–307.

Durkheim, E. & Mauss, M. (1963) *Primitive Classification* (translation by R. Needham). London, Cohen and West.

Fairhurst, E. (1993) Caring for the elderly in the community: home and the documentation and re-documentation of a normal environment. Paper presented at the *International Conference on Caring for the Elderly in the Community*, University of Plymouth, April.

Fairhurst, E. (1997a) What is home? In: D. Skidmore (ed.) *Community Care: Initial training and beyond.* London, Arnold, pp. 43–57.

Fairhurst, E. (1997b) 'Recalling life': analytical issues in the use of memories. In: A. Jamieson, S. Harper & C. Victor (eds) *Critical Approach to Ageing and Later Life.* Buckingham, Open University Press, pp. 63–73.

Fairhurst, E. (2000) Utilising space in sheltered housing or fitting a quart into a pint pot: perspectives of architects and older people. *Society and Space* **18** (6): 761–776.

Fairhurst, E. (2005) Memories, objects and older people's worlds: continuities with the past? Paper given to the *5th International Symposium on Cultural Gerontology, Current and Future Pasts*, Open University, Milton Keynes, 19–21 May.

Fairhurst, E. (2007) Theorising sleep practices and later life: moving to sheltered housing. *Sociological Research Online* **12** (5). www.socresonline.org.uk/12/5/10 [accessed 11 July 2007].

Fairhurst, E. & Vilkko, A. (2004) Defining risk in the context of home: comparisons from Finland and England. Paper given at the *7th ESA Conference*, Torun, Poland, 9–12 September.

Garfinkel, H. (1967) *Studies in Ethnomethodology.* New York, Free Press.

Goffman, E, (1966) *Asylums.* New York, Doubleday.

Gubrium, J. & Sankar, A. (eds) *The Home Care Experience: Ethnography and policy.* London, Sage Publications.

Hazan, C. (1989) Continuity and change in a tea-cup: on the symbolic nature of tea-related behaviour among the aged. *Sociological Review* **28** (3): 417–516.

Higgins, J. (1989) Defining community care: realities and myths. *Social Policy and Administration* **23**: 3–16.

Imrie, R. (2004) Disability, embodiment and the meaning of home. *Housing Studies* **19** (5): 745–763.

Kelly, M. & Charlton, B. (1995) The modern and the post-modern in health promotion. In: R. Burrows, S. Nettleton & R. Burrows (eds) *The Sociology of Health Promotion.* London, Routledge, pp. 78–90.

Kontos, P. (1998) Resisting institutionalization: constructing old age and negotiating home. *Journal of Aging Studies* **12**: 167–184.

Lee, J. & Watson, D.R. (1992–3) Regards et habitudes des passants. *Les Annales de la Recherche Urbaine* **57/58**: 101–109.

Luff, D., Nicholl, J., O'Cathain, A., Munro, J. & Paisley, S. (2000) *Patient Preferences. Annex C, the National Bed Inquiry.* London, HMSO.

Mallett, S. (2004) Understanding home: a critical review of the literature. *Sociological Review* **52** (1): 62–89.

McCreadie, C. & Tinker, A. (2005) The acceptability of assistive technology to older people. *Ageing and Society* **25**: 91–110.

Oldman, C. & Beresford, B. (2000) Home sick home: using the housing experience of disabled children to suggest a new theoretical framework. *Housing Studies* **15**: 429–442.

Park, R. (1952) *Human Communities: The city and human ecology.* New York, Free Press.

Peace, S. & Holland, C. (2001) Homely residential care: a contradiction in terms? *Journal of Social Policy* **30** (3): 393–410.

Percival, J. (2002) Domestic spaces: uses and meanings in the daily lives of older people. *Ageing and Society* **22**: 729–749.

Raynes, N., Temple, B., Glenister, C. & Coulthard, L. (2001) *Quality at Home for Older People: Service users in defining home care specifications.* London, Polity Press.

Richman, J. (1980) *Ethnography of the Street.* Manchester, Manchester University Press.

Sankar, A. (1986) Out of the clinic and into the home: control and patient–physician communication. *Social Science and Medicine* **22**: 973–982.

Saunders, P. & Williams, P. (1988) The constitution of the home: towards a research agenda. *Housing Studies* **3**: 81–93.

Schutz, A. (1964) *Collected Papers II: Studies in social theory.* The Hague, Martinus Nijhoff.

Scott, S. & Williams, G. (1992) Introduction. In: S. Scott, G.H. Williams, S.D. Platt & H.A. Thomas (eds) *Private Risk and Public Danger.* Aldershot, Avebury, pp. 1–12.

Sullivan, C. (2000) Space and the intersection of work and family in homeworking households. *Community Work and Family* **3** (2): 185–205.

Tambiah, S.J. (1969) Animals are good to think and good to prohibit. *Ethnology* **8**: 423–459.

Ward-Griffin, C. & McKeever, P. (2000) Relationships between nurses and family caregivers: partners in care? *Advances in Nursing Science* **22** (3): 89–103.

Willcocks, D., Peace, S. & Kellaher, L. (1987) *Private Lives in Public Places.* London, Tavistock Publications.

Chapter 10

Cultural competence in service delivery

Margaret Presho

Key points

- Exploring the notion of cultural competence in health and social care practice
- Valuing the importance of patient's health beliefs
- Acknowledging the diversity of patient's needs and not assuming that specific cultures will conform to traditional conventions
- The importance of critical reflection on one's own practice
- The impact of health inequalities and health inequity on patient's health outcomes

Dreher and MacNaughton (2002) assert that cultural competence is actually synonymous with nursing competence and after examining some of the key issues that nursing and allied health professional literature have defined as necessary for cultural competence, this statement would seem to be a reasonable conclusion. This chapter explores how factors that influence culture often influence health and consequently, to best manage long term conditions in a culturally sensitive way, health care practitioners need to respond appropriately and be proactive advocates for patients from different cultures with whom they come into contact. Those interpersonal and communication skills required for culturally sensitive practice are to a great extent tantamount to those skills required for competent practice as a health care practitioner. The term 'culture' is used throughout this chapter to define those of different age, gender, race, ethnicity, social class, physical or mental ability to that of the practising health practitioner.

Culture and ethnicity

The overseas-born proportion of the population has doubled in the last 30 years to 8.1% of the total population, meaning that the ethnic mix of the UK population has changed with a greater mix of Asian, African, Chinese and other ethnic minority groups growing alongside the expanding native British population (National Statistics, 2004). It is important to acknowledge that cultural values may well have an important role to play in the way that people feel about and manage their lives when living with a long term condition, especially as response to and collaboration with professional carers may hinge upon inherent health beliefs. Health beliefs may have a strong impact on a person's ability to manage ill health, particularly within the context of long term conditions because, as Krause and Miller (1995) highlight, those beliefs may affect the person's ability to instigate or even envisage change. I refer in particular to lay health beliefs, which should be considered of no less importance than those health beliefs (perspectives) held by practitioners. Lay health beliefs as defined by Watson (1996), may be considered as the person's individual response to the way in which the body functions (or not) and the decision to seek professional help as an option amongst other potential courses of action.

Danish researchers, Povlsen et al. (2005), suggest that it should be emphasized that working with ethnic minority patients and clients calls for flexible health care professionals who are active, supportive and open to new and possibly different procedures and solutions. This latter aspect can be particularly significant, Eshiett and Parry (2003) argue, as many immigrants are not especially future orientated and thus can be less open to acknowledging the consequences of chronic diseases. As a response to this philosophy, health education programmes and health care interventions will need to be adapted to the individual's background, taking into consideration their culture, health beliefs and level of education. Culture is taken within this context to imply a shared set of values, beliefs and attitudes common to a particular group of people with the same national or ethnic origin. However, it should not be forgotten that culture can also be construed as a social construct that may encompass gender, religion, level of education, age, socioeconomic status or any other demographic aspect that impacts on the life of individuals (Kai, 2003). Adhering to cultural values is not a static phenomenon but rather a dynamic process in which individuals may totally and wholly engage in certain situations or not engage at all due to prevailing health beliefs. Health beliefs may in fact dictate that seeking medical attention is inappropriate even in serious circumstances and that needs would be better served by calling upon the assistance of friends and family, complementary and alternative medicine, environmental sources or deities.

The concept of the psychosocial impact on health is not confined to Western belief systems; a study by Papadopoulos et al. (2004) found that Ethiopian migrants believe that happiness is a prerequisite to and an indication of healthiness. Additionally, in this study, a majority believed that sickness results from disease and mental illness can be due to both supernatural and psychosocial causes. Thus pharmacological and behavioural therapies alone may be insufficient in addressing the needs of some ethnic minority groups within the context of mental health issues. Involvement of faith leaders may prove a valuable resource within some situations, although it should not be assumed that those from ethnic minorities will subscribe to any given faith codes and conventions, nor are people from ethnic minorities a homogeneous group.

Tools for practice

The extended use of professional interpreters in order to overcome linguistic as well as comprehensibility problems is an increasing feature of practice for some health professionals. However, as Richardson et al. (2006) recognize, it can be potentially difficult to work with interpreters as well as family members, both of whom could be reluctant to translate important information particularly where there are culturally sensitive issues involved. For example, Siriwardena and Clark (2004) highlight some of the concerns that centre around end of life care for people from minority ethnic groups. A preference for more aggressive care, cynicism of the hospice movement, mistrust of the medical profession, a belief that spiritual aspects of care are as important as the physical aspects, as well as a preference for family-orientated decision-making may provide potential areas for conflict between practitioners and ethnic minority patients. Such potential for conflict outlines the significance of skills in risk identification, managing mental impairment and well-being, end of life care, and professional practice and leadership – all of which are of such importance in the development of care managers, community matrons and other community-based practitioners. Those practitioners working in the acute sector may argue that these issues are equally important features of their practice and this notion is not in dispute. However, when caring for patients out of their own environment, the traditional power balance is in favour of the health care practitioner despite attempts at inclusivity; whereas in community practice, the traditionally accepted power base is reversed. The underpinning philosophy of community practice is that patients be consulted, not in a tokenistic manner, but rather in a way that enables them to become an integral part of the decision-making process as defined by Hills and Mullett (2000).

It appears that there is an implication that the onus is on those providing the direct care to familiarize themselves with the customs and culture of a wide and diverse range of ethnic groups. In practice this may be both unrealistic and unnecessary, not only because individual patients may not subscribe to particular culturally embedded traditions but also because practitioners may only come into contact with specific ethnic or other culturally focused groups. Being familiar with the customs, traditions and generic health beliefs of given ethnic or culturally located populations, with whom day-to-day contact is likely, is a more realistic proposition. At the same time, it should not be assumed that the individual patient will be conformist; it is always best to ask. Abrums (2000) even goes so far as to suggest that practitioners abandon traditional racial or class categories as they may contribute to stereotyping, blame laying and other forms of albeit unintentional oppression. Administratively this may prove difficult as many practitioner–patient encounters require demographic information, including postcodes, primarily to be collected for the purpose of organizational care planning. Such administrative protocol, however, should not impede subsequent practitioner–patient relationships by relying on the postcode or ethnic code as a foundation for beginning the consultation. Otherwise one may be led into thinking that health is synonymous with behaviour and that poor health is a direct result of bad or non-conformist behaviour rather than environmental, political or socioeconomic circumstances that lie beyond the control of the individual.

Action Learning Point

- Examine your practice profile, community profile or visit http://www.statistics.gov.uk/ and click on the 'neighbourhood' section to determine which ethnic minority groups populate your practice area.
- Using this information, determine the prevailing health beliefs within the context of long term conditions.
- Ensure that you and any new members of your team are familiar with the process of initiating interpreting and support services.

The burden of illness

Statistical and epidemiological data demonstrate how some ethnic groups are more prone to certain long term conditions. For example Pakistani and Bangladeshi men have a 70% greater risk of cardiovascular disease; Indian men have a 25% greater risk, Pakistani women a 45% greater risk and Bangladeshi women a 43% greater risk of cardiovascular disease than the general populace (Naqvi, 2003). Gender, genetics and ethnicity clearly have a role to play here, but equally poverty, with its associated environmental and socioeconomic conditions, has a part in this too. This is illustrated by Acheson (1998) who detailed how 17% of professional men lived with a long term illness compared to 48% of unskilled men. The statistics outlined above indicate how not only ethnic aspects but also class aspects impact on health outcomes. Both of these have a bearing on culture, as both class and ethnic origin may determine the frame of reference to which individuals will subscribe, although, of course, these two elements are not the only determinants of cultural identity nor the basis for holding particular health beliefs.

In the clinical practice arena it would be prudent to familiarize oneself with dominant lay perspectives on prevalent conditions given that patient co-operation and concordance may hinge on the professional understanding and application of such discourses. Concordance is concerned with shared decision-making rather than the patient complying with the wishes and direction of the health care professional. There is no such entity as a non-concordant patient, as concordance does not rely on the patient behaving in a specific manner. Non-concordance may, however, be an agreement to differ on an aspect of care or treatment and the discussion may be revisited at subsequent consultations should circumstances change or new perspectives be considered. Concordance is a particularly important concept within the context of health beliefs and managing, or living with, long term conditions as circumstances constantly change and new experiences may well alter a person's perspective.

Traditionally, health care professionals have paid minimal attention to lay health beliefs, possibly because to do so would present a challenge to their authority and knowledge but also perhaps because the public have accepted health professional knowledge, perspectives (beliefs) and action as authentic. A number of highly publicized events have challenged this authority such as the Royal Liverpool Children's Inquiry (Redfern, 2000), Bristol Royal Infirmary Inquiry (Kennedy, 2001) and Shipman Inquiry (Smith, 2005). Additionally, the concept of the 'expert patient' (Department of Health (DOH), 2001a), subsequent government policy documents and practice-based initiatives have also advocated the notion of patient choice and concordance in place of health professional direction and patient compliance (Weiss & Britten, 2003; DOH, 2004a, 2006a). If the large majority of patients are to be expected to take an active role in the care and management of their own long term conditions as indicated by the Department of Health (2004b), then lay health beliefs and health professional awareness of those beliefs will become an increasingly important feature of practice. Total knowledge of all health belief concepts would, as previously mentioned, be an impossible task for any practitioner, but a rational starting point for those new to this field of practice may be knowledge of those beliefs in relation to the most prevalent conditions seen in community practice. Of course as practitioners build, discharge and rebuild their caseloads, then a repertoire of knowledge can be drawn upon to influence planned and ad hoc responses and actions to patient concerns.

The Department of Health (2004b: p. 3) states that asthma, diabetes, chronic obstructive pulmonary disease, arthritis and mental health problems constitute the major preventable causes for contact with health care professionals. Additional problems underpin the reasons why 8.8 million of those with long term conditions find themselves severely limited in their ability to cope with one or more conditions and subsequently find themselves requiring frequent contact with health care professionals. The greater the number of simultaneous long term conditions that a person must cope with, the less is their ability to do so effectively. People from marginalized cultures are doubly disadvantaged as their likelihood of engaging with service provision is diminished due to a number of reasons. For example, language differences, low levels of education, non-recognition of symptoms, mistrust of health care practitioners, low levels of income (which may affect their ability to obtain medication, attend appointments or act upon advice offered) and, as identified by Morris et al. (2004), a perceived and actual smaller likelihood of achieving appropriate referral or having expectations met.

The migrant ethnic population of the UK is predominantly white with a mix of European, Australian, New Zealand and Canadian immigrants, the second and third largest immigrant populations come from India and Pakistan, closely followed by black Africans then Afro-Caribbean people (National Statistics, 2005). Despite common racial origins within these sub-groups of people, a mixture of language, religion, customs and culture are found amongst groups and between individual people just as would be expected within the indigenous British population. Most immigrants will be young people with the possible exception of the Afro-Caribbean and Irish populace due to their long-established links and UK immigration patterns.

Social class and ethnicity, in addition to gender and genetics, will determine the extent to which some groups and individuals are likely to experience long term health problems. Additionally, cultural factors will, to a great extent, influence levels of engagement and ability to communicate with dissimilar communities. Whilst interpreters and translated health information materials can be useful resources to aid communication during patient consultations, these resources are not always available, helpful or appropriate; particularly the latter resource if the patient is illiterate or sight impaired. Additionally, the current financial crisis within the health service has resulted in some Primary Care Trusts withdrawing funding for interpreter services at very short notice, leaving GPs to bear the cost – that in some practices will be disproportionately high due to the ethnic mix of the population and refugee and asylum-seeker dispersal policies (Clewes, 2007).

Ethical problems and intended meaning inaccuracies may be also be experienced when engaging in the practice of using relatives as third party communicators, especially where that person is a child or partner of the patient. As Clewes (2007) highlights, if service providers take on responsibility for the provision of interpreter services, albeit indirectly, then those providing the service will become responsible for the quality of the service and any problems arising from translation inaccuracies. Communication difficulties as a barrier to providing effective care are well documented and there are no easy solutions, although as Richardson et al. (2006) observe, involving senior family members in discussion and decision-making processes within some Asian cultures may be considered normal cultural practice. The difficulties arise where it is the senior family member that is experiencing the health problem. In a litigation-conscious health arena, health practitioners of all levels will be looking for guidance from the professional, statutory, regulatory bodies.

Whilst toolkits, or what Richardson et al. (2006: p. 98) term 'fact files', may be useful to health care professionals in learning about traditional customs of certain cultural groups (particularly ethnic minority groups), not every individual or family will necessarily subscribe to that traditional practice. Learning to ask is perhaps the best means of addressing the issue. This is especially so since the majority of patient contact time will not be spent managing specific events such as death, but rather engaging in the day-to-day rapport that is usually established with patients who are learning to cope in changing circumstances. Toolkits have a tendency to be universal and concept-focused whilst care provision has an obligation to be individually tailored, largely pragmatic and applied in changing situations and circumstances.

Self-awareness: becoming a reflective practitioner

One important aspect of learning to address concerns raised by those from different cultures is for the practitioner to reflect upon their own biases and prejudices centred on caring for people from other cultures. Whilst Health Care Trusts and other organizations will have policies in place to theoretically address equality within the context of race and culture, individual practitioners may well carry their own 'baggage'. Critical reflection on practitioner–patient consultations is a key aspect of learning to care for people from a diverse range of backgrounds. Perhaps the mnemonic 'SHENA' may prove useful in helping to structure a reflection on one's own practice within the context of cultural competence (Box 1).

Box 1: SHENA as a model for critical reflection in the context of cultural competence

S   Self-awareness of one's own prejudices and bias towards cultural differences within the context of race, ethnicity, gender, age, class and disability (if present)

H   Health beliefs as an important consideration for consultation and health education approaches

E   Engaging with clients on their terms and treating them with respect as expert patients by asking their opinions

N   Non-verbal cues as triggers for moderating consultations, taking into consideration the patient's concomitant emotional, physical and mental status

A   Awareness of key cultural influences that when practised unconditionally or in certain situations may impact on individual health outcomes

---

Consideration of the aspects outlined in Box 1 is not a paper exercise but rather is ingrained in the principles outlined by the National Service Frameworks for Mental Health, Coronary Heart Disease, Diabetes, Older People and Long Term Conditions (DOH, 1999: p. 4; 2000a: p. 5; 2001b: p. 5; 2001c: p. 12; 2005: p. 13) Those same principles are also the foundation for standard 2 of the *NHS Plan: A plan for investment, a plan for reform* (DOH, 2000b). These policy documents highlight how practitioners should plan their service delivery by acting as guiding principles that underpin everyday practice and form the basis of clinical governance. For the future, in terms of practice-based commissioning (DOH, 2006b: item 2.19), it may be that services will be selected or rejected by commissioners on the strengths or weaknesses of the service provider's ability to demonstrate that these same principles are being adhered to. Outcome measures will inevitably be drawn up by those commissioning services, and monitoring and review exercises, including regular audit and patient surveys, will be carried out to ensure that these target outcome measures are being met. For example, the Department of Health (2006b) 'Partnerships for older people's project pilot scheme' (POPPS) is being rolled out across the country, and those bidding to provide services to address the needs of older people need to make explicit within their applications how services and interventions funded by the project will positively contribute to supporting and maintaining the physical and mental well-being and independence of the older population. In addition, those bidding for funds must also detail how there will be meaningful and continuous involvement of older people in identifying, developing and evaluating service provision. The focus of POPPS is on quality of life, choice and control and freedom from discrimination for older people – all key elements of cultural competence in practice with an emphasis on anti-ageism.

Action Learning Point

- Find out about local POPPS projects in your area.
- What kind of services can patients expect?
- How do patients access service provision and are there any gaps in the provision of services that would best meet the needs of the local populace of older people?

Codes of practice: cause for concern

The focus on identified elements required for anti-ageist practice could also be equally applied to preventing oppression and discrimination in the presence of other culturally defined differences as highlighted by Kelleher and Hillier (1996). Health care practitioners cannot plead ignorance of the factors that contribute to oppression and discrimination as they have a duty of care outlined by their codes of professional conduct (Royal Bristol Infirmary Inquiry, 2001; Health Professions Council, 2007; Nursing and Midwifery Council, 2004). They are also bound by law to treat all equally and without oppression through the Sex Discrimination Act 1975, Race Relations Act 1976, Race Relations Amendment Act 2000, Disability Discrimination Acts 1995 and 2005 and Carers (Equal Opportunities) Act 2004. However, health care professionals do have concerns regarding the practicalities involved in applying those identified principles in practice and some of those concerns are outlined below.

One easily identifiable cause for practitioner concern is that difficulties in communication may extend the time needed to be spent with patients of differing cultural backcloth. This is time not devoted to hands-on care but rather time taken in delivering or communicating options, addressing patient and family concerns, or seeking consent to implement treatment or care pathways. Arguably this necessity for lengthy consultation is a legitimate concern given heavy caseloads and finite resources associated with modern day health care practice. It would be false economy not to invest time in getting the basics right, given that future consultations will inevitably be judged on the patient's first encounter. Where English is spoken as a second language or where the patient's accent or dialect is different from that of the health care professional, it should be remembered that the spoken word is not the only means of communication. Each person in their everyday speech consciously or unconsciously uses body language as well as paralinguistic features of speech to assist in communication. Paralinguistic features of speech include aspects such as intonation, rhythm or vocabulary. Henley and Schott (1999) highlight how paralinguistic features of a patient's mother tongue may remain even when spoken English is well managed, and may differ greatly in its meaning to each party thus leaving the conversation open to misinterpretation by all. Misunderstanding by either party is even more likely where the person is ill, in pain or frightened by the circumstances in which they find themselves. One such example of cultural misunderstanding resulting in misinterpretation that I have personally experienced is detailed in Case study 1.

Case study 1

As student nurse I trained with a colleague from Nigeria and frequently felt upset following conversations with her because I wrongly assumed that she was not interested in anything that I had to say, nor did she appear by her body language to believe or trust in me. My rationale for this assumption was that every time I spoke to her, she turned away or looked at the floor even whilst replying to me. This practice was observed for at least 12 months, then one day the opportunity arose for me to challenge her behaviour during a classroom-based exercise on communication. It transpired that the reason that my colleague had left herself open to accusations of aloofness and disengagement was that it was considered impolite in her native society to maintain eye to eye contact during conversation with a person not of her own family; hence she considered it necessary to look elsewhere rather than maintain eye contact when having conversations. She herself had been unaware that her actions caused offence or misunderstanding as she believed that she was merely being polite. New knowledge gained enabled her to modify her actions (with some difficulty) to meet the demands of Western conversational practice. Had I asked the question in the first place, it would have saved such misunderstanding.

When caring for someone with a long term condition, there is likely to be frequent contact over a prolonged period of time, thus establishing a rapport with patients and their carers is an important aspect of the health professional role. An essential aspect of care provision that is open to misinterpretation by lay carers and health care professionals is that people from ethnic minority groups and people from a working class backcloth are more inclined to care for their relatives themselves, rather than to delegate responsibility to professionals (Henley & Schott, 1999; Katbamna et al., 2000; Crisp, 2005). Women especially may be regarded by health care professionals as more likely to want to become primary carers regardless of the gender or age of, or social relationship with, the patient in need. One reason that such misunderstanding can arise is because some ethnic minority and socially deprived communities do not like to disclose the full extent of the difficulties that they may be experiencing. This is because they may perceive that others regard the person's illness or disability as their fault, with mental impairment being perceived a greater social stigma than physical disability. Conversely, seeking support from those outside of the family unit may be regarded by family members and local communities as disloyal, uncaring or 'sponging from society'. Discussion with the person experiencing the long term condition and, where appropriate, the family, is essential for determining the criteria acceptable for the establishment, continuity and, when required, increased levels of support from outside agencies and individuals. Perhaps it is important to note at this juncture, given the UK adaptation of the Evercare system (Gravelle et al., 2007) for community case management, that some North American research papers indicate that people from black and ethnic minorities, as well as those from deprived areas, are less likely to want referral to secondary care or for consultant appointments (Wong et al., 2004). Whilst this may well be so, the rationale behind this decision-making may have more connection with the potential cost implications inherent in the US care system than mistrust of the efficacy and ability of community-based service provision. Additionally, women from some ethnic minority and less affluent communities may find it more difficult to articulate their perspectives on becoming or remaining a primary carer because of their own perceived social standing within their family and community. Alternatively, they may consider it to be their duty to be the primary family carer and be unaware that options for support are available to them.

The same but different?

Social constructs of disability have an important role to play in determining people's attitudes to chronic illness. The medical model of health reinforces the fear that people may harbour in being associated with impaired health, the connotation being that health equates with disease and disease is contagious. Other explanations for linking poor health with blame are highlighted by Richman (1987), who details how some health belief systems attribute health deficits as being a reciprocal result of angering or upsetting a third party or deity. Hence to steer clear of the affected person is the wisest policy and, consequently, shifting the burden of care to a third party is the preferred course of action.

Divine influence has an equally important role to play in the way in which some people respond to the diagnosis of a particular condition or its prognosis. For example, those who follow the laws of Islam may well believe that everything that they experience within the context of ill health is the will of Allah. To endure the problem and its consequences may be regarded as a test of faith. Even where their faith does not restrict certain behaviours that would, if practised, perhaps ameliorate the effects of ill health, their own personal code will not allow that individual to behave in a manner that defies their personal belief system (Karmi, 1996). A useful example from practice may be that someone with diabetes would be exempt from fasting during Ramadan according to the laws of Islam, but because personally held beliefs may perceive not fasting as being sacrilegious, then that person may continue to fast and in doing so put their health at increased risk. Perhaps a role for the health care professional in this scenario would be to encourage the individual to take advice from a respected faith leader to assist them in seeking personal goals to exemplify their religious fervour that would not put their health at risk.

Self-efficacy is a person's estimate of their own ability to reach a specific goal. One example from practice that encapsulates the role of health beliefs in the context of self-efficacy is illustrated by Greenhalgh et al. (1998) who highlight how research participants with diabetes interviewed from a Bangladeshi community in London considered illness to be due to extracorporeal agents and thus beyond their control. Health was considered synonymous with youth and plumpness and degeneration of the body and its functions concomitant with the ageing process. The latter aspect does not seem unreasonable from a Western health belief perspective, except that amongst the research participants interviewed, the micro- and macrovascular complications associated with diabetes tended to be ignored as an inevitable consequence of the ageing process rather than an aspect of health that could be addressed by personal action. Asking patients about their beliefs, expectations and aspirations during initial and subsequent consultations may be helpful in reducing concerns and assisting patients in achieving optimal health status. Dreher and MacNaughton (2002) advocate documenting that this aspect has been addressed during the assessment process and whenever the issue is revisited. Self-efficacy may also be positively or negatively influenced by a person's belief in what fate may have in store for them. As fate or destiny is beyond the control of the individual then it may well be considered that, despite changes in lifestyle, pharmacological interventions or health professional support, good or bad events and outcomes will happen as planned by forces beyond their control. Henley and Schott (1999) refer to this perspective as a belief in good or bad luck and it may help to explain why some patients unexpectedly recover or deteriorate in circumstances where health professionals would normally expect the opposite outcome to be the end result.

One man's meat is another man's poison

An example from practice regarding health beliefs, this time within the context of social class, is given in Case study 2.

Case study 2

When working as a general practice nurse in a deprived practice within the northwest of England, I had a consultation with an elderly gentleman and his wife. The man had been diagnosed with diabetes and had been sent a letter of invitation to attend the practice with his partner to discuss the management of his newly diagnosed condition. The discussion proceeded focusing on the dietary aspects of diabetes. I asked the gentleman, who was in fact clinically obese, if he considered that he had a good diet; before he could reply, his wife interjected that he had a very good diet with only fresh food because she personally baked fresh pies for him each day. Clearly she believed that I intended to cast aspersions on her ability to look after her husband and was keen to disabuse me of that notion. Much tact and diplomacy was required to assure her that her culinary skills were not being undermined; on the contrary the benefits of fresh produce were well documented but some amendment to portion size and fat content was required to best meet her husband's changed health needs.

A further issue for consideration, that is closely related to both divine intervention and health beliefs and that has a potential impact on the care and management of people from different ethnic groups, is the practice of consulting traditional healers. The principle of consulting traditional medicine practitioners is not problematic, especially as a person's quality of life and response to the changing effects of long term health conditions may be more positive and their ability to cope more effective when engaging with familiar concepts and practice. However, there may be unintended side effects to traditional medicine when used concomitantly with Western medicine. Traditional medicine may also, sometimes, incorporate some toxic elements such as toxic metals, as described by Karmi (1996). Conversely, some products used in Western medicine may be unacceptable or harmful to some ethnic minority communities. For example, many South Asians are lactose intolerant (Karmi, 1996) and the use of pork derivatives or alcohol-based products for Muslims is forbidden, thus oral medication may be accepted but not taken when prescribed. Health practitioners unaware of these issues may regard the individual patient as unco-operative whereas, in reality, the patient is living within their faith code whilst trying to 'please the practitioner'. Flagging those issues up during initial assessment and subsequent medication reviews is a functional means of management and will open the door or 'give the patient permission' to discuss medication concerns and preferred routes of administration.

Some long term conditions such as hypertension, diabetes and chronic renal disease require that patients adhere to certain dietary guidelines to maintain optimal health and to prevent the early onset of complications associated with the primary condition. For some patients, perceived and actual dietary changes necessary for optimal health are more problematic than adjusting to, accepting and living with the condition itself. Food consumption in many societies means more than meeting energy requirements – eating is often seen as a social event when the family come together to discuss family business, a means of celebration such as on feast days or a means of preventing ill health by eating foods that are attributed with certain properties. In the West, for example, garlic is considered by many to be beneficial to the heart in reducing cholesterol, although this notion is contested by Hooper (2001) who states that the evidence is equivocal. In some Asian cultures certain properties are attributed to certain types of food which, if consumed, may positively or negatively influence a person's health according to the existing condition of the body. As Chopra and Kendra (2002) explain, Ayurvedic medicine is a 4000-year-old Indian method of healing that includes the use of certain foods, herbal preparations and other natural therapies. These components, used in the correct combination, are considered to restore harmony of body, mind and spirit, essential for well-being. Such a notion of health makes the World Health Organization (1948) definition of health seem embryonic by comparison. The harmony of body and spirit may not be possible to achieve if certain foods are consumed at inappropriate times or in inappropriate combination. Whilst practitioners would not necessarily need to know the correct combinations or even the properties attributed to different food products, an understanding that those considerations need to be taken into account when discussing dietary concerns with patients would be a good starting point.

The incidence and prevalence of diabetes in black and ethnic minority groups is six times greater than that found in the general population (All Parliamentary Group for Diabetes & Diabetes UK, 2006). Within that population, the principles concerning Ayurvedic medicine may be of some significance for some patients originating from South Asia. In addition, some patients may regard certain food products as indicative of their status within society. For example Asian colleagues inform me that to cook with 'ghee' (clarified butter) is considered a sign of wealth, thus even patients who can ill afford to buy ghee will endeavour to obtain and use it despite its contribution to the problems associated with obesity; ghee is also considered to be beneficial to health in terms of balancing stomach acid and improving learning, memory and recall. Similarly, some patients from deprived communities, especially older people, may consider a diet rich in red meat to be of benefit to their health; attributing prevention of anaemia and improvement in muscular strength to its frequent consumption. Discussing dietary habits as an integral part of consultation visits can be a relatively easy topic to introduce given the social connotations of food. Advice regarding a balanced diet – consisting of all food groups in moderation, and a reduction in salt, refined sugars and saturated fat intake – can be woven into consultations. This also offers an opportunity to raise the issue of alcohol and cigarette consumption, even in cultures where alcohol is forbidden but may be consumed if people do not wholly subscribe to all tenets of a given faith. Supporting literature can be used to illustrate and reiterate verbal advice. There are also booklets, videos and DVDs provided by charitable and other organizations, which patients may find useful in helping to understand and assimilate advice offered by health care professionals, some of which have resources available in languages other than English. The British Heart Foundation, Heart UK, Diabetes UK, Age Concern, CORE (Digestive Disorders Foundation), Coeliac UK, Food Standards Agency, Weight Wise and Caroline Walker Trust are a few examples of organizations that provide patient support resources. Giving patients an opportunity to discuss their dietary habits in a non-threatening, open environment will also allow the practitioner an opportunity to negotiate referral to support organizations where patients may be struggling to lose weight or adjust long-held habits that may be detrimental to their health. It should, however, be remembered that dietary intake is not always a matter of choice but rather what is affordable and available, as discussed in greater detail below.

Action Learning Point

- Consider your own views on complementary medicine; are there any specific beliefs that you subscribe to or actively reject within this context?
- What level of advice could you offer in terms of healthy eating to different patient groups that is practicable and affordable?
- Are there any food co-operatives or healthy eating clubs in your practice area, and if so, how do patients access them?
- What can you do as a practitioner to improve dietary intake and self-help for patients where nutrition is an important aspect of their care management plans?

Living on the fringes: the reality of social exclusion

Those from disadvantaged communities that experience health, economic and educational deprivation – as well as those from marginalized groups such as people with learning disabilities, the elderly living alone or in residential care, those with severe mental illness, and black and ethnic minority groups – are more likely to experience conditions such as diabetes, epilepsy, cancer and heart disease. This is because those conditions are much more prevalent in these population groups (All Parliamentary Group for Diabetes & Diabetes UK, 2006; Disability Rights Commission, 2006; Szaflarski et al., 2006). An important issue within this context is that these population groups are less likely to be known to mainstream services, are known to find access to health care provision difficult, and may not have the economic or educational means to identify and address health care needs especially with reference to the management of long term conditions. As a consequence of these identified health inequity issues, the complications of conditions are more prevalent, more complex and inevitably require more resource intensiveness. The All Parliamentary Group for Diabetes and Diabetes UK (2006) cite heart disease, cardiovascular disease and renal complications as being three and half times higher in socioeconomically deprived groups. In terms of case management, it is individuals from the above population groups that should be actively considered as a priority when 'case finding' for care planning and case management in community practice.

Food combinations and inappropriate timing of food consumption have already been identified as potential problems for some cultural groups. However, individuals from these same groups, as well as those from deprived communities, may find the purchase of healthy food options an unattainable goal. Older people with limited incomes and long-established dietary habits may also find dietary changes difficult to adjust to. In addition, those with long term conditions may have limited mobility, both to purchase food and to prepare and cook it. When people are on a limited income, decisions about food purchase may be determined by local availability and what is filling yet least expensive, rather than what is healthy. If transport is not easily available to visit supermarkets and the local environment is not conducive to walking or taking public transport for food shopping, then local produce, which may be limited in range and nutritional value, may be the only option – as identified by Acheson (1998). For those with limited mobility and dexterity, low levels of education, mental health problems or learning disabilities, culinary skills may be limited. Sometimes there is a perception that special foods need to be purchased, much in the same way as a prescription for medication is required. This latter aspect is particularly applicable to diabetes where many patients consider that they need to buy special diabetic products, rather than eat a balanced healthy diet that would be suitable for other family members. The Food Standards Agency and Diabetes UK (2001) have specified that there is no benefit to 'special diabetic foods' and that they are often more expensive than conventional foods.

Community practitioners have an important role to play in tailoring dietary health education to individual patients, taking into consideration some of the issues raised above. Other aspects that may be taken into account when supporting patients in achieving dietary changes are local food co-operatives, healthy cooking clubs, on-line shopping, expert patient groups and other condition-specific support groups, organized shopping trips facilitated by a health care professional or health advisor, referral to a dietician for initial or ongoing assessment, or participation in local weight management initiatives provided by general practice or private organizations. The latter, of course, can prove expensive and it is recognized that where weight reduction is an issue, ongoing support is necessary to sustain weight loss and to maintain target weight (Drinkwater, 2002; DOH, 2004a; National Obesity Forum, 2005).

Lifestyle and health

Smoking

Accepted social customs within some cultural groups may contribute to poor health outcomes and subsequent development of long term conditions, although participation in any identified detrimental social customs is not necessarily common to all members of specific groups. The detrimental effects of smoking have long been acknowledged (DOH, 1998; Raw et al., 1999) and individual and community-based efforts to diminish smoking have been supported by government policy (Health Act 2006). Watson (1996) highlights how ethnic minority groups may be less susceptible to health education messages, both due to language barriers and to prevailing health beliefs. For example, some South Asians may engage in practices such as chewing betel nuts and their associated products ('pan') – this, in combination with chewing tobacco, is known to contribute to such conditions as oral and stomach cancers. Heavy smoking is also known to be more prevalent in deprived communities and amongst Bangladeshi and Chinese men (Karmi, 1996; West Midlands Public Health Observatory, 2004). Additional individually tailored advice and support may therefore be necessary to encourage reduced participation in and abstention from such practices.

Encouraging risk reduction in those with long term conditions will possibly not have an effect on the condition itself but may well contribute to the secondary prevention of early-onset complications such as the micro- and macrovascular complications associated with diabetes or cardiovascular conditions. Harm reduction strategies will also prevent premature deterioration of a patient's health in the presence of chronic obstructive pulmonary disease, asthma and congestive heart failure. Research on smoking reported by the Arthritis Research Council (2001) also demonstrates how smoking can contribute to the development of rheumatoid arthritis and Evidence Based Health Care (2004) reports how smoking leads to reduced bone mass and delayed bone union following surgery or injury. All of these circumstances are more likely in a person already affected by a long term condition and more particularly so in the older population. Older Asian women have a less dense bone mass than their Caucasian or African sisters and are therefore at much greater risk of osteoporosis, falls and fractures – an issue to bear in mind when tailoring health education advice (National Collaborating Centre for Women's and Children's Health, 2005) and in aiming to prevent admission to hospital with orthopaedic fractures and their subsequent sequelae. Some smoking cessation products may not be acceptable to some cultural groups for a number of reasons. Some ethnic minority groups are mistrustful of oral medication, preferring injectable products instead, much in the same way that the indigenous population are suspicious of rectal products and have a preference for oral pharmaceutical products (Karmi, 1996; Henley & Schott, 1999). However, there are no injectable delivery routes for smoking cessation products. The cost of smoking cessation products may be prohibitive for younger patients on low incomes who do not qualify for free prescriptions. In practice, it has been observed that many GPs require that patients attend smoking cessation groups before they will prescribe smoking cessation products. If patients are housebound, have transport difficulties, find mixed sex groups unacceptable, or dislike group activities then purchasing smoking cessation products may be the only alternative and this can be an expensive option. Additionally, trying to quit alone requires a lot of will power and if patients do not regard smoking cessation as a priority then the habit and the addiction are difficult to overcome. In deprived communities, peers and family are more likely to be smokers (Honjo et al., 2005), therefore passive smoking and increased temptation to restart may also contribute to the difficulties that patients have in trying to quit. Offering support to the whole extended family as an outreach target group for smoking cessation may be an alternative approach to address smoking cessation.

Alcohol consumption

Another custom that needs to be addressed, within the context of managing long term conditions and improving both health outcomes and life expectancy by behaviour modification, is alcohol consumption. Exploration of demography and the index of multiple deprivation (Social Disadvantage Research Centre, 2004) illustrate how people from deprived communities are more likely to have higher levels of alcohol consumption and are less likely to participate in physical activity. The index of multiple deprivation takes into consideration seven domains, which relate to income deprivation, employment deprivation, health deprivation and disability, education, skills and training deprivation, barriers to housing and services, living environment deprivation and crime. Multiagency collaboration, including input from health care practitioners, is required to help address the needs of deprived communities so as to improve health outcomes associated with access to health care as well as improving the social conditions detailed above that concomitantly impact on the quality of people's lives. Health care practitioners caring for and co-ordinating care for those living with long term conditions can improve people's health by negotiating acceptable direct care interventions. They can also raise patients' awareness of, and facilitate access to, social, psychological, financial and physical support services that may otherwise be invisible or perceived as inaccessible to those most in need of them.

Alcohol Concern (2002) report how alcohol misuse amongst the older population (those over 65 years of age) has been underestimated. This is perhaps due to the fact that older people may regard some alcohol intake as necessary for medicinal purposes, thus they do not report that portion of alcohol intake when questioned about alcohol consumption. Older single men, men from deprived communities (including homeless people) and Indian-born men who are Asian Muslims, Sikhs and Hindus but living in Britain (Cochrane & Bal, 1990) are all more likely than the general populace to consume alcohol in excess of that recommended as safe. Alcohol-related morbidity rather than mortality is an issue for concern amongst those over 65 and that same group is more likely to be affected by one or more long term conditions (DOH, 2004b). Alcohol abuse trigger factors such as bereavement, social isolation and loss of social status are also more prevalent in those of post-retirement age and in some ethnic minority, recent refugee and asylum-seeker communities. In addition to the above there is a very real concern for practitioners that concomitant use of alcohol and prescribed medication can expedite the detrimental effects of each substance whilst contributing to other risk factors such as dizziness, falls and organic mental health disorders.

The Department of Health (2006c: p. 15) advocates tailored interventions for marginalized groups, particularly where there is a greater potential for religious or cultural sensitivity; home visits by specialist team members may be one option to consider. However, community practitioners, including case managers and community matrons, will be commissioned to deliver at least tier one services that involve screening and referral, brief interventions and support as well as risk identification and appropriate responsive action (Skills for Health, 2002). Apposite skills development, both in mental health and substance misuse recognition (including alcohol screening), will now be considered a requisite on the learning agenda of community practitioners, in particular for effective engagement with those considered most at risk. Involving family members and initiating referral to self-help agencies, where appropriate, as well as forming professional relationships with specialist support teams – whilst maintaining patient confidentiality and working within the relevant codes of professional conduct – will become essential components for community practice. Alcohol screening and risk assessment will also need to be considered when conducting medication reviews of those with long term conditions. There should also be a recognition that the range of people adversely affected by alcohol is diverse, and assumptions should not be made by practitioners regarding the likelihood of abstinence or indulgence according to a person's cultural backcloth.

Physical activity

The Department of Health (2004a) also advocates community-based health trainers, indigenous to the communities in which they practice, to support people in leading healthier lifestyles. Community health professionals may collaborate with health trainers to support people with long term conditions to improve their health outcomes by leading healthier lifestyles including participation in physical activity. Some older people with limited mobility and some women in purdah from Muslim and Hindu communities may find participation in organized exercise regimes unacceptable. For those women who want to be segregated, recruitment of health trainers from local communities may be a helpful means of addressing the issue. However, organized activities are not the only means of achieving the recommended 30 minutes of physical activity five times per week that the government would have people aspire to if the annual premature death rate is to be reduced by 20–30% (DOH, 2004c). Household and other domestic activities such as vacuuming, mopping, painting and decorating, walking upstairs or gardening, as well as yoga-style exercises, can all contribute to involvement in physical activity. As there is no requirement to travel beyond the boundaries of the home, little or no cost is incurred, nor is there any need to abandon purdah.

Discussion with individual patients will enable their potential for increased physical activity to be determined and a plan of activity can be negotiated. This is especially important where weight reduction is a planned therapeutic intervention. Delay in onset of osteoporosis, improvement in insulin sensitivity, prevention of falls in older people, halt in progression of osteoarthritis, and improvement in psychological well-being are also attributed to participation in physical activity (DOH, 2004c). Where available, patients may prefer to be involved in prescribed exercise activities. Such participation may have a two-fold benefit as patients will also have the opportunity to meet people in situations similar to themselves, thus reducing their sense of social isolation. Older people may also be interested in activities such as sequence dancing, bowling or, as advocated by Health for Asylum Seekers and Refugees Portal (2003), purchasing and cultivating an allotment, as the concept of exercise in some cultures may not be a familiar one. It should, of course, be recognized that land in the UK is expensive and therefore allotment rental, let alone purchase, may be beyond the means of those with reduced incomes.

Hitting where it hurts most

Financial concerns can, especially with reduced health status, strongly impact upon psychological well-being and a person's ability to cope in changed circumstances. Signposting patients to agencies and organizations that can offer practical support as well as alerting patients to their rightful benefit entitlements is an important aspect of the community practitioner role. Patients with increasingly complex needs regardless of their demography may be entitled to benefits such as the attendance allowance. This benefit is available for those aged over 65 years at two different rates dependent upon whether night-time assistance is also required, and can be paid even if patients remain in employment, have savings, have not paid National Insurance contributions or are in receipt of other benefits. Patients who are in receipt of palliative care will have their claims met as a priority. As this benefit is mainly unconditional, those accepted as refugees in the UK are also able to apply. If patients require the services of a full-time carer (for 35 hours per week or more) then the carer may be able to claim a carer's allowance if the patient is already in receipt of a middle or higher band disability living allowance. The carer's allowance is not payable for those already receiving a state pension but claims may still be worth applying for as additional premiums and bonuses may be provided. If the carer's allowance is claimed, this may have an impact on the benefits that the patient is allowed to obtain. Carers who concomitantly work can also claim the carer's allowance but there is a limit to the amount that can be earned. Carers undertaking part-time study may also be able to claim.

Patients under the age of 65 can claim a disability living allowance if they have limited mobility or require social care after more than three months and for greater than six months. The disability living allowance does not impact on other benefits, income or savings. Those in receipt of this benefit may also seek or be in employment. Incapacity benefit, income support and family tax credit are also available for people aged less than 60 years provided that certain criteria are met. Pension credit may also be available for those aged over 60 years to enable them to receive the minimum state pension. For those aged over 65 years, even with savings, a savings credit may be payable to bring their pensions in line with the minimum state pension. Some patients may also be eligible to receive help for costs incurred with NHS appointments including dental and ophthalmic services, fuel, housing and council tax costs, or motability costs; the latter being available for those in receipt of the higher band disability living allowance. Further information is available from Motability (www.motability.co.uk), local social security offices, Jobcentre Plus or the Department for Work and Pensions (www.dwp.gov.uk). Also, practitioners may advise patients to call the Benefit Enquiry Line on 0800 88 22 00 (Textphone 0800 24 33 55).

Alternatively, community practitioners may wish to act in an advocacy role for their patients and seek advice on benefits on behalf of their patients, especially where English is a second language for the patient.

Free prescriptions are available for those aged over 60 and under 16 (up to 19 years for those in full-time education), but those aged under 60 and over 16 will also be entitled to free NHS prescriptions if they experience some long term conditions. For example, those with a stoma, diabetes, thyroid disease, epilepsy, adrenal conditions, myaesthenia gravis, in receipt of a war pension or with very limited mobility. Surprisingly, despite the continuous need for pharmacological intervention, patients with coronary heart disease, asthma and chronic obstructive pulmonary disease are not entitled to free prescriptions unless they are concomitantly unemployed or on a low income that already entitles them to other benefits. Patients on low incomes and not otherwise entitled to benefits may find prescription payment certificates helpful in saving money, especially where multiple medication is a feature of their condition(s).

It has been observed in practice that in some older, deprived and South Asian communities (Henley & Schott, 1999), the man may be considered the head of the household and have total control particularly where finances are concerned. If that person becomes incapacitated physical or mentally, either temporarily or permanently, then other family members may not have access to income for daily provision. The potential for this should be considered and raised sensitively, especially where patients have progressive conditions that permit forward planning. Asylum seekers, including those appealing or awaiting deportation, and those granted refugee status or exceptional leave to remain are all entitled to free medical treatment under the NHS (DOH, 2006d).

Action Learning Point

- Consider two patients who have need of financial support – they may be fictitious for the purpose of this exercise.
- What financial benefits and social support may they be missing out on and how can you help them to access those resources?
- What barriers might you face in obtaining increased support both from the system and from patients (or carers) themselves?

Living with long term conditions is an experience shared by many people within the UK: 60% of adults from a total population of more than 59 million people report living with a long term condition (DOH, 2004b). Whilst both the indigenous and immigrant population have their share of long term conditions, the burden of ill health is unequally distributed amongst the older population (DOH, 2004b), the ethnic minority population and those from deprived communities (All Parliamentary Group for Diabetes & Diabetes UK, 2006). The ability to cope with the consequences of a long term condition is determined by the resources available to an individual and their capability in utilizing those resources in a meaningful and structured manner. Where support from family and friends is available and where a degree of independence remains, then the ability to cope is much more likely. For those who are already marginalized from society, have limited human or material resources to employ, and envisage rapidly advancing dependence on others outside of the family unit, living with one or more long term conditions becomes an increasingly traumatic and debilitating experience that can have additional consequences for the mental health of those affected. It is clear to see that those least likely to have the intrinsic and extrinsic resources for managing long term conditions are the most likely to experience them. Sidell (2001) explains how, in Western society, people are valued for their competence, in other words, for what they are able to do and contribute. As living with one or more long term conditions impacts on a person's ability both to be fully independent and to contribute to society, they begin to generate a sense of worthlessness as they spiral towards invalid status. Consequently their poor health status becomes synonymous with being invalid (of no value). This sense of invalidity may well deter people from expressing their needs even to those closest to them. Where supportive networks are already scarce the potential for expressing needs is reduced, and the effect of this is greater where structural barriers to communication already exist. Robinson (2002) highlights how involving link workers and community leaders in determining the needs of such groups can sometimes be a positive experience for those from marginalized groups in marshalling the resources required to improve life where structural barriers to communication exist. He does, however, add a cautionary note that link workers and community leaders can sometimes act in a gate-keeping role when their views do not represent those of the communities which they are intended to serve.

An inadequate knowledge of services available and thus poor take up of service provision amongst marginalized groups can pose a double problem. Where service provision remains invisible to its target population, those individuals continue to carry the burden alone, and where take up of service provision is low, funding may be withdrawn in a climate of budget deficits and competition for dwindling resources. Health literacy is concerned with having the knowledge, understanding, motivation and application to use information in a health-enhancing manner (Sihota & Lennard, 2004). For those who are disadvantaged in communication either through disability or communication deficit (different language or low basic literacy skills), health literacy is liable to be lacking. The older person, people from disadvantaged communities and some ethnic minority groups (particularly women), refugee and asylum-seeker populations are more disadvantaged in terms of health literacy. This deficit contributes both to their poorer health status and their inability to access resources that may enhance health outcomes, including preventative care. It is also recognized that even those with apparently good spoken English may have poor health literacy (Sihota & Lennard, 2004). The Moser Report (Department for Education and Employment, 1999) highlighted how 7 million adults living in England have difficulties with basic numeracy and literacy. However, failing eyesight, English as a foreign language, existing learning disability and concomitant long term conditions will also negatively impact on a person's ability to be literate or be articulate, particularly within the context of health. The role of the community practitioner in improving health access and acting as an advocate for such individuals and groups is therefore an important role aspect to fulfil.

Advocacy and the rights of the patient

Gates (1994) highlights how practitioners acting as advocates can be viewed with hostility by colleagues, especially in closed or hostile environments. Closed environments comprise clinical arenas that view collaborative work as a necessary evil and, where this does take place, outside agencies and individuals are viewed with suspicion and any engagement is approached defensively. Hostile environments have been illustrated by high profile cases where 'whistle blowing' is regarded as traitorous and patient rights constitute a low priority in the concept of patient care. Such environments are still possible within health care environments where there are competing agendas, finite resources and a dominance of the medical model of care. The latter predicates paternalism and offers little room for patient choice or preference. Consideration of how the wider determinants of health may disadvantage a patient, as well as how their condition(s) may disable their health literacy or self-determination, should be taken into account. As advocacy is concerned with defending and supporting the rights of patients (Vaartio & Leino-Kilpi, 2005), those taking on an advocacy role need to be assertive, knowledgeable about the rights and needs of patients, have well developed interpersonal, negotiating and influencing skills, and be confident and articulate – in short, many of the skills recognized as those required for leadership. Novice community practitioners will benefit from adopting a role model, engaging in continuing professional development and seeking out clinical supervision. Seasoned practitioners will also benefit from engaging in clinical support networks and actively participating in continuing professional development. It is recognized that engaging with such supportive frameworks may enhance the practitioner's clinical knowledge, raise standards of practice, motivate staff, improve the quality of patient care and prevent staff burnout (Canham, 1998; Playle & Mullarkey, 1998; Scottish Intercollegiate Guidelines Network, 2002; Royal College of Nursing, 2003).

Concluding on advocacy and 'empowerment'

Advocacy is based upon empowering the patient rather than the health care practitioner (Teasdale, 1998). I am rather reluctant to use the word 'empowerment' as the word has been used indiscriminately by health care professionals and often implies information giving rather than its original meaning. The original context is to support patients in acquiring health literacy and decision-making skills, then assisting patients in using that knowledge to pursue their own personal goals and health outcomes rather than meeting agendas defined by health care professionals or the organizations that they represent. A key component of empowering patients is to recognize the potential unequal power base that practitioners may hold and to desist from coercing or persuading patients by presenting information in such a way that the practitioner's values and ideas are not more favourably represented. Where language barriers exist, advocacy can become more problematic as a third party may need to be involved in interpreting the patient's needs and, as previously identified, those needs can be inadequately addressed where there are value conflicts between the patient and the interpreter.

Conclusions

In conclusion, cultural competence in health care provision can be considered as an integral part, rather than an adjunct, of the practitioner's role within present day practice. An increasing older population, a widening gap between affluent and non-affluent communities and individuals, a diverse mix of cultures and ethnicities, an increasing learning disabled and physically disabled population due to advances in medical technology and increased life expectancy, as well as an expanding population living with one or more long term conditions, means that health care practitioners need to adjust their skills in cultural competence to meet the day-to-day needs of their patient populations. Finite resources and a trend towards health care provision rationing means that front-line practitioners are often expected to meet the needs of their patients without the practical support that would ideally be required. The health care practitioner role demands a multiskilled individual who is resourceful, flexible, knowledgeable and assertive. Advanced communication skills as identified by the Department of Health (2000b) are certainly a prerequisite to role fulfilment. Continuing professional development and collaborative working are necessary to enable safe practice that meets the needs of patients and supports the notion of patient choice as purported by a series of government policy initiatives (DOH, 2001a, 2001b, 2001c, 2004a, 2005, 2006a, 2006b, 2006d). Additionally, patients have increased expectations partly as a result of government initiatives and because the media have brought to public attention what is expected from the health care provider organizations and their employees. Clinical competence in all its manifestations equates with cultural competence and there is no opt-out clause for modern day health care practitioners.

References

Abrums, M. (2000) Jesus will fix it after a while. *Social Science and Medicine* 50: 89–105.

Acheson, D. (1998) *Independent Inquiry into Inequalities in Health Report*. London, HMSO.

Alcohol Concern (2002) *Acquire: Alcohol Concern's Quarterly Information and Research Bulletin*, No. 34. London, Alcohol Concern.

All Parliamentary Group for Diabetes & Diabetes UK (2006) *Diabetes and the Disadvantaged: Reducing health inequalities in the UK. World Diabetes Day 14 November 2006*. London, All Parliamentary Group for Diabetes and Diabetes UK.

Arthritis Research Council (2001) Heavy Smoking Can Lead to Rheumatoid Arthritis. http://www.arc.org.uk/newsviews/press/feb2001/smoke.htm [accessed 12 February 2007].

Canham, J. (1998) Educational clinical supervision: meeting the needs of specialist community practitioner students and professional practice. *Nurse Education Today* 18: 394–398.

Chopra, D. & Kendra, J. (2002) *Grow Younger, Live Longer: 10 steps to reverse ageing*. London, Rider and Co.

Clewes, G. (2007) PCT dumps GPs with costs of interpreting. *BMA News* 17 February: 6.

Cochrane, R. & Bal, S. (1990) The drinking habits of Sikh, Hindu, Muslim and white men in the West Midlands: a community survey. *Addiction* 85 (6): 759–769.

Crisp, N. (2005) Improving People's Health Perceptions. http://www.esrc.ac.uk/ESRCInfo-Centre/about/CI/CP/the_edge/issue13/improvingpeoples.aspx?ComponentId=2616&SourcePageId=6473 [accessed 12 February 2007].

Department for Education and Employment (1999) *A Fresh Start – Improving literacy and numeracy*. London, Department for Education and Employment.

Department of Health (1998) *Smoking Kills: A White Paper on tobacco*. London, HMSO.

Department of Health (1999) *National Service Framework for Mental Health*. London, Department of Health.

Department of Health (2000a) *National Service Framework for Coronary Heart Disease*. London, Department of Health.

Department of Health (2000b) *The NHS Plan: A plan for investment, a plan for reform*. London, Department of Health.

Department of Health (2001a) *The Expert Patient: A new approach to chronic disease management for the 21st century*. London, Department of Health.

Department of Health (2001b) *The National Service Framework for Diabetes: Standards*. London, Department of Health.

Department of Health (2001c) *The National Service Framework for Older People*. London, Department of Health.

Department of Health (2004a) *Health Choices: Making healthy choices easier*. London, Department of Health.

Department of Health (2004b) *Chronic Disease Management: A compendium of information*. London, Department of Health.

Department of Health (2004c) *At Least Five a Week: Evidence on the impact of physical activity and its relationship to health. A report from the Chief Medical Officer*. London, Department of Health.

Department of Health (2005) *The National Service Framework for Long Term Conditions*. London, Department of Health.

Department of Health (2006a) *Our Health, Our Care, Our Say: A new direction for community services*. London, Department of Health.

Department of Health (2006b) *Practice Based Commissioning: Practical implementation*. London, Department of Health.

Department of Health (2006c) *Models of Care for Alcohol Misusers (MoCAM)*. London, Department of Health.

Department of Health (2006d) *Entitlement to NHS Treatment*. London, Department of Health.

Disability Rights Commission (2006) Health Inequality Enquiry Panel Visits Wales. http://www.drc-gb.org/about_us/drc_wales/newsroom/health_inequality_enquiry_pane.aspx [accessed 13 February 2007].

Dreher, M. & MacNaughton, N. (2002) Cultural competence in nursing: foundation or fallacy? *Nursing Outlook* 50 (5): 181–186.

Drinkwater, C. (2002) *A Randomised Controlled Trial Evaluating Three Methods to Promote Physical Activity: In a primary care setting*. London, Department of Health.

Eshiett, M. & Parry, E. (2003) Migrants and health: a cultural dilemma. *Clinical Medicine* 3: 229–231.

Evidence Based Health Care (2004) NSAIDs, coxibs, smoking and bone. *Bandolier Extra* **March**: 1–7. http://www.jr2.ox.ac.uk/bandolier/booth/painpag/wisdom/NSB.pdf [accessed 12 February 2007].

Food Standards Agency & Diabetes UK (2001) Diabetic foods: Joint statement on 'diabetic foods' from the Food Standards Agency and Diabetes UK. http://www.diabetes.org.uk/About_us/Our_Views/Position_statements/Diabetic_foods/ [accessed 14 February 2007].

Gates, B. (1994) *Advocacy; A nurses' guide*. London, Scutari Press.

Gravelle, H., Dusheiko, M., Sheaff, R. et al. (2007) Impact of case management (Evercare) on frail elderly patients: controlled before and after analysis of quantitative outcome data. *British Medical Journal* 334: 31–34. doi:10.1136/bmj.39020.413310.55.

Greenhalgh, T., Helman, C. & Chowdhury, A.M. (1998) Health beliefs and folk models of diabetes in British Bangladeshis: a qualitative study. *British Medical Journal* **316**: 978–983.

Health for Asylum Seekers and Refugees Portal (HARP) (2003) Nutrition and Staying Well. http://www.harpweb.org.uk/content.php?section=women&sub=w13 [accessed 23 February 2007].

Health Professions Council (2007) *Standards of Conduct, Performance and Ethics*. London, Health Professions Council.

Henley, A. & Schott, J. (1999) *Culture, Religion and Patient Care in a Multi-Ethnic Society: A handbook for professionals*. London, Age Concern.

Hills, M. & Mullett, J. (2000) Community-based research: creating evidence based practice for health and social change. Paper presented at the *Qualitative Evidence-based Practice Conference*, Coventry University, 15–17 May 2000. http://www.leeds.ac.uk/educol/documents/00001388.htm [accessed 8 February 2007].

Honjo, K., Tsutsumi, A., Kawachi, I. & Kawakami, N. (2005) What accounts for the relationship between social class and smoking cessation? Results of a path analysis. *Social Science and Medicine* **62**: 317–328.

Hooper, L. (2001) *Dietetic Guidelines: Diet in secondary prevention of cardiovascular disease*. Birmingham, British Dietetic Association.

Kai, J. (ed.) (2003) *Ethnicity, Health and Primary Care*. Oxford, Oxford University Press.

Karmi, G. (1996) *The Ethnic Handbook: A factfile for health care professionals*. Oxford, Blackwell Science.

Katbamna, S., Padma, B. & Parker, G. (2000) Perceptions of disability and care-giving relationships in South Asian Communities. In: W.I.U. Ahmad (ed.) *Race, Health and Social Care: Ethnicity, disability and chronic illness*. Buckingham, Open University Press, pp. 12–27.

Kelleher, D. & Hillier, S. (eds) (1996) Researching cultural differences in health. London, Routledge.

Kennedy, I. (2001) *The Report of the Public Inquiry into Children's Heart Surgery at the Bristol Royal Infirmary 1984–1995: Learning from Bristol*. London, HMSO.

Krause, I.B. & Miller, A.C. (1995) Culture and family therapy. In: S. Fernando (ed.) *Mental Health in a Multi-ethnic Society: A multi-disciplinary handbook*. London, Routledge, pp. 150–171.

Morris, S., Sutton, M. & Gravelle, H. (2004) Inequity and inequality in the use of health care in England: an empirical investigation. *Social Science and Medicine* **60** (6): 1251–1266.

Naqvi, H. (2003) *Access to Primary Health Care Services for South Asian Cardiovascular Disease Patients: Health care professional perspective*. Bristol, Bristol Primary Care Trust Avon HImP Performance Scheme.

National Collaborating Centre for Women's and Children's Health (2005) *Long-acting Reversible Contraception: The effective and appropriate use of long-acting reversible contraception*. London, National Institute of Health and Clinical Excellence.

National Obesity Forum (2005) Obesity Care Pathway Toolkit. http://nationalobesity forum.org.uk/content/blogcategory/18/170/ [accessed 14 February 2007].

National Statistics (2004) Census 2001 People and Migration: Overseas born and ethnic population. http://www.statistics.gov.uk/cci/nugget.asp?id=767 [accessed 1 December 2004].

National Statistics (2005) Census 2001 People and Migration: Foreign born and ethnic population. http://www.statistics.gov.uk/cci/nugget.asp?id=1312 [accessed 8 February 2007].

Nursing and Midwifery Council (2004) *Code of Professional Conduct: Standards for conduct, performance and ethics*. London, Nursing and Midwifery Council.

Papadopoulos, I., Lees, S., Lay, M. & Gebrehiwot, A. (2004) Ethiopian refugees in the UK: migration, adaptation and settlement experiences and their relevance to health. *Ethnicity and Health* **9** (1): 55–73.

Playle, J.F. & Mullarkey, K. (1998) Parallel process in clinical supervision: enhancing learning and providing support. *Nurse Education Today* 18: 558–566.

Povlsen, L., Olsen, B. & Ladelund, S. (2005) Educating families from ethnic minorities in type 1 diabetes – experiences from a Danish intervention study. *Patient Education and Counselling* 59 (2): 164–170.

Raw, M., McNeil, A. & West, R. (1999) Smoking cessation: evidence based recommendations for the health care system. *British Medical Journal* 318: 182–185.

Redfern, M. (2000) *The Royal Liverpool Children's Inquiry*. Liverpool, HMSO.

Richardson, A., Thomas, V.N. & Richardson, A. (2006) 'Reduced to nods and smiles': experiences of professionals caring for people with cancer from black and ethnic minority groups. *European Journal of Oncology Nursing* 10: 93–101.

Richman, J. (1987) *Medicine and Health*. London, Longman.

Robinson, M. (2002) *Communication and Health in a Multi-Ethnic Society*. Bristol, Policy Press.

Royal Bristol Infirmary Inquiry (2001) *The Report of the Public Inquiry into Children's Heart Surgery at the Bristol Royal Infirmary 1984–1995. Learning from Bristol*. Norwich, HMSO.

Royal College of Nursing (2003) *Clinical Supervision in the Workplace; Guidance for occupational health nurses*. London, Royal College of Nursing.

Scottish Intercollegiate Guidelines Network (2002) *Continuing Professional Development: A manual for SIGN guideline developers*. Edinburgh, Scottish Intercollegiate Guidelines Network.

Sidell, M. (2001) Understanding chronic illness. In: T. Heller, R. Muston, M. Sidell & C. Lloyd (eds) *Working for Health*. London, Open University Press/Sage Publications.

Sihota, S. & Lennard, L. (2004) *Health Literacy: Being able to make the most of health*. London, National Consumer Council.

Siriwardena, A.N. & Clark, D.H. (2004) End-of-life care for ethnic minority groups. *Clinical Cornerstone. Diversity in Medicine* 6 (1): 43–49.

Skills for Health (2002) Drugs and Alcohol National Occupational Standards (DANOS). http://www.skillsforhealth.org.uk/view_framework.php?id=61 [accessed 22 February 2007].

Smith, J. (2005) *Sixth Report – Shipman: The final report*. Norwich, HMSO.

Social Disadvantage Research Centre (2004) *English Indices of Deprivation Summary; 2004 (revised)*. Oxford, Neighbourhood Renewal Unit.

Szaflarski, M., Szaflarski, J.P., Privitera, M.D., Ficker, D.M. & Horner R.D. (2006) Racial/ethnic disparities in the treatment of epilepsy: what do we know? *Epilepsy and Behavior* 9: 243–264.

Teasdale, K. (1998) *Advocacy in Health Care*. Oxford, Blackwell Science.

Vaartio, H. & Leino-Kilpi, H. (2005) Nursing advocacy – a review of the empirical research 1990–2003. *International Journal of Nursing Studies* 42 (6): 705–714.

Watson, N. (1996) Health promotion and lay health beliefs. In: N. Cooper, C. Stevenson & G. Hale (eds) *Integrating Perspectives in Health*. Buckingham, Open University Press, pp. 87–97.

Weiss, M. & Britten, N. (2003) What is concordance? *Pharmaceutical Journal* 271 (7270): 493.

West Midlands Public Health Observatory (2004) *Smoking across Birmingham: Health Equity Audit*. Birmingham, South Birmingham Primary Care Trust.

Wong, M.D., Asch, S.M., Andersen, R.M., Hays, R.D. & Shapiro, M.F. (2004) Racial and ethnic differences in patient's preferences for initial care by specialists. *American Journal of Medicine* 116: 613–620.

World Health Organization (1948) World Health Organization Constitution. http://www.who.int/about/en/index.html [accessed 13 February 2007].

Chapter 11

Policy and practice

Margaret Presho

Key points

- Outlining the National Service Frameworks
- Discussing the requirement for change in the way that health and social care is provided within the community
- Exploring the effect of the General Medical Services contract on community practice
- Identifying the demise in conformation to the medical model of care
- Changing perceptions of the public, government and practitioners on health outcomes and health and social care service provision
- Addressing health inequalities and health inequity
- Raising the political consciousness of practitioners

It is interesting that the National Service Framework (NSF) for Long Term Conditions (Department of Health (DOH), 2005a) focuses on neurological conditions when respiratory conditions took up more than 2.6 million bed days in 2004 (Information Centre for Health and Social Care, 2005). Additionally, chronic obstructive pulmonary disease combined with asthma accounts for more than 5.5 million patients, yet there is no National Service Framework to guide practice in caring for those with respiratory conditions. The government purports that the NSF for Long Term Conditions (DOH, 2005a) can be used as a template for any long term condition and that the most important aspect of managing long term conditions is to:

> 'improve health outcomes for people with long term conditions by offering a personalised care plan for vulnerable people most at risk'. (DOH, 2005a: p. 3)

However, effective care plans should comprise more than medical care plans, they need to detail social care, service entitlements and options for choice (Coalition of Health Bodies, 2005). Co-ordinating the provision of such a diverse range of services will be a complex task and should be carried out in collaboration with individual patients and, where appropriate, with their families and carers. Case managers and, in some Primary Care Trusts (PCTs), community matrons have been identified as the most appropriate individuals to co-ordinate service input and other supportive mechanisms. Recognition that support is fragmented and requires organization is a step in the right direction. Conversely, it is acknowledged that the infrastructure to support service co-ordination does not really exist (DOH, 2004a) despite alleged political will to put the patient at the centre of service delivery as evidenced by the plethora of recent health-related policies (DOH, 2003a, 2004b, 2004c, 2006a). It is possible that in the near future practice-based commissioning will enable the infrastructure required to scaffold a new style of service delivery (DOH, 2006b, 2006c), although UK community practitioners may be slow in adapting to a new style of service delivery given the hasty manner in which the decommissioning of PCT roles and responsibilities has been implemented. Moreover, health and social care service providers have never been happy bedfellows, with each having their own distinctive philosophies, agendas and budgets. Managed care pathways have long been a feature of USA practice, but then again the philosophy of the American health care system is not directly comparable with that of the British NHS. Also, the concept of patients determining and procuring their own health care needs is alien not only to practitioners but also to the general public.

The systems are working against patients

Saville et al. (2005) advocate a 'one stop shop' style group appointment system within primary care as this would obviate the requirement for frequent, asynchronous, inconvenient appointments with various service providers. Whilst the above concept is laudable, the target-driven NHS, reinforced by the implementation and amendment of the General Medical Services (GMS) contract (NHS Confederation & British Medical Association (BMA), 2003; BMA & NHS Employers, 2006), does not constructively support such an approach to service delivery within the context of general practice. Additionally, a focus on targeted service delivery highlights continued preponderance with the medical model and directs attention away from the quality of life or well-being experienced by those living with long term conditions.

There is more to health than health care and a series of government policy documents focusing on health inequalities (as well as health access inequity) draws attention to this fact (Acheson, 1998; DOH, 2001a, 2002a; Wanless, 2003). Furthermore, having 'one stop shop' clinics will not address the needs of those housebound by their conditions any better than having numerous hospital-based clinic appointments with arranged NHS transport. It should be noted at this point that the revised GMS contract (BMA & NHS Employers, 2006) contains a caveat regarding 'exceptions'. This caveat means that if patients are invited for review of their long term condition and do not attend on three occasions, then the practice can make an exception of those patients, which implies that the practice need not count them in their percentage rates for payment calculation for the next 12 months and will not be penalized for the patient's not having received the planned review under the Quality and Outcomes Framework (QOF). As a result the practice will have no vested interest in trying any further to encourage or arrange for those patients to attend until the following year.

Consequently, if the patient is not known to the practice as being housebound and not in contact with any other health and social care service provider, they ultimately become invisible. Clinical reviews as detailed above are, of course, a necessary feature of some therapeutic interventions, but social support networks and practical measures to enhance daily living for those most affected by long term conditions are equally important, in particular for those who are housebound by their condition.

Action Learning Point

- Examine your practice profile, community profile or go to http://www.statistics.gov.uk/ and click on 'neighbourhood statistics'.
- How many elderly people live in your area of clinical practice who are aged 85 years or more?

What additional support mechanisms are in place to ensure that they receive adequate health and social care?

If possible, find out what your local general practices do to monitor the health of this vulnerable age group and see if there are facilities within a local Carers' Centre to encourage independence and provide a voice to articulate their needs.

Care planning to address patient needs

American evidence suggests that 45% of those living with a long term condition are likely to have more than one condition and that this factor rises to 70% for people aged over 65 years. UK evidence supports these statistics and makes explicit that more than a quarter of those people living with long term conditions endure three or more concomitant long term problems (DOH, 2005a: p. 4). Whilst the NSF for Older People (DOH, 2001b) offers some guidance for practice, the apparent complexity of living with such multiple concerns signifies the importance of health professionals' having clear guidance for practice in supporting people across a diverse age range living with a range of long term conditions. To some extent, at least for those people living with less complex chronic health problems, the notion of guidance for support has been addressed by the Expert Patient initiative (DOH, 2001c) (see Chapter 3), but for those with composite issues, solutions are much more ambiguous.

The NHS Institute for Innovation and Improvement (2006) alleges that between 6% and 13.2% of hospital costs are due to 19 ambulatory conditions that would be preventable if appropriate care were instigated within PCTs. They also assert that developing community services to target those conditions would reduce hospital admissions with a potential saving of £94 million to the NHS. The implication is that community case managers and community matrons should therefore be focusing their attention on patients with the following conditions (the conditions are listed in order of frequency of attendance): chronic obstructive pulmonary disease (COPD), angina, ear, nose and throat infections, epilepsy, congestive heart failure, asthma, influenza and pneumonia, gastroenteritis, cellulitis, diabetic complications, pylonephritis, iron deficiency anaemia, bleeding gastric ulcers, dental conditions, hypertension, gangrene, pelvic inflammatory disease, vaccine preventable conditions and nutritional deficiencies. As previously stated within this chapter, there is no NSF for any respiratory condition despite the NHS cost of hospital admissions with COPD and asthma amounting to £253 million and £64 million, respectively (NHS Institute for Innovation and Improvement, 2006). In the absence of a NSF, practitioners must be guided by the National Institute for Health and Clinical Excellence (NICE) (2004a) and British Thoracic Society Guideline Development Group (2007) guidelines regarding COPD, and the British Thoracic Society/Scottish Intercollegiate Network (2005) guideline on the management of asthma. These clinically focused guidelines are very useful practical directives for practitioners on the clinical management of both conditions. However, they do not address the potential inequalities in health and inequity in health access experienced by patients with these conditions because it is not within the remit of the guidelines to address the infrastructure required to support standards of service provision.

One element of the role of community case managers and community matrons is to drive for the reorientation of services within the community to facilitate improved care for patients with long term conditions. The World Health Organisation (1986) first identified the need for reorientation of service provision as a means to improving public health by addressing the total needs of the individual as a whole person. The implication of this is that the health of an individual is not merely dependent on the presence or absence of disease but rather on the sum of the factors that impinge on a person's quality of life. For example, dyspnoea is in itself distressing but it also will impact on a person's ability to be independent. Dependency may well lead on to social isolation, depression and loss of self-esteem, especially where there are limited social networks that the individual with dyspnoea may call upon to support them in their daily life. Assessment therefore of a person with a long term condition must take into account the social factors that may impact on the individual patient's condition and, where possible, mobilize services and other supportive networks to address those factors that could expedite deterioration of the patient's condition.

The single assessment process

The single assessment process (SAP) addresses social issues that impact upon patients, but Ferriter et al. (2006) argue that utilization of this tool has led to impaired clinical communication between practitioners due in part to the lengthy nature of the tool and also its greater potential for illegibility and loss of meaningful information. However, the traditional focus on the medical model of health relegates social issues that have an equal impact on the quality of a person's life to the back burner. According to Sargent and Boaden (2006) community matrons and, by implication, community practitioners need to consider the patient from a more holistic perspective. In fact such an approach is imperative if the patient is not to be reduced to a series of symptoms to be addressed without consideration of the quality of life for themselves, their families and where applicable their carers. The wider determinants of health that contribute to the social model of health incorporate both the medical perspective and the psychosocial aspects that contribute to a person's well-being. Thus despite the criticisms of the SAP, the assessment of a person's health needs should have equal focus on both medical and environmental factors. The latter will take into account issues such as housing, social support networks, financial resources, transport issues, level of patient education and access to health and social care resources. Case management is in effect not about disease management in isolation but rather about resolving complex issues in patients with multiple health concerns. A further response to the critique of the SAP is that nurses are obliged to ensure that their documentation is contemporaneous, apposite, permanent, signed, dated and legible (Nursing and Midwifery Council, 2005). The same criteria will apply to other practitioners under the auspices of clinical governance and risk management strategies. In the near future, on-line completion of SAP documentation is an emerging possibility that has already come to reality in Sheffield, so arguments regarding illegibility and complexity would no longer be viable (NHS Connecting for Health, 2007).

Action Learning Point

- To what extent does your clinical practice area employ the single assessment process?
- Have any adaptations been made to the documentation to better meet the needs of the local population being served?
- Is there a focus on health care interventions or are social care interventions afforded equal standing?
- How much collaborative or partnership practice exists between different service providers? For example, are budgets, agendas and philosophies similar or polemic?
- Which evidence-based assessment tools contribute to the assessment process?

Is the policy drive for case management working?

Latour et al. (2007) identified that case management will improve patients' quality of life but not reduce emergency bed admissions and this opinion is supported by an earlier report by Gravelle et al. (2006). However, Gravelle et al. (2006) do acknowledge that the case management system may well be identifying previously unknown patients that would otherwise have been subject to very poor life quality. The arguments about the benefits of case management as a policy for managing patients with the most complex long term conditions does not rest there because NHS Employers (2006) stated in their report that of the 26 teams across 66 organizations engaged in reducing emergency bed days, 80% had reported success with 70% of those same teams implementing community matron or case manager roles in the provision of services. Perhaps case managers and community matrons really are making a difference but the debate lies in where the difference is being made and for the benefit of whom. In fairness, the study by Gravelle et al. (2006) was completed in early 2005 and therefore may not have taken into account the reduction in emergency bed admissions highlighted by NHS Employers (2006) in their pilot studies.

Anderson et al. (2007) identify how only 13% of the 2 million new referrals to social service providers came from the primary care sector in 2005/6; this figure puts referral from primary health care professionals on a par with friends and family referrals, at 14%, compared to 29% and 24% of referrals instigated by clients and secondary care providers, respectively. These statistics may indicate that primary care practitioners are not recognizing the psychosocial and economic needs of clients that they themselves consider important aspects of coping with long term conditions. The same source cites how over 70% of those in receipt of social care services or packages of care were aged more than 65 years, with those opting for receipt of direct payments rising by 50% from 2004/5. Conversely, those requesting nursing care packages were down by 4% on previous years, despite a rise in community care assessments of 2% on the previous year. Perhaps the patients are becoming experts in their own care due to increased information technology, media involvement in and promotion of self-help measures, and increasing realization that health care professions are not quite as expert as they once considered themselves to be (BC Partners for Mental Health and Addictions Information, 2003–2006; BBC, 2006; Dyer, 2006).

Nursing care is not the only intervention

An alternative explanation for patients' opting for social care rather than nursing care packages may be found in studies from Europe as well as studies from the United Kingdom. Mohseni and Lindstrom (2007) found that those with poor perceptions of their own health had little trust in health care systems, perhaps due to earlier experiences which had led them to delay in seeking help. Those same people also experienced low self-esteem and had lower levels of education; similarly Pattenden et al. (2007) in their British study on patients living with chronic heart failure found that those with less socioeconomic resources found it harder to cope with their condition and perceived a lack of rehabilitation services and psychosocial support that heavily impacted on the physical and mental health of both patient and carer. The impact was greater on families from ethnic minority communities as they sometimes had the additional barrier of language and consequent communication difficulties to overcome. An added element of difficulty was that some ethnic minority patients and their carers held different health beliefs about their condition to those of their formal care providers, thus conflict about the best means of condition management impeded the formal caring process (see Chapter 10). Current economic conditions and their negative impact on service provision, with subsequent cuts in service delivery, even where their input is shown to have positive outcomes for patients (Scottish Intercollegiate Guidelines Network, 1999; DOH, 2003b), will not have escaped patients and carers due to the high profile media attention given to the NHS budget deficit. People may be reluctant to ask for services that they perceive can not be delivered.

Fagerstrom et al. (2006) in their Swedish study found that patients become anxious and less able to manage their health-related problems even before their activities of daily living become impaired, especially when they have no social support networks. Thus even before nursing input is deemed to be required, there is an impact on patients' quality of life due to poor life satisfaction and low self-esteem incurred by a lack of social support networks. In Italy, where COPD is the third most common cause of death and the fourth most common reason for admission to hospital, and heart failure the most common cause of hospitalization in older adults, a study by Aimonino et al. (2008) found that a multidisciplinary approach to managing patients at home with COPD and heart failure not only improved the patients' quality of life but also reduced six-month hospital readmission rates. It should be added that the potential cause for readmission in those previously treated in the hospital rather than at home may be due to iatrogenic impact and that the Italian model of home care involved not only nurses but also social workers and counsellors, as well as physiotherapists and doctors. Reorientation of health service provision, rather than increased service provision, may well be a key to improved patient outcomes for those living with long term conditions, but equally important are notions of social justice and social capital.

Social justice is predicated from the concept of those with least resources being provided with greater opportunities and access, whilst social capital is concerned with achieving effective levels of personal interaction based on mutual trust, reciprocity and improved outcomes through collective action. Those with least resources – material, physical or psychosocial – may be less able to effectively engage in health-promoting behaviours or to have any input into how and what service provision they most need. Thus policies that actively promote equity of access and equity of opportunity are more likely to engender social capital. The Disability Discrimination Act 1995 and 2005 are policies that put the onus on public bodies such as the NHS to promote equality of opportunity for, and prevent discrimination towards, people with a disability including those with multiple sclerosis, cancer and human immunodeficiency virus (HIV). Of course not all people living with long term conditions, even those most severely affected, will be registered as disabled. Therefore the onus is on practitioners to promote social justice and build upon social capital by providing services that are concomitantly equitable, accessible and best meet the needs of those they serve within the confines of the resources available to them. Those needs may not be best served by nursing interventions but rather by providing access to support for those requiring financial help that would enable them to remain independent from managed or institutionalized care, for example: support in accessing community care grants or interest-free budgeting loans from the Social Fund, the carer's allowance, the disability living allowance, and help with NHS costs or obtaining a crisis allowance. More information about these and other fiscal resources is available from the UK Government (2007) at www.directgov.uk.

Reorienting health services: rhetoric or reality?

District nursing colleagues have questioned how the role of the community case manager or community matron differs from that provided by district (community) nurses. This is a difficult nut to crack given that community service provision has not radically altered with the introduction of the new roles, but perhaps the focus is on a psychosocial rather than a nursing or medical approach. It has been observed, in practice, that although the Department of Health defined in their document *Best Practice Guidance* what commissioners and practitioners (and patients) should expect from those practising within the domain of the new roles and how the community matron role differed from that of the community case manager, those guidelines have not been adhered to (NHS Modernisation Agency & Skills for Health, 2005). Budget deficits may well be responsible for people being designated as case managers rather than matrons; the latter having and applying advanced clinical skills. Or it may be that it had already been recognized by service providers that psychosocial rather than nursing interventions are what is required by patients. One fundamental problem with the new role of community case managers is that it was introduced coterminously with the public service agreement to reduce emergency hospital bed days and improve health outcomes for those living with long term conditions. Subsequently, existing practitioners, regardless of their field of clinical practice, had experienced little or no education or training to prepare them for that role transition. Whereas in the USA, the Commission for Case Manager Certification conducts a quinquennial review into the role and functions of the case manager both to facilitate educational programmes and to define the criteria for the examination of case managers as preparation for practice (Hussein, 2005). Mental health practitioners and health visitors may argue that they have engaged in case management for a considerable number of years. However, it is also true that their caseloads have constituted a very specific client group and that their work has been impeded by limited availability of, or restricted access to, services that would have benefited their client group in terms of psychosocial support as well as prevented them from being subject to the competing agendas between health and social care service providers. These deficits have resulted from poor communication between service providers and competition for resources. This latter statement is evidenced by high profile cases and reports such as *On the State of the Public Health: Annual report of the Chief Medical Officer 2005* (DOH, 2006c), *Clearing the Air* (Commission for Health Care Audit and Inspection, 2005), the Victoria Climbie Inquiry (Laming, 2003) and the Clunis Inquiry (Ritchie, 1994).

One of the government's latest attempts to reorientate health services and amalgamate service provision provided by the health and social care sectors is *Our Health, Our Care, Our Say* (DOH, 2006a), a government White Paper. However, one year after its inception stakeholders are still regarding joint planning of health and social care and other services as a top priority, indicating that this aspect still has some way to go if targets are to be met. It is also interesting to note that more support for carers continues to be the second most important aspect for attention in terms of improving health outcomes for the nation and, in particular, those with long term conditions (DOH, 2007a). Demographic statistics provide evidence that the population is ageing and with an ageing population comes a potential increase in those living with long term conditions. More than a quarter of a million people reported living with a long term condition that restricted their ability in Great Britain in 2001 (National Statistics, 2007a, 2007b).

As a consequence of the ageing population and the impact of long term conditions, with a concomitant rise in the age of both lay and formal carers (see Chapter 4), more services will need to be established that contribute to the prevention of ill health and to promote and sustain the maintenance of independence in those affected by long term conditions. It is much easier for health care professionals and the government to blame the state of the nation's health on poor lifestyle choices, but many people do not have a choice and their actions are largely dominated by the circumstances in which they find themselves. Poverty rather than lifestyle choice is a major factor in determining the health of the most deprived sectors of the population, particularly in major cities (Irving, 2004). Consequently, 50 years since its inception, the NHS remains a 'national sick service' with public health largely remaining a concept and one that is the first aspect to be axed in the face of economic stringency. The potential for cuts in service provision is reflected in the academic and publishing world with the acclaimed national journal *Public Health News* being axed due to falling revenues in July 2006. However, one national project in the UK that aims to address the balance in promoting independence, focusing on the older and less able population, and incorporating a public health stance is currently undergoing a series of pilot studies between 2006 and 2008. The aims of the 'Partnerships for older people project' (POPPS) are to establish sustainable, innovative approaches to prevention work in order to improve health outcomes for older people. A sum of £60 million has been released by the government over two years through a process of bids to help achieve the desired outcomes. An important element of these projects is that they are intended as a joint partnership between PCTs and Councils with Responsibility for Social Services. A key stipulation of the funding body (Department of Health) is that older people must be involved in the planning, implementation and evaluation process. The grand plan is, in effect, a reorientation of services away from institutionalized care and a cultural shift towards early intervention and uptake of preventative approaches. The outcome measures for the older population amount to demonstrated improvements in the wider determinants of health with a particular focus on improved quality of life and economic well-being. Should these pilot projects prove successful, and early indications do point to their success, then this will be a landmark move towards reorientation of services as intended by the Ottawa Charter more than 20 years ago.

As previously indicated, quality of life and a sense of well-being are not totally dependent on absence from disease and access to health service provision. The focus of health promotion is that all people regardless of their status in life should have equal opportunities and access to resources that will enable them to maximize their fullest health potential. Factors that influence health can be political, cultural, environmental, economic, social, behavioural or biological. The government, local communities and individuals must work in partnership to address these factors if the health of the nation is to improve. Particular emphasis needs to be directed to those who are most vulnerable and disadvantaged, as advocated by Acheson (1998) and Wanless (2003). The government has already, and continues to put into place policies that make an attempt to address inequalities in health and inequity of access, as evidenced throughout this chapter. However, policies are often given little time to be evaluated for effect before a further policy is introduced that appears to countermand what has come before. One such example of this phenomenon is the introduction of the National Strategy for Sexual Health and HIV (DOH, 2001d); two of the main intentions of this policy were to reduce the transmission and prevalence of HIV and sexually transmitted infections (STIs), with the plan to make service provision more accessible by moving services into the primary care sector, in particular into general practice. However, the new GMS contract (BMA & NHS Employers, 2006) barely acknowledges sexual health service provision, thus acting as a disincentive towards supporting people living with HIV (a recognized long term condition) or preventing the transmission of HIV (and STIs). The funding provided by the government for the reorientation of service provision was not ring-fenced and therefore has disappeared into the black hole that is the funding pot for PCTs. Meanwhile record numbers of people continue to be diagnosed with HIV, with the biggest rise being seen in the heterosexual population – all of whom will need access to antiretroviral therapy (Health Protection Agency, 2006).

Everyone is equal but some are more equal than others

Where prescribed therapy forms part of the management plan for any long term condition, those with the relevant conditions should have equal access to prescribed therapy. However, this is not the case: while those with diabetes and thyroid conditions have a right to free prescriptions regardless of their socioeconomic status, those with asthma or COPD are not entitled to free prescriptions unless they are already exempt due to age or very low income status. This anomaly is disturbing, especially given the high volume of those with COPD and the fact that mismanaged asthma may well result in irreversible airways damage, producing symptoms similar to COPD (Tsoumakidou et al., 2004). It is also grossly unfair, especially to disadvantaged populations with long term conditions in England, that since 1 April 2007 people in Wales are entitled to free prescriptions, wigs and appliances regardless of their socioeconomic status. Additionally, those in Wales who have obtained pre-payment certificates for reduced price prescriptions are being refunded for those, even if they are registered with an English GP but living in Wales (Welsh National Health Service, 2007). Those most affected by ineligibility for free prescriptions are people receiving minimum wages in occupations that offer unstable employment conditions, where the requirement for possession of occupational entry criteria is very low or non-existent. In fact people who have long term conditions are more likely, when employed, to be in such low paid positions. This is due to the prevalence of long term conditions in economically and socially disadvantaged populations and the difficulties associated in obtaining and remaining in paid employment when experiencing one or more long term health problems (Bishop, 2003; Arthritis Care, 2006; Varekamp et al., 2006).

Action Learning Point

- How might you support younger people with long term conditions in gaining employment or assist older people in regaining a sense of purpose and value to themselves and their communities?
- Find out if there are any active patient support groups in your area and visit them to discover their advice on becoming an active citizen when living with a long term condition. Note that these voluntary and charitable organizations will be separate from the Expert Patient initiatives, which are now 'not for profit' community interest companies.

Whilst this chapter makes clear that those with long term conditions remain socially and economically disadvantaged despite some attempts by government policy to address some of the issues raised, one group of people with a high prevalence of long term conditions remains doubly disadvantaged. That group constitutes those with learning disabilities. The seminal White Paper *Valuing People* (DOH, 2001e: p. 15) estimates that there are around 210 000 people with severe learning disabilities and about 1.2 million people with mild to moderate learning disabilities in England. Those with learning disability are more likely to come from socially and economically disadvantaged backgrounds and are much more liable to experience a range of health care problems than the general populace. Conditions such as epilepsy, neurological and physical disabilities, chronic dental disease, and heart and respiratory dysfunction are much more prevalent in the learning disabled population. Inequity in access to health care, poor health outcomes and lower life expectancy are also dominant features of life for those living with a learning disability. Consequently, low levels of educational achievement and poor employment prospects make it almost impossible for the learning disabled person to lift themselves out of the spiral of ill health, thus ensuring that they remain on the margins of society. Although not a homogeneous group of people, those with learning disability are also apt to concomitantly suffer from mental health problems, hence confounding their marginalized health status and poor employment prospects.

Government policies that target at risk communities for behaviour change are unlikely to have an impact on those affected by learning disabilities given that changing behaviour is dependent upon recognizing that personal health is at risk (Prochaska & DiClemente, 1983; DOH, 2007b). People with learning disability have a tendency to be less well endowed in the self-efficacy stakes. Self-efficacy requires that a person be able to cope well, with confidence, in situations that would normally induce risk-taking behaviour – not an easy task for anyone, let alone someone who is cognitively impaired by learning disability (Bandura, 1982). Despite good intentions, as evidenced by the launch of *Valuing People* (DOH, 2001a), those with learning disability are still being treated as second class citizens, particularly in the health stakes, and dying unnecessarily due to neglect or poor understanding on behalf of health care professionals (Mencap, 2007). Additionally, the Disability Rights Commission (2006a) published the findings of their report that investigated how people with learning disabilities and common mental health problems are treated inequitably in primary care. The report is a stark reminder to community health care professionals that those with learning disabilities and mental health problems are less likely to be afforded evidence-based care for acute or long term health problems and as a result have greater morbidity and mortality than the general populace with associated reduction in life expectancy. The Disability Rights Commission (2006b) made 11 recommendations as to how the inequalities experienced should be addressed. Furthermore, the Commission for Health Care Audit and Inspection (2007) found that people with learning disabilities were given less respect, afforded less dignity and were subject to poor health and social care practices that were detrimental to their physical and mental health. This was due in part to poor staff training and education, inadequate management and leadership, poor communication skills, inadequate staffing levels and lack of patient advocacy. It is clear that the government consultation document *Independence, Well-being and Choice: Our vision for the future of social care for adults in England* (DOH, 2005b) did not have the impact on care providers that was intended in seeking to improve the quality of life for those with learning disability, despite the notions of inclusion, choice and greater control over the quality of people's lives being at the heart of the Green Paper.

A key aspect of the Green Paper (DOH, 2005b) was to increase the capacity of direct payments for vulnerable adults to enable them to decide which care packages would best suit them and to allow them to directly purchase those services. This concept is in itself a major exercise in risk management given that vulnerable adults, especially people with learning disabilities, may be easily manipulated, which could lead to their funding being misappropriated and the individuals being exploited. It was not until the murder of Holly Wells and Jessica Chapman that the subsequent Bichard Inquiry (Bichard, 2004) recommended that a register be established for people who wish to work with vulnerable adults (or children). Prior to this event and report, employers routinely investigated the background of those working with children through the Criminal Records Bureau system but no such requirement was in place for those working with vulnerable adults. Police forces across the country were not obliged to share records with other forces or key agencies on offences committed until the implementation of the recommendations of the Bichard Inquiry in December 2005. Some of the recommendations made were, in fact, not put in place until April 2007.

Action Learning Point

- How many patients on your caseload or within your sphere of clinical practice have a learning disability?
- How do you as a practitioner facilitate their health?
- Do you consider that this group of patients are disadvantaged compared with other patient groups?
- How might you address this and what resources does your PCT have to support you in effectively working with this patient group and engaging in health facilitation?

Vulnerable patients: policy plethora and punitive practices

The bureaucratic process that enables policy to become reality can be a slow and cumbersome beast and, in the clinical arena, is reliant on efficient leadership and management to disseminate information and translate concepts into the reality of practice. Students often comment that they were unaware of particular guidelines or contemporary evidence regarding various aspects of practice until they were formally introduced to them during taught units of study. This is particularly so if the guideline is not directly relevant to their usual field of practice. However, health care professionals cannot plead ignorance as a form of defence and must endeavour to keep their knowledge and skills up to date in order to practise lawfully (Health Professions Council, 2003: p. 5; Nursing and Midwifery Council, 2004: p. 6.1). This premise is especially applicable where patients and clients are least able to challenge formal carers regarding aspects of their care or management; those with learning disability are, of course, one such vulnerable group, but equally vulnerable are those with mental health problems.

The Mental Health Bill 2006 seeks to replace the Mental Health Act 1983 and is to some extent contentious in that it intends to detain people who do not have the capacity to consent to care or treatment but in whose best interest it is to deprive them of their liberty. The government argue that only a small minority of people will be affected by this change, citing figures of 1250 people being detained at any one time, yet they have initially made provision for 21 000 such assessments to be carried out. The Mental Health Foundation have campaigned for two years to have the Mental Capacity Act 2005 amended so that the 'Bournewood Provisions' (DOH, 2006d) will be taken into consideration to safeguard the rights of the people most likely to be affected by the new bill. Those safeguards arose from a case taken to the European Court of Human Rights (ECHR) in 2004, whereby the detention of the man concerned was judged to have contravened Article 5(4) of the ECHR. The Mental Capacity Act 2005 came into force in April 2007.

The government's apparent capacity for churning out policy documents seems unending and, as commented upon earlier in this chapter, there is often little time to assimilate and apply the policy in practice before a new and sometimes contradictory policy is made. Additionally, policy documents contain concepts for practice rather than means of enactment in the real world of practice. Implementation guidelines are often left to local interpretation, which results in discrepancies in practice and non-standardization of care and treatment leading to inequity of access to service provision and diverse inclusion and exclusion criteria. Such inconsistencies inevitably lead to a postcode lottery in the context of care provision, just the situation that the government intended to avoid when introducing the NSFs. The NSFs focus on the best-evidence care and management for a range of long term conditions and incorporate the plans for the infrastructure that would enable the NSFs to work in practice, regardless of the individual patient's geographical location. Given that long term conditions are the focus of the majority of NSFs so far published, it seems odd that the government then published the NSF for Long Term Conditions as a separate entity (DOH, 2005c). It should also be pointed out that the Department of Health website now refers to the above document as the NSF for Long Term (Neurological) Conditions, perhaps a reflection of the critique that this NSF focused only on neurological conditions yet was referred to by the government as a blueprint for managing long term conditions in general. The hard copy of the published document states only *National Service Framework for Long Term Conditions*.

By early 2007, six NSFs had been published, those being for Mental Health (DOH, 1999a) Coronary Heart Disease (DOH, 2000a), Diabetes (DOH, 2001f), Older People (2001b), Children, Young People and Maternity Services (DOH, 2004e) and Long Term Conditions (2005a). These topic areas address two of the major public health concerns identified by the incumbent government in *Saving Lives: Our healthier nation* (DOH, 1999b), these being mental health and coronary heart disease. However, there is no NSF for cancer but there is *The NHS Cancer Plan: A plan for investment, a plan for reform* (DOH, 2000b), a long term strategy that attempts to address the inequity in access to service provision and standards of care previously experienced by some of the 200 000 people each year that are diagnosed with cancer. The plan focuses on standards of prevention, screening, diagnosing, treating and caring for those with or with a potential for cancer. It also sets out to improve standards of care delivery by addressing staff training and improving equipment, drugs and patient information systems. Despite all of the effort and funding invested in the strategy, the condition will still be there in the future and, as Cancer Research UK (2006) point out in their campaign, further investment will be required in the future if cancer is to be effectively combated. In November 2006, Patricia Hewitt (Health Secretary) bowed to pressure from the campaigners and announced a Cancer Reform Strategy for England to build upon the success of the preceding Cancer Plan. Two of the key criteria that Cancer Research UK (2007) highlight in their priorities for the strategy are service reconfiguration and prioritizing cancer prevention. These two aspects of service reorientation and preventative approaches are recurring themes, both in the management of long term conditions and in the public health approach to service delivery.

Most practitioners and the public are generally not focused on prevention as a means of health service provision; practitioners possibly because aside from encouraging lifestyle changes, they feel disempowered by the community development approaches favoured by the public health movement. The public on the other hand have been led to believe that their ill health can be cured by improvements in medical technology, genetic manipulation and drug treatments that act like magic bullets and get directly to the root cause of the problem. Lifestyle changes are difficult on an individual level and also possibly beyond the scope of those who would perhaps be most advantaged by them. For example *The NHS Cancer Plan: A plan for investment, a plan for reform* (DOH, 2000b) advocates people eat five portions of fruit and vegetables each day both to prevent obesity and to reduce the risk of cancer. However, those from disadvantaged backgrounds may be unfamiliar with fruit and vegetable consumption and find adjusting their taste difficult. Additionally, people who are on a limited budget may find purchase of fruit and vegetables too expensive or they may not have easy access to large supermarkets where those products can be bought in bulk at reduced cost. When hungry it is easier to fill up on foods high in fat content and a lifetime diet of refined, processed food may make fruit and vegetables difficult to digest. Practitioners advising patients to increase their consumption of fruit and vegetables should take into account these aspects if there is to be any progress made on lifestyle change. Additionally, in a nation that has become familiar with fast food and ready meals, the culinary skills necessary to prepare some vegetables and other healthy food options may be lacking.

Perhaps the only recent policy document that has taken a pragmatic stance on lifestyle change when addressing public health concerns is *Choosing Health: Making health choices easier* (DOH, 2004d). Prior to this, public health concerns had been repeatedly raised and ongoing issues such as health inequalities and health inequity identified but no attempt was made within previous policy documents to outline how these issues could be tackled on a practical level. The documents tended to make broad statements and present a strategic perspective but did not address operational issues that practitioners require to help them turn policy into practice. Previous public health publications comprise *Report on Independent Inquiry into Inequalities in Health* (Acheson, 1998), *Saving Lives: Our healthier nation* (DOH, 1999b), *Tackling Health Inequalities: Cross cutting review* (DOH, 2002b), and *Securing Good Health for the Whole Population: Final report* (Wanless, 2004). Perhaps one good reason for the lack of implementation guidance on delivering health improvement was, as Wanless (2004) highlights, the dearth of evidence on what improves health. Health is a very subjective issue and some people consider themselves to be healthy in the face of quite debilitating conditions, whereas others may feel themselves to be greatly restricted even by minor, self-limiting health problems. Sidell (2001) purports that the way in which people cope with and adapt to living with a long term condition is to a great extent dependent on their network of social support and the economic resources available to them. This perspective reinforces the earlier point regarding the probability of people making lifestyle changes.

Choosing Health: Making healthy choices easier (DOH, 2004d), in a structure similar to other government documents, uses a series of case studies to illustrate best practice. However, there is no real way of knowing how representative those case studies are and whether or not there were competing priorities for the funds and resources available. Interestingly, there have been concerns highlighted by the national media that funds intended to operationalize *Choosing Health* have been diverted to make up budget deficits within trusts. Additionally, general practice is considered the cornerstone of primary health care delivery within the community but much of the work that goes on within the general practice arena is strongly linked to the GMS Contract (BMA & NHS Employers, 2006). As a consequence, public health work is serendipitous as general practice core staff focus on activities that attract points (and funding) under the auspices of the GMS contract. For example, some of the public health concerns targeted for address within *Choosing Health* (DOH, 2004d), such as accident reduction, reduction in alcohol consumption, improving physical activity levels and tackling substance misuse, do not attract any points under the GMS contract. These issues therefore receive scant attention during consultation, despite the role of excess alcohol consumption in some cancers, obesity and cardiovascular conditions. Improving sexual health and addressing obesity levels attract only minimum points, two and eight points, respectively, with the latter only being added to the terms of the GMS contract when revised in 2006. This anomaly is surprising given the contribution of obesity to the rising levels of type II diabetes and the fact that all STIs are on the increase. In fact, addressing the transmission of sexually-acquired infections, including HIV, is not mentioned at all within the GMS contract and obesity is only considered an issue once the patient's body mass index has reached 30 – hardly a preventative approach to care management!

Meeting targets or meeting needs?

Whilst the GMS contract is to be commended for standardizing the quality of care provided by general practice, it does focus rather heavily on the medical model approach to care and does not take account of the underlying wider determinants of health that may contribute to the conditions on which it focuses. In practice, the GMS contract has also been criticized as data collection for its own sake, even though the contract clearly states that data should only be collected when useful to patient care and never merely for audit purposes. However, as long as the NHS remains target driven, practitioners and managers will concentrate on meeting the targets rather than upon the real needs of the patients. Additionally, tailored care may well fall by the wayside if the directive is to standardize care delivery rather than respond to the needs of the patient whilst working within the constraints of the resources available.

As discussed earlier, an additional problem that still requires satisfactory address within general practice is the quality of care delivered to those with long term conditions who are housebound. There is no standard practice for visiting housebound patients with long term conditions and general practice nurses may or may not include home visits within their practice, depending on the terms and conditions of their employment. Likewise district nurses may not agree to visit housebound patients for preventative activities such as smoking cessation advice or influenza and pneumoniococcal vaccinations unless the individual patient is already known to them and is on their current caseload. Furthermore, the clause within the GMS contract on exception reporting (BMA & NHS Employers, 2006: p. 58) could potentially be detrimental to the housebound patient, as detailed previously.

Perhaps the move towards practice-based commissioning within primary care will enable more tailored care for those who are housebound with long term conditions, as GPs will be able to request holistic care of such patients as part of their commissioning specification. Discussion with community case managers and district nursing teams has demonstrated how GPs are having more influence on the service specifications offered by community nursing teams, including case managers. This situation has arisen as service managers are anxious that GPs may well purchase their services elsewhere should they be dissatisfied with local provision.

Earlier in this chapter it was identified that those with a learning disability are more likely than the general populace to have one or more concomitant long term conditions and that they fare less well than other members of the population in accessing service provision. Unfortunately the GMS contract does little to improve the situation since as a category under the Quality and Outcomes Framework (QOF), learning disability attracts only four points. Those points are awarded to practices for establishing a register of those in the practice population aged over 18 years with a learning disability. Footnotes in the QOF that accompany the rationale for including those with learning disability focus on the potential range of learning disability diagnosis. Whilst it is highlighted that people with a learning disability are amongst the most vulnerable members of the population, there is nothing within the QOF criteria that contributes to facilitating better health outcomes for this group.

The GMS contract appears to have many negative aspects but, in fairness, the medical care afforded to those with a range of long term conditions has been improved by the GMS contract. This has been done by focusing attention on those conditions and some others, such as epilepsy, which were perhaps previously neglected within general practice. The National Collaborating Centre for Primary Care (2004) acknowledges within their guidelines that the care of patients with epilepsy is less than optimal and that more work needs to be done on improving clinical standards. Moret-Hartman et al. (2006) in their Dutch study found that, despite guidelines being in place for the management of epilepsy, if the guidelines were not congruent with the beliefs of practitioners regarding the management of the condition, then evidence-based practice was less likely to occur. This, of course, will have an impact on patient management and potentially on health outcomes for patients. The Dutch researchers argue that for policies (clinical standards) to be implemented in practice, then those who work in that field of practice need to be involved in the policy-making process. Of course this rationale does not only apply to epilepsy management but to the management of all long term conditions. Therefore, not only does there need to be a partnership between patients and practitioners, but also between patients, practitioners and policy-makers. Organizations and agencies such as eGuidelines and NICE, with responsibility for operational policy generation, regularly advertize inviting practitioners to contribute to planned policies or policy revisions. Practitioners working with patients with long term conditions should take up those opportunities to help make policy applicable in the real world of practice. In collaborating with policy-makers, practitioners can act as patient advocates by presenting the patient's perspective for incorporation in policies that will directly affect patient care. Despite earlier critique of the GMS contract, Shohet et al. (2007) have demonstrated in their UK study that inclusion of epilepsy within the QOF of the GMS contract has resulted in reduced emergency bed admissions for those over the age of 16 with epilepsy. They argue that their positive findings were a direct result of the QOF epilepsy indicator number 4 being included in the practice remit as shown below:

'Epilepsy 4. The percentage of patients aged 16 and over on drug treatment for epilepsy who have been seizure free for the last 12 months recorded in the last 15 months.' (NHS Confederation & BMA, 2003: p. 51)

This indicator is now known as Epilepsy 8 within the revised 2006 contract and applies to those patients aged 18 or over (BMA & NHS Employers, 2006: p. 65). Shohet et al. (2007) in presenting these findings demonstrate that the QOF indicators can be much more than a paper exercise of tick boxes to generate practice points and subsequent income. The quality indicators really can make a difference to the quality of life for patients with a range of long term conditions. This is especially so where applied to those conditions that had previously been given a less than high profile within primary care.

Including the excluded

The consequences of being invisible to primary care services are that not only are your views not represented and therefore taken into consideration but also that there is one less means of support in managing your condition. Earlier in this chapter it was demonstrated that a person's ability to cope with long term health problems directly correlates with the network of social support (and financial support) available to that individual and also the person's ability to make sense of their lives when living with that health status. Where that ability to cope is diminished due to social deprivation – be that due to isolation or material or educational deprivation – Curtis et al. (2004) purport that cognitive behavioural therapy (CBT) would be of great benefit. They suggest that take up of social support resources, adopting appropriate coping strategies and a reduction in stress and depressive symptom levels associated with long term health problems are all possible with CBT. However, access to this support mechanism is not only dependent on a person being in touch with health and social care service providers but is also dependent on the service being available as a local resource as well as formal care providers recognizing the symptoms contributing to poor quality of life.

The Royal College of Nursing (2007) have cited job losses of more than 22 000 in the last year across the NHS. With such radical cutbacks in service personnel and service provision, the potential for obtaining access to in-demand services when those with established enduring mental health problems are experiencing difficulty with access, is becoming increasingly less likely. Patient organizations such as Patient UK (2005) also comment that despite approval by NICE (2004b), GPs are reluctant to refer patients for CBT because prescribing pharmacological interventions is cheaper and quicker, referral pathways are ambiguous and the potential for CBT is not well understood by GPs. There are computer-assisted programmes for CBT, but for many with a complex array of long term conditions, the ability to use a computer in a therapeutic manner, gain access to computing facilities and have the motivation to engage with such a self-directed support mechanism may be beyond their means. Depression is a well recognized feature of life for many living with a long term health problem, as identified by researchers and patient representative groups (de Souza & Dalgado, 2006; Arthritis Care, 2006; Diabetes UK, 2006; Whooley et al., 2007), with a greater proportion of adverse health outcomes being associated with concomitant depression in those with long term conditions. Community practitioners need to be aware of the potential for depression in patients with long term health problems and act swiftly to manage this where identified. Simple screening tools that involve asking patients about mood and interest can prove effective in identifying those in need of referral, as advocated by NICE (2004b: p. 14):

> 'During the last month, have you often been bothered by feeling down, depressed or hopeless?'

> 'During the last month, have you often been bothered by having little interest or pleasure in doing things?'

However, with cutbacks in staff training and education (Royal College of Nursing, 2007), despite the edict of clinical governance and its cornerstone of evidence-based practice, many community staff are ill prepared to recognize depressive symptoms. As a result patients may not gain access to the care that they require to improve their quality of life. In clinical practice practitioners have mistaken depressive symptoms for attention-seeking behaviour, particularly where social support networks are limited and family visits sparse or intermittent. The responsibility for these issues lies directly with central government, as the Royal College of Nursing (2007: p. 3) identifies: 83% of nurses believe that training budgets have been affected by financial pressures within the NHS, 86% of nurses believe that patients are at increased risk as a result of those financial cutbacks, 36% of nurses have had study leave cancelled and 54% of nurses have had training requests refused. With 47% of PCTs forecasting a budget deficit and a total NHS deficit of £1318 billion, the future of primary care, quality care for patients and service provision free for all at the point of contact appears to be in jeopardy. The Chief Medical Officer in his annual report on public health (DOH, 2006c) acknowledges that there has been an inordinate amount of waste in terms of resources, time and finances within the NHS and is seeking a means of reducing that level of waste to minimize harm to patients, improve poor health outcomes and address lost opportunities. He plans to disinvest in outmoded treatment and treatments that have no proven value. However, one problem with such an approach is that judgement of value tends to be based on only those interventions that can be objectively measured. It is notoriously difficult to measure quality of life as it can be so subjective and based, as previously discussed, on the person's ability to cope in the face of long term health problems.

A pill for every ill

One particular drain on the NHS resources is the cost of medicines. Choonara (2006) highlights how pharmaceutical companies have been conspiring to push up the cost of drugs sold to the NHS by preventing cheaper generic brands becoming available through the use of patenting laws. Public demand for pharmacological interventions as a quick fix option over 'wait and see' or other care management alternatives contributes to the rising cost of medicinal products supplied by the

NHS. In practice it has been observed that those with long term conditions often have an array of prescribed medicinal products littering bathroom cabinets and medicine chests that have expired long before they are used and many of which patients do not understand how to use effectively. UK European MPs have rejected a proposal that would allow direct-to-consumer advertising of prescription drugs that is commonplace within the United States. Labour's health spokesperson Catherine Stihler is quoted as stating that:

> 'Europe was at a crossroads and had to decide if it wanted to go down the "slippery slope" towards hard sell drug advertising as seen in the US.' (Meek, 2003: p. 2)

The Association of the British Pharmaceutical Industry (ABPI) (2006a) has a code of practice and within that code is a clause (clause 2) that specifies how promotional materials must never discredit or reduce confidence in the pharmaceutical industry. Note the focus, nothing about compromising the patient. However, since the publication of the Chief Medical Officer's annual report (DOH, 2006c), the ABPI has responded by producing a manifesto that states its intent to provide value for money and fairness with patient welfare as the key component (ABPI, 2006b). This is a reassuring development given the *New England Journal of Medicine* editorial (Angell, 2000) that highlighted how many doctors are so intrinsically tied to pharmaceutical companies through sponsorship, research and consultancy that the risks and benefits of those associations must be thoroughly scrutinized to prevent potential for misconduct. It is true that all medical schools provide guidelines for students on association with pharmaceutical companies but those guidelines are generally only loosely applied. As more nurses become prescribers and engage in entrepreneurial activities under the auspices of direct enhanced services and practice-based commissioning, they too must make themselves aware of the potential risks associated in fraternizing with the pharmaceutical industries. Most PCTs already have policies in place to prohibit such associations but practitioners must also have self-awareness within this context.

Medication reviews are a key component of practitioner activity within community practice, as poor concordance with pharmacological interventions can result in poor health outcomes including unnecessary hospital admission and premature death. Reviews may be instigated on four different levels, as advocated by Shaw et al. (2002), and a target of good medicine management is to review all those over the age of 75 annually, with those on four or more medicinal products being reviewed every six months. The key objectives of such reviews are to ensure appropriateness of treatment and patient safety. An optimal review consists of face-to-face contact with the patient giving them an opportunity to ask questions, clarify their understanding of their care and treatment, and to establish a true partnership between patient and practitioner thereby improving concordance and health outcomes for the patient. Shaw et al. (2002) report on one pilot study on medication review that took place in Huntingdon PCT. This demonstrated that half of the patients reviewed did not know or understand why they were taking one or more of their medicines, almost half considered themselves to be experiencing side effects and almost a third of patients were confused about which medicine to take and when. Clearly these issues could be addressed by community practitioners during planned contact visits, and there is room for further development within this context. An evaluation of *Room for Review* (Shaw et al., 2002) demonstrates that less than 10% of all PCTs were undertaking level 3 reviews in 2005 (Celino et al., 2005), with GPs claiming to be the instigators of medication reviews, closely followed by PCT-employed pharmacists, and nurses taking third place. The outlook is set to improve for patients in terms of medication review given that review is part of the QOF arrangements (BMA & NHS Employers, 2006). Review can also be considered as part of enhanced services through contracts with pharmacists under the practice-based commissioning process.

Practice-based commissioning: the road to redemption?

Practice-based commissioning (PBC) has had a rocky start, partly because the implementation process has not been made clear from the outset and some practice managers have stated that the paperwork associated with this process is mountainous. One aspect of care delivery that should be improved by the implementation of practice-based commissioning is that services can be tailored to meet the needs of local practice populations. This should be similar to the service configurations possible under the auspices of personal medical services-based care delivery, this being another mode of service delivery that many practices were deterred from taking up because of the paper mountain overload. In PCTs known as 'Super output areas', due to high levels of deprivation and subsequent demand on services, service delivery can be enhanced by profiling practices located within that area and pooling resources to commission services that best meet the needs of the populations to be served.

A recent criticism of immigration policy has been that essential services such as medical services, particularly in pressured, less affluent areas, are being compromised by the high influx of migrant populations with diverse and complex needs (Byrne cited by Johnston & Holt, 2007). Practice-based commissioning would enable practices to be adequately funded for the diversity and demand on services that such areas require. Ethnic minority groups, in particular those who have recently migrated, may be traumatized by war, famine or poverty or by the journey experienced in travelling to the UK. Additionally, ethnic minority groups have disproportionate levels of long term health problems and may require intensive support until they acquire refugee status and become settled into the areas to which they have been dispersed (Craig et al., 2006). Mental health issues are high on the agenda of problems experienced by such groups of people. Language barriers resulting in communication difficulties can compound their problems, and with PCTs seeking to reduce costs, vital services can be lost including translation and interpretation services. This can lead to reduced health outcomes for those affected and increased pressures on service providers. The indigenous population in those same less affluent areas will also be negatively affected by the reduced service provision and this could become a contentious issue for both sections of the community involved.

Conclusions

In seeking to provide adequate services for a diverse population with complex health needs, the government must focus their efforts on reorienting services to meet the needs of the population instead of producing conceptual policy documents that are not rooted in the real world of practice. Community practitioners need to take up opportunities to contribute to policies that are both evidence based and applicable in the real world within the constraints of the resources available to them. I do not suggest that all practitioners adapt their mindset to a Lindis Percy perspective (BBC, 2005), but rather that they become politically aware and recognize how policy impacts on practice and endeavour to act as advocates for their patient groups by becoming involved beyond an operational level of practice.

For those who may not be familiar with the campaigns of Lindis Percy, she is a health visitor who is actively engaged in campaigning for nuclear disarmament. Lindis holds such strong beliefs on this subject that she has been arrested on several occasions for trespassing on government defensive property, chaining herself to boundary fencing and generally making her voice and opinions heard by the military hierarchy. She argues that if prevention of nuclear engagement between nations is not part of the health visitor's remit in reducing potential harm to the population then she does not know what the role of the health visitor is or should be. Clearly this is not how many practitioners would choose to practise in an advocacy role, but by becoming politically aware and making a good attempt to actively participate in strategic as well as operational roles, then practitioners are better placed to direct some of the policy decisions that directly affect their patient/client groups. Those working within the health and social care sectors are not renowned for political astuteness, but in aiming towards achieving political awareness and participating in the policy-making process, practitioners can make a real difference for the people whom they are intended to serve.

References

Acheson, D. (1998) *Report on Independent Inquiry into Inequalities in Health*. London, HMSO.

Aimonino, R., Tibaldi, V., Leffe, B., Scarrafiotti, C., Marinello, R., Zanocchi, M. & Malaschi, M. (2008) Substitutive 'hospital at home' versus inpatient care for elderly patients with exacerbations of chronic obstructive pulmonary disease: a prospective randomized, controlled trial. *Journal of the American Geriatrics Society* 56 (3): 493–500.

Anderson, K., Sylvester, C., Archer, S. & Alamdari, A. (eds) (2007) *Adult Social Services Statistics*. London, the Information Centre, part of the Government Statistical Service.

Angell, M. (2000) Is academic medicine for sale? *New England Journal of Medicine* 342 (20): 1516–1518.

Arthritis Care (2006) *A New Deal for Welfare: Empowering people to work. Consultation response from Arthritis Care*. London, Arthritis Care.

Association of the British Pharmaceutical Industry (2006a) *Code of Practice for the Pharmaceutical Industry (2006)*. London, Association of the British Pharmaceutical Industry.

Association of the British Pharmaceutical Industry (2006b) *The Right Medicine, the Right Patient, the Right Time: A manifesto from the ABPI*. London, Association of the British Pharmaceutical Industry.

Bandura, A. (1982) Self-efficacy mechanism in human agency. *American Psychologist* 37: 122–147.

BBC (2005) No ASBO for protest grandmother. *BBC News* 17 May, http://news.bbc.co.uk/1/hi/england/humber/4555131.stm [accessed 24 April 2007].

BBC (2006) Mental Health and Emotional Health. http://www.bbc.co.uk/health/conditions/mental_health/emotion_esteem.shtml [accessed 23 March 2007].

BC Partners for Mental Health and Addictions Information (2003–2006) Here to Help: Mental Disorders Toolkit. http://www.heretohelp.bc.ca/helpmewith/mdtoolkit.shtml [accessed 23 March 2007].

Bichard, M. (2004) *The Bichard Inquiry Report*. London, HMSO.

Bishop, M. (2003) Determinants of employment status among a community-based sample of people with epilepsy: implications for rehabilitation interventions. *Rehabilitation Counseling Bulletin* **47** (2): 112–121.

British Medical Association & NHS Employers (2006) *Revisions to the GMS Contract 2006/07: Delivering investment in general practice*. London, British Medical Association and NHS Employers.

British Thoracic Society Guideline Development Group (2007) Intermediate Care – Hospital-at-home in chronic obstructive pulmonary disease: British Thoracic Society guideline. http://www.brit-thoracic.org.uk [accessed 11 March 2007].

British Thoracic Society/Scottish Intercollegiate Network (2005) Guideline on the Management of Asthma. http://www.brit-thoracic.org.uk [accessed 11 March 2007].

Cancer Research UK (2006) Cancer 2020: Latest news. http://www.cancercampaigns.org.uk/cancercampaigns/ourcampaigns/cancer2020/ [accessed 8 April 2007].

Cancer Research UK (2007) *Cancer Research UK Policy Statement. Priorities for the cancer reform strategy. February 2007*. London, Cancer Research UK and Policy and Public Affairs Team.

Celino, G., Dhalla, M. & Levenson, R. (2005) *Implementing Medication Review: An evaluation of the impact of 'Room for Review': Executive briefing*. London, Medicines Partnership.

Choonara, J. (2006) How the drug giants overcharge the NHS. *Socialist Worker Online* October 2006: 2022. http://www.socialistworker.co.uk/article.php?article_id=9926 [accessed 22 April 2007].

Coalition of Health Bodies (2005) *17 Million Reasons: Improving the lives of people with long-term conditions*. London, NHS Confederation.

Commission for Health Care Audit and Inspection (2005) *Clearing the Air*. London, Commission for Health Care Audit and Inspection.

Commission for Health Care Audit and Inspection (2007) *Investigation into the Service for People with Learning Disabilities Provided by Sutton and Merton Primary Care Trust*. London, Commission for Health Care Audit and Inspection.

Craig, T., Jajua, P. & Warfa, N. (2006) Mental healthcare needs of refugees. *Psychiatry* **5** (11): 405–408.

Curtis, R., Groarke, A.M., Coughlan, R. & Gsei, A. (2004) The influence of disease severity, perceived stress, social support and coping in patients with chronic illness: a 1 year follow up. *Psychology, Health and Medicine* **9** (4): 456.

Department of Health (1999a) *National Service Framework for Mental Health: Modern standards and service models*. London, Department of Health.

Department of Health (1999b) *Saving Lives: Our healthier nation*. London, Department of Health.

Department of Health (2000a) *National Service Framework for Coronary Heart Disease*. London, Department of Health.

Department of Health (2000b) *The NHS Cancer Plan: A plan for investment, a plan for reform*. London, Department of Health.

Department of Health (2001a) *Valuing People: A new strategy for learning disability for the 21st century*. London, Department of Health.

Department of Health (2001b) *National Service Framework for Older People*. London, Department of Health.

Department of Health (2001c) *The Expert Patient: A new approach to chronic disease management for the 21st century*. London, Department of Health.

Department of Health (2001d) *Better Prevention, Better Services, Better Sexual Health: The National Strategy for Sexual Health and HIV.* London, Department of Health.

Department of Health (2001e) *Valuing People: A new strategy for learning disability for the 21st century.* London, HMSO.

Department of Health (2001f) *National Service Framework for Diabetes: Standards.* London, Department of Health.

Department of Health (2002a) *Health and Neighbourhood Renewal Guidance from the Department of Health and the Neighbourhood Renewal Unit.* London, Department of Health.

Department of Health (2002b) *Tackling Health Inequalities: Cross cutting review.* London, Department of Health.

Department of Health (2003a) *Building on the Best: Choice, responsiveness and equity in the NHS.* London, Department of Health.

Department of Health (2003b) *Developing Services for Heart Failure.* London, Department of Health.

Department of Health (2004a) *Chronic Disease Management: A compendium of information.* London, Department of Health.

Department of Health (2004b) *The NHS Improvement Plan: Putting people at the heart of public services.* London, Department of Health.

Department of Health (2004c) *Better Information, Better Choices, Better Health: Putting information at the centre of health.* London, Department of Health.

Department of Health (2004d) *Choosing Health: Making healthy choices easier.* London, Department of Health.

Department of Health (2004e) *Core Standards: National Service Framework for Children, Young People and Maternity Services.* London, Department of Health and Department for Education and Skills.

Department of Health (2005a) *National Service Framework for Long Term Conditions.* London, Department of Health.

Department of Health (2005b) *Independence, Well-being and Choice: Our vision for the future of social care for adults in England.* London, Department of Health.

Department of Health (2005c) *National Service Framework for (Neurological) Long Term Conditions.* London, Department of Health.

Department of Health (2006a) *Our Health, Our Care, Our Say: A new direction for community services.* London, Department of Health.

Department of Health (2006b) *Practice Based Commissioning: Early wins and top tips.* London, Department of Health.

Department of Health (2006c) *On the State of the Public Health: Annual report of the Chief Medical Officer 2005.* London, Department of Health.

Department of Health (2006d) *Bournewood Briefing Sheet – June 2006.* London, Department of Health.

Department of Health (2007a) *Our Health, Our Care, Our Say: One year on, end of day report.* London, Department of Health.

Department of Health (2007b) *Small Change, Big Difference.* London, Department of Health.

Diabetes UK (2006) Diabetes and Depression. http://www.diabetes.org.uk/Guide-to-diabetes/Living_with_diabetes/Coping_with_diabetes/Depression_and_diabetes/ [accessed 22 April 2007].

Disability Rights Commission (2006a) *Equal Treatment: Closing the gap; a formal investigation into physical health inequalities experienced by people with learning disabilities and/or mental health problems.* Stratford-upon-Avon, Disability Rights Commission.

Disability Rights Commission (2006b) *Report of the DRC Formal Inquiry Panel to the DRC's Formal Investigation into the Inequalities in Physical Health Experienced by*

People with Mental Health Problems and People with Learning Disabilities. Stratford-upon-Avon, Disability Rights Commission.

Dyer, C. (2006) Media's treatment of Roy Meadow was 'unfair', says High Court judge. *British Medical Journal* 332: 196. doi:10.1136/bmj.332.7535.196-a. [accessed 4 July 2007].

Fagerstrom, C., Holst, G. & Hallberg, I. R. (2006) Feeling hindered by health problems and functional capacity at 60 years and above. *Archives of Gerontology and Geriatrics* 44 (2007): 181–201.

Ferriter, K., Gangopadhyay, P. & Nilforooshan, R. (2006) Quality of referrals to old age psychiatry following introduction of the single assessment process. *Psychiatric Bulletin* 30 (12): 452–453.

Gravelle, H., Dusheiko, M., Sheaff, R. et al. (2006) Impact of case management (Evercare) on frail elderly patients: controlled before and after analysis of quantitative outcome data. *British Medical Journal* 334: 31–34. doi:10.1136/bmj.39020.413310.55 [accessed 5 April 2007].

Health Professions Council (2003) *Standards of Conduct, Performance and Ethics: Your duties as a registrant: 2003*. London, Health Professions Council.

Health Protection Agency (2006) *England HIV Diagnosis Surveillance Tables: Data to the end of September 2006*. London, Health Protection Agency.

Hussein, T. (2005) *Essential Activities and Knowledge Domains of Case Management*. New York, Quality and Performance Excellence International.

Information Centre for Health and Social Care (2005) Hospital Episode Statistics 2003–2004. http://www.ic.nhs.uk/default.asp?sID=1174661299260.

Irving, S. (2004) Poor deal. *Public Health News* 17 September.

Johnston, P. & Holt, R. (2007) Immigration has 'deeply unsettled' Britain. *Telegraph* 19 April. http://www.telegraph.co.uk/news/main.jhtml?xml=/news/2007/04/18/nmigrants118.xml [accessed 23 April 2007].

Laming, H. (2003) *The Victoria Climbie Inquiry: Report of an Inquiry by Lord Laming*. Norwich, HMSO.

Latour, C.H.M., van der Windt, D.W.A.W.M., de Jonge, P., Riphagen, I.I., de Vos, R., Huyse, F.J. & Stalman, W.A.B. (2007) Nurse-led case management for ambulatory complex patients in general health care: a systematic review. *Journal of Psychosomatic Research* 62 (2007): 385–395.

Meek, C. (2003) *Direct-to-Consumer Advertising (DTCA) of Prescription Medicines: Fourth quarterly update – October to December 2002*. London, Royal Pharmaceutical Society.

Mencap (2007) *Death by Indifference: Following up the Treat Me Right! report*. London, Mencap.

Mohseni, M. & Lindstrom, M. (2007) Social capital, trust in the health-care system and self-rated health: the role of access to health care in a population-based study. *Social Science and Medicine* 64: 1373–1383.

Moret-Hartman, M., Knoester, P.D., Hekster, Y.A. & van der Wilt, G.J. (2006) Non-compliance on the part of the professional community with a national guideline: an argumentative policy analysis. *Health Policy* 78 (2006): 353–359.

National Collaborating Centre for Primary Care (2004) *The Diagnosis and Management of the Epilepsies in Adults and Children in Primary and Secondary Care*. London, National Institute for Clinical Excellence.

National Institute for Health and Clinical Excellence (2004a) *Chronic Obstructive Pulmonary Disease: Management of chronic obstructive pulmonary disease in adults in primary and secondary care*. London, National Institute for Health and Clinical Excellence.

National Institute for Clinical Excellence (2004b) *Depression: Management of depression in primary and secondary care*. London, National Institute for Clinical Excellence.

National Statistics (2007a) Ageing. www.statistics.gov.uk [accessed 5 April 2007].

National Statistics (2007b) Health and Well-being. www.statistics.gov.uk [accessed 5 April 2007].

NHS Confederation & British Medical Association (2003) *Investing in General Practice: The New General Medical Services Contract.* London, NHS Confederation and British Medical Association.

NHS Connecting for Health (2007) Electronic Single Assessment Process (SAP) Starts to Revolutionise Community Nursing in Sheffield. http://www.connectingforhealth.nhs.uk/factsandfiction/nhscasestudies/sap [accessed 23 March 2007].

NHS Employers (2006) *Improving Services for People with Long-term Conditions through Large-scale Workforce Change.* London, NHS Employers.

NHS Institute for Innovation and Improvement (2006) *Delivering Quality and Value. Focus on: productivity and efficiency.* Coventry, Department of Health.

NHS Modernisation Agency & Skills for Health (2005) *Case Management Competences Framework.* Bristol, Skills for Health.

Nursing and Midwifery Council (2004) *The NMC Code of Professional Conduct: Standards for conduct, performance and ethics protecting the public through professional standards.* London, Nursing and Midwifery Council.

Nursing and Midwifery Council (2005) *Guidance on Records and Record Keeping.* London, Nursing and Midwifery Council.

World Health Organisation (1986) Ottawa Charter for Health Promotion. First International Conference on Health Promotion. Ottawa, 21 November 1986. WHO/HPR/HOP/95.1.

Patient UK (2005) Cognitive and Behaviour Therapies. http://www.patient.co.uk/showdoc/40000658/ [accessed 22 April 2007].

Pattenden, J.F., Roberts, H. & Lewin, R.J.P. (2007) Living with heart failure; patient and carer perspectives. *European Journal of Cardiovascular Nursing* 6 (4): 273–279. doi:10.1016/j.ejcnurse.2007.01.097 [accessed 4 May 2007].

Prochaska, J.O. & DiClemente, C.C. (1983) Stages and processes of self-change of smoking: toward an integrative model of change. *Journal of Consulting and Clinical Psychology* 51: 390–395.

Ritchie, J. (1994) *The Report of the Inquiry into the Case and Treatment of Christopher Clunis.* London, HMSO.

Royal College of Nursing (2007) *Our NHS – Today and tomorrow: a Royal College of Nursing commentary on the current state of the National Health Service and the steps needed to secure its future.* London, Royal College of Nursing.

Sargent, P. & Boaden, R. (2006) Implementing the role of the community matron. *Nursing Times* 102 (23): 23–24.

Saville, M., Humphrey, C. & Mama, J. (2005) Supporting patients with long term conditions. *Practice Nursing* 16 (10): 488–491.

Scottish Intercollegiate Guidelines Network (1999) *Diagnosis and Treatment of Heart Failure due to Left Ventricular Systolic Dysfunction.* SIGN Guideline No. 35. Edinburgh Scottish Intercollegiate Guidelines Network.

Shaw, J., Seal, R. & Pilling, M. (2002) *Room for Review: A guide to medication review: the agenda for patients, practitioners and managers.* London, Medicines Partnership.

Shohet, C., Yellolly, J., Bingham, P. & Lyratzopoulos, G. (2007) The association between the quality of epilepsy management in primary care, general practice population deprivation status and epilepsy-related emergency hospitalizations. *Seizure* 16: 351–355.

Sidell, M. (2001) Understanding chronic illness. In: T. Heller, R. Muston, M. Sidell & C. Lloyd (eds) *Working for Health.* London, Sage Publications, pp. 255–264.

de Souza, E.A.P. & Dalgado, P.A.C. (2006) A psychosocial view of anxiety and depression in epilepsy. *Epilepsy and Behavior* 8 (2006): 232–238.

Tsoumakidou, M., Tzanakis, N. & Kyriakou D. (2004) Inflammatory cell profiles and T-lymphocyte subsets in chronic obstructive pulmonary disease and severe persistent asthma. *Clinical Experimental Allergy* **34** (2): 234–240.

UK Government (2007) Health and Well-being. www.directgov.uk [accessed 4 April 2007].

Varekamp, I., Verbeek, J. & Dijk, F.J. (2006) How can we help employees with chronic diseases to stay at work? A review of interventions aimed at job retention and based on an empowerment perspective. *International Archives of Occupational and Environmental Health* **80** (2): 87–97.

Wanless, D. (2003) *Securing Good Health for the Whole Population: Population health trends*. London, HMSO.

Wanless, D. (2004) *Securing Good Health for the Whole Population: Final report*. London, HMSO.

Welsh National Health Service (2007) NHS Prescription Charges. www.wales.nhs.uk [accessed 6 April 2007].

Whooley, M.A., Caska, C.M., Hendrickson, B.E., Rourke, M.A., Ho, J. & Ali, S. (2007) Depression and Inflammation in Patients with Coronary Heart Disease: Findings from the heart and soul study. doi:10.1016/j.biopsych.2006.10.016. http://www.sciencedirect.com/science?_ob=MImg&_imagekey=B6T4S-4NH6CWR-1-3&_cdi=4982&_user=4801305&_orig=search&_coverDate=04%2F16%2F2007&_sk=999999999&view=c&wchp=dGLbVlz-zSkzk&md5=1e561ecf4d3c813037238368afc34ab7&ie=/sdarticle.pdf [accessed 22 April 2007].

Index

Page numbers in *italic* represent figures, those in **bold** represent tables